Contents

Acknowledgements

Reviewers of the UK edition

Marion Johnson, RNMH, BSc (Hons), MSc, PG Cert. (Ed.), ENB 998, LPE, ONC Med. Lab. Sciences
Senior Lecturer/BSc Branch Coordinator
Birmingham City University
UK

Gillian Lim, RNT Cert. (Ed.), RN/Adult., RN/Mental Health, RM, BSc, MSc, Dip. Nursing (London)
Mental Health Programme Leader/Senior Lecturer
Kingston University and St George's London University
UK

Tennyson Mgutshini, RMN, BSc (Hons), MSc, PG Dip. (Ed.), PhD, Dip. (HE) Nursing,
Associate Professor in Nursing
Indiana State University
USA

Andy Young, RMN, PG Cert. (Hed.), LLB (Hons), LLM
Senior Lecturer
Sheffield Hallam University
UK

A Framework for Capable Practice (p. 11) reproduced with permission from The Sainsbury Centre for Mental Health.

made INCREDIBLY

Mental Health Nursing

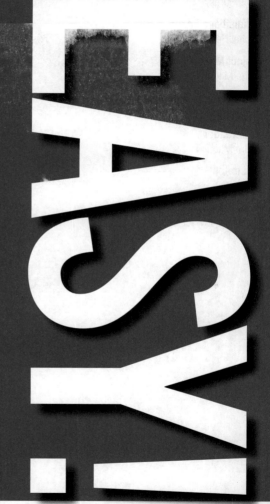

EASY!

Adapted for the UK by

Debbie Evans, PhD, MPhil, BSc (Hons), RMN, RGN

Head of Applied Social Sciences
Institute of Health and Society
University of Worcester

and

Helen Allen, PhD, MPhil, BSc (Hons), RMN, RGN

Practice Facilitator (Mental Health)
Worcestershire Mental Health Partnership
NHS Trust

First UK Edition

Wolters Kluwer | Lippincott Williams & Wilkins
Health
Philadelphia · Baltimore · New York · London
Buenos Aires · Hong Kong · Sydney · Tokyo

SWNHS

C2162511

Withdrawn

Staff

Director, Global Publishing
Cathy Peck

Production Director
Chris Curtis

Acquisitions Editor
Rachel Hendrick

Project Manager
Laura Maguire

Academic Marketing Executive
Alison Major

Proofreader
Laura Maguire

Illustrator
Bot Roda

Text and Cover Design
Designers Collective

The clinical treatments described and recommended in this publication are based on research and consultation with nursing, medical, and legal authorities. To the best of our knowledge, these procedures reflect currently accepted practice. Nevertheless, they can't be considered absolute and universal recommendations. For individual applications, all recommendations must be considered in light of the patient's clinical condition and, before administration of new or infrequently used drugs, in light of the latest package-insert information. The authors and publisher disclaim any responsibility for any adverse effects resulting from the suggested procedures, from any undetected errors, or from the reader's misunderstanding of the text.

Printed and bound by Euradius in The Netherlands. Typeset by Macmillan Publishing Solutions, New Delhi, India.

For information, write to Lippincott Williams & Wilkins, 250 Waterloo Road, London SE1 8RD.

British Library Cataloguing in Publication Data. A catalogue record for this book is available from the British Library.

ISBN-13: 978-1-901831-10-8
ISBN-10: 1-901831-10-8

Contributors and consultants to the UK edition

Graham Alexander, RMN, RGN, PhD (Pharmacology)
Non-medical Prescribing Lead Mental Health
Worcestershire Mental Health Partnership NHS Trust
UK

Pat French, RMN, BA (Hons), PG Cert. (Eating Disorders and Mental Health Act)
Clinical Manager
Eating Disorders Team
Worcestershire Mental Health Partnership NHS Trust
UK

Kay Lobo, RMN, RGN, BSc (Hons) (Eating Disorders)
Senior Eating Disorders Practitioner
Worcestershire Mental Health Partnership NHS Trust
UK

Margaret Shannon, RMN (Disorders of the Elderly)
Day Hospital Manager
Worcestershire Mental Health Partnership NHS Trust
UK

Foreword

Experienced mental health nurses, those new to the field and students beginning their mental health nursing clinical placements will discover *Mental Health Nursing Made Incredibly Easy!* to be a rare find. This handy reference book introduces the reader to the complex field of mental health nursing and discusses specific mental disorders and the latest therapeutic nursing interventions.

What makes this book exceptionally useful is the transformation of complex topics (such as service user and family advocacy, mental health promotion, psychopharmacology, multidisciplinary care and ethical and legal issues) into a focused, concise and accessible form. Light-hearted cartoons encourage and support the nurse's progress through each topic. Numerous quick-scan tables, flow charts and illustrations enable the reader to quickly identify and focus on key information.

Another helpful feature is the use of special graphic logos throughout the text to highlight specific information and opportunities for self-assessment. These logos include:

Advice from the experts – offers tips and how-to's from experienced mental health nurses.

Myth busters – distinguishes facts from fantasy about people with mental illness and the proper treatment for these service users.

Bridging the gap – offers overviews of unique beliefs and needs of specific cultural groups.

Meds matters – focuses on pharmacological and herbal remedies for mental health problems.

Mental Health Nursing Made Incredibly Easy! is organised into 13 chapters, beginning with an introductory chapter that provides descriptions of the mental health nurse's scope of practice, areas of concern, the nursing process, communication techniques, multidisciplinary care, patient and family rights, advocacy and ethical and legal issues. Seventy specific disorders, such as depression, substance abuse and bulimia, are presented in the next 12 chapters, including two chapters that address disorders experienced by children, adolescents and older adults.

For each disorder, the text presents a brief introduction, typical symptoms, possible causes, diagnostic methods, treatment approaches and nursing interventions. Research findings and the latest pharmacological advances are also included where appropriate.

A 'continuum of care' philosophy, carried throughout the book, reflects the current trend towards brief hospitalisation for acute episodes followed by ongoing outpatient treatment. The mental health nurse's participation in 'collaborative management' for the person who has a mental illness reflects current clinical practice.

Nurses are in a strategic position to intervene on behalf of people with mental illness and to promote mental health in all settings. *Mental Health Nursing Made Incredibly Easy!* presents information in efficient, effective ways to increase understanding of mental health nursing and optimal nursing interventions for people, their families and friends who are dealing with specific mental disorders.

Mental Health Nursing Made Incredibly Easy! will fill a void for experienced and novice mental health nurses as well as for nursing students beginning their mental health nursing clinical placements. It will become a valuable resource in your professional library.

Debbie Evans, PhD, MPhil, BSc (Hons), RMN, RGN
Head of Applied Social Sciences
Institute of Health and Society
University of Worcester
Henwick Grove
Worcester WR2 6AJ

Helen Allen, RMN, BA (Hons)
Practice Facilitator (Mental Health)
Worcestershire Mental Health Partnership NHS Trust
220 Newtown Road
Worcester WR5 1DD

Contributors and consultants to the US edition

C. Judith Birger, RN, CS, MS
Clinical Nurse Specialist
South Central Human Service Center
Jamestown, N.D.

Barbara Broome, RN, PhD, CNS
Assistant Dean and Chair Community/
Mental Health
University of South Alabama College of
Nursing
Mobile

**Colleen C. Burgess, RN, MSN, APRN, CS,
NCSAC**
Director of Nursing
Catawba Valley Community College
Hickory, N.C.

Linda Carman Copel, RN, PhD, CS, DAPA
Associate Professor
Villanova University College of Nursing
Villanova, Pa.

**Joseph T. DeRanieri, RN, PhD, BCECR,
CPN**
Assistant Professor
Thomas Jefferson University
Philadelphia, Pa.

Candace Furlong, RN, MSN, CNS
Professor
American River College
Sacramento, Calif.

Sudha C. Patel, RN, MN, MA, DNS
Assistant Professor
University of Louisiana at Lafayette, La.

Barbara C. Rynerson, RNC, MS, CS
Independent Clinical Consultant
Chapel Hill, N.C.

Matthew Sorenson, RN, PhD
Nursing Research Fellow
Edward Hines Jr. Veterans Affairs Hospital
Hines, Ill.

Phyllis Hart Tipton, RN, MSN
ADN Instructor
McLennan Community College
Waco, Tex.

Kathleen Tusaie, RNCS, PhD
Assistant Professor
University of Akron
Advance Practice Nurse
William Beckett & Associates
Akron, Ohio

**E. Monica Ward-Murray, SRN, RMN,
BSN, MA, EdD**
Assistant to the Dean for Research and
Assistant Professor
North Carolina Agricultural and Technical
State University
Greensboro, N.C.

1 Introduction to mental health nursing

Just the facts

In this chapter, you'll learn:

♦ the nurse's role in mental health care

♦ ways to enhance communication with service users

♦ therapies used to treat mental health disorders

♦ components of the mental health nursing assessment

♦ ethical and legal issues in mental health care.

A look at mental health nursing

In any clinical setting, you'll encounter service users with mental and emotional problems. Even if you never work in a mental health unit, you'll inevitably care for service users with depression, anxiety or thought disorders, or dementia, to name just a few common mental health problems.

To provide effective care for any service user, you must consider both the psychological and physiological aspects of health. Many medical conditions are linked to or lead to emotional and mental distress.

> You don't need to work on a psychiatric unit to encounter people with psychiatric problems.

The psychology of chest pain

Take the case of chest pain: not only can such pain *cause* anxiety and depression if the service user fears he's having a heart attack, but chest pain also can *result from* acute anxiety. Recognising such problems and how they affect the service user's overall health is crucial.

Goal: More beautiful minds

Various social, economic and professional forces have brought dramatic changes in the mental health field. Health care professionals are now much more knowledgeable about mental health and its link to physical health. Accordingly, mental health programmes have grown in number and diversity.

At the same time, a host of community mental health programmes have been established – everything from family advocacy programmes, substance abuse rehabilitation programmes and stress-management workshops to bereavement groups, victim assistance programmes and domestic violence shelters. Most public education systems also offer classes and other information programmes on mental health issues.

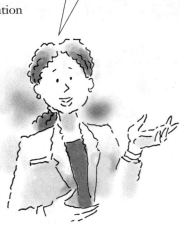

Scientists are learning more and more about what makes our minds tick.

A real page-turner

Media attention to mental health has increased, too. At any given time, best-seller lists typically include at least one book on self-help or coping. Mental health has become a standard topic on television, too.

Upgrading our understanding

Meanwhile, advances in neurobiology have revolutionised our understanding of the physiological basis of mental functioning and emotional states. These advances have improved the diagnosis and treatment of mental health disorders, especially in the realm of drug therapy for acute disorders.

Like other mental health professionals, mental health nurses need to stay abreast of the rapid changes taking place in neurobiology.

Holism in the house

In addition, an increasing focus on holistic health care has created closer ties between psychiatry and medicine. With more health care professionals recognising the emotional basis and implications of physical disorders, more hospitalised service users are now benefiting from mental health consultations.

Social factors

Some researchers attribute today's seemingly increased incidence of mental and emotional disorders to social changes that have altered the traditional family structure and contributed to loss of the extended family.

These changes have led to greater numbers of single parents, dysfunctional families, troubled children and homeless people – many of whom have meagre support systems. Combat veterans, rape victims and child abuse victims also struggle to cope with the trauma they've experienced.

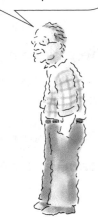

Elderly, fearful and isolated – Boy, am I depressed!

People who need people

Loss of effective support systems strains a person's ability to cope with problems. A single mother, for instance, may lack the necessary support to meet the demands of her job, children and home. If she views herself as ineffective in these roles, her self-esteem will falter and her stress level will rise. (See *Links between stress and disease*, page 3.)

Links between stress and disease

Hans Selye, a pioneer in stress research, found a link between the environment and biological response. He noted that emotional and physical stress cause a pattern of responses that, unless treated, lead to infection, illness, disease and eventually even death. Selye called this set of responses the general adaptation syndrome and identified three stages – alarm reaction, resistance and exhaustion.

Alarm reaction

During this stage, any type of physical or mental trauma triggers immediate biological responses designed to counter the stress. These responses depress the immune system, which lowers resistance and makes the person more susceptible to infection and disease. Unless the stress is severe or prolonged, though, the person recovers rapidly.

Resistance

This stage begins when the body starts to adapt to prolonged stress. The immune system shifts into high gear to meet increased demands. At this point, the person becomes more resistant to illness.

However, the perception of a threat lingers, so the body never reaches complete physiological equilibrium. Instead, it stays aroused, which places stress on body organs and systems.

Because adaptation appears to work initially, a person in the resistance stage may become complacent and assume he's immune to the effects of stress – and thus fail to take steps to relieve it.

Exhaustion

With chronic stress, adaptive mechanisms eventually wear down, and the body can no longer meet the demands of stress. Immunity and resistance decline dramatically and illness is likely to set in. The point at which exhaustion occurs differs among individuals.

Interrupting the stress response

Selye's work laid the groundwork for the use of relaxation techniques in interrupting the stress response, thereby reducing susceptibility to illness and disease.

Angst through the ages

Mental disorders occur at all ages and socioeconomic levels. The rates of teenage depression and suicide have more than tripled in the past 20 years. Alcohol and substance abuse are proliferating – and taking younger victims.

Among the elderly, isolation, fear of violent crime and loneliness have contributed to a similar rise in depression.

Classifying mental disorders

To care for service users with mental health problems, you need to be familiar with how mental disorders are classified and diagnosed. A popular system of classification and diagnosis is the American Psychiatric Association's (APA) *Diagnostic and Statistical Manual of Mental Disorders*.

In 2000, the APA published the fourth edition of its *Diagnostic and Statistical Manual of Mental Disorders*, Fourth Edition, Text Revision (*DSM-IV-TR*). This edition emphasises observable data while placing less importance on subjective and theoretical impressions. (See *Understanding the DSM-IV-TR*, page 4.)

The *DSM-IV-TR* is a must-read for all mental health nurses.

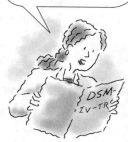

Understanding the *DSM-IV-TR*

The American Psychiatric Association's *Diagnostic and Statistical Manual of Mental Disorders,* Fourth Edition, Text Revision *(DSM-IV-TR)* defines a mental disorder as a clinically significant behavioural or psychological syndrome or pattern associated with at least one of the following criteria:

- current distress (a painful symptom)
- disability (an impairment in one or more important areas of functioning)
- a significantly greater risk of suffering, death, pain and disability
- an important loss of freedom.

The syndrome or pattern must not be merely an expected, culturally sanctioned response – such as grief over the death of a loved one. Whatever be its original cause, it must currently be considered a sign of behavioural, psychological or biological dysfunction.

Five axes

For greater diagnostic detail, the *DSM-IV-TR* uses a multiaxial approach, which specifies that every service user be evaluated on each of five axes.

- *Axis I: Clinical disorders* – mental disorders comparable to general medical illnesses

- *Axis II: Personality disorders and mental retardation* – personality disorders and traits as well as mental retardation
- *Axis III: General medical conditions* – general medical illnesses or injuries
- *Axis IV: Psychosocial and environmental problems* – life events or problems that may affect diagnosis, treatment and prognosis of the mental disorder
- *Axis V: Global assessment of functioning (GAF)* – level of functioning, reported as a number from 0 to 100 based on the service user's overall psychological, social and occupational function

Multiaxial diagnosis

After being evaluated on these five axes, a service user's diagnosis may look like this example:

- Axis I: adjustment disorder with anxious mood
- Axis II: obsessive-compulsive personality
- Axis III: Crohn's disease, acute bleeding episodes
- Axis IV: recent remarriage, death of father
- Axis V: GAF = 83.

Role of mental health nurses

NHS carers state that mental health nursing is one of the most complex and demanding areas of nursing. As many as one in three people are thought to suffer some form of mental health problem. For many, mental illness is brought on by a crisis in life, which they can't cope with, such as depression after the death of a partner. A mental health nurse may be part of a team working with people who may have been excluded from services through drug or alcohol abuse.

The range of conditions is vast: neuroses, psychoses and psychological and personality disorders all come under the broad heading of mental health.

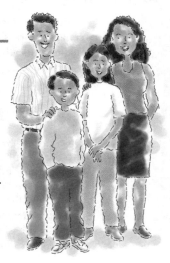

What does it involve?

The key role and challenge is to form therapeutic relationships with mentally ill people and their families. Most mentally ill people are not cared for in hospital but in the community.

You might be based in a community health care centre, day hospital and outpatient department or specialist unit. You will need to have a good understanding of the theories of mental health and illness.

What are the special demands?

Your main tool as a mental health nurse will be the strength of your own personality and communication skills. You will need to empathise with the people you are dealing with and show warmth and care about them. Regrettably, there is still some stigma attached to mental illness. Combating this and helping the individuals and their families deal with it is a key part of the job.

The danger of violence is often associated with this branch of nursing and one of the special skills required to spot a build-up of tension and defuse it.

Dealing with the human mind and behaviour is not an exact science. The job of helping people back to mental health is every bit as valuable and satisfying as caring for those with a physical illness.

Starring role

The nurse's role in helping emotionally troubled service users has grown considerably. Besides carrying out the traditional task of administering prescribed drugs and monitoring drug effects, a nurse may act as primary therapist in certain types of therapy, or may direct behaviour therapies.

Using an interpersonal approach, mental health nurses promote, maintain, restore and rehabilitate individual, family and community mental health and functioning. Their skills draw on the psychosocial and biophysical sciences as well as theories of personality and human behaviour.

Impressive clientele

Mental health nurses may work with individual service users, families, groups or even entire communities.

Settings and skills for mental health nurses

Mental health nurses practise in diverse settings – mental health hospitals, community mental health centres, general hospitals, community health agencies, outpatient clinics, homes, schools, prisons, health maintenance organisations, primary care practices, private practices, crisis units and industrial centres.
In these settings, nurses may serve in various roles. (See *The versatile nurse*.)

Order out of chaos

To care for mental health service users, you'll need to develop a practical, orderly way of dealing with problems that can be as diverse and complex as humanity itself. Besides planning, implementing and evaluating care, the mental health nurse must establish a meaningful therapeutic relationship with service users.

The versatile nurse

Depending on her skills and the setting, a mental health nurse may take one of the following roles:

- staff nurse
- primary care provider
- administrator
- consultant nurse
- in-service educator
- clinical practitioner
- researcher
- programme evaluator
- liaison between the person and other health care team members.

Wanted: Soul searcher

Working as a mental health nurse calls for some serious soul searching. To deal effectively with mental health problems, you must first develop a keen awareness of your own attitudes and feelings. Otherwise, frustration may impede your efforts to help your service users.

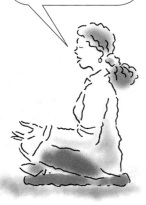

Searching your own soul will help you deal with people's mental health problems.

Scope of practice

There are five fundamental themes.
- The Nursing & Midwifery Council (NMC) code of conduct (2008)
- The capable practitioner
- The national service framework for mental health
- The 10 essential shared capabilities
- The National Institute for Clinical Excellence (NICE) guidelines

The NMC code of conduct

To work in the UK, all nurses, midwives and specialist community public health nurses must register with the NMC and renew their registration annually.

The NMC regulates entry into the profession and defines the legal limits of nursing practice. It also developed the code – standards of conduct, performance and ethics for nurses and midwives – which states that the people in your care must be able to trust you with their health and well-being.
- Make the care of people your first concern, treating them as individuals and respecting their dignity.
- Treat people as individuals.
- Respect people's confidentiality.
- Collaborate with those in your care.
- Ensure you gain consent.
- Maintain clear professional boundaries.
- Work with others to protect and promote the health and well-being of those in your care, their families and carers, and the wider community.
- Share information with your colleagues.
- Work effectively as part of a team.
- Delegate effectively.
- Manage risk.
- Provide a high standard of practice and care at all times.
- Use the best available evidence.
- Keep your skills and knowledge up to date.
- Keep clear and accurate records.
- Be open and honest, act with integrity and uphold the reputation of your profession.
- Act with integrity.
- Deal with problems.
- Be impartial.
- Uphold the reputation of your profession.
- Be accountable. As a professional, you are personally accountable for actions and omissions in your practice and must always be able to justify your decisions.

The code

Standards of conduct, performance and ethics for nurses and midwives

The people in your care must be able to trust you with their health and well-being.

To justify that trust, you must:

- make the care of people your first concern, treating them as individuals and respecting their dignity
- work with others to protect and promote the health and well-being of those in your care, their families and carers and the wider community
- provide a high standard of practice and care at all times
- be open and honest, act with integrity and uphold the reputation of your profession.

As a professional, you are personally accountable for actions and omissions in your practice and must always be able to justify your decisions.

You must always act lawfully, whether those laws relate to your professional practice or personal life.

Failure to comply with this code may bring your fitness to practise into question and endanger your registration.

This code should be considered together with the Nursing & Midwifery Council's (NMC) rules, standards, guidance and advice available from www.nmc-uk.org.

Make the care of people your first concern, treating them as individuals and respecting their dignity

Treat people as individuals

- You must treat people as individuals and respect their dignity.
- You must not discriminate in any way against those in your care.
- You must treat people kindly and considerately.
- You must act as an advocate for those in your care, helping them to access relevant health and social care, information and support.

Respect people's confidentiality

- You must respect people's right to confidentiality.

- You must ensure people are informed about how and why information is shared by those who will be providing their care.
- You must disclose information if you believe someone may be at risk of harm, in line with the law of the country in which you are practising.

Collaborate with those in your care

- You must listen to the people in your care and respond to their concerns and preferences.
- You must support people in caring for themselves to improve and maintain their health.
- You must recognise and respect the contribution that people make to their own care and well-being.
- You must make arrangements to meet people's language and communication needs.
- You must share with people, in a way they can understand, the information they want or need to know about their health.

Ensure you gain consent

- You must ensure that you gain consent before you begin any treatment or care.
- You must respect and support people's rights to accept or decline treatment and care.
- You must uphold people's rights to be fully involved in decisions about their care.
- You must be aware of the legislation regarding mental capacity, ensuring that people who lack capacity remain at the centre of decision making and are fully safeguarded.
- You must be able to demonstrate that you have acted in someone's best interests if you have provided care in an emergency.

Maintain clear professional boundaries

- You must refuse any gifts, favours or hospitality that might be interpreted as an attempt to gain preferential treatment.
- You must not ask for or accept loans from anyone in your care or anyone close to them.
- You must establish and actively maintain clear sexual boundaries at all times with people in your care, their families and carers.

(continued)

The code (*continued*)

Work with others to protect and promote the health and well-being of those in your care, their families and carers and the wider community

Share information with your colleagues

- You must keep your colleagues informed when you are sharing the care of others.
- You must work with colleagues to monitor the quality of your work and maintain the safety of those in your care.
- You must facilitate students and others to develop their competence.

Work effectively as part of a team

- You must work cooperatively within teams and respect the skills, expertise and contributions of your colleagues.
- You must be willing to share your skills and experience for the benefit of your colleagues.
- You must consult and take advice from colleagues when appropriate.
- You must treat your colleagues fairly and without discrimination.
- You must make a referral to another practitioner when it is in the best interests of someone in your care.

Delegate effectively

- You must establish that anyone you delegate to is able to carry out your instructions.
- You must confirm that the outcome of any delegated task meets required standards.
- You must make sure that everyone you are responsible for is supervised and supported.

Manage risk

- You must act without delay if you believe that you, a colleague or anyone else may be putting someone at risk.
- You must inform someone in authority if you experience problems that prevent you working within this Code or other nationally agreed standards.

- You must report your concerns in writing if problems in the environment of care are putting people at risk.

Provide a high standard of practice and care at all times

Use the best available evidence

- You must deliver care based on the best available evidence or best practice.
- You must ensure any advice you give is evidence based if you are suggesting health care products or services.
- You must ensure that the use of complementary or alternative therapies is safe and in the best interests of those in your care.

Keep your skills and knowledge up to date

- You must have the knowledge and skills for safe and effective practice when working without direct supervision.
- You must recognise and work within the limits of your competence.
- You must keep your knowledge and skills up to date throughout your working life.
- You must take part in appropriate learning and practice activities that maintain and develop your competence and performance.

Keep clear and accurate records

- You must keep clear and accurate records of the discussions you have, the assessments you make, the treatment and medicines you give and how effective these have been.
- You must complete records as soon as possible after an event has occurred.
- You must not tamper with original records in any way.
- You must ensure any entries you make in someone's paper records are clearly and legibly signed, dated and timed.
- You must ensure any entries you make in someone's electronic records are clearly attributable to you.
- You must ensure all records are kept confidentially and securely.

The code (continued)

Be open and honest, act with integrity and uphold the reputation of your profession

Act with integrity

- You must demonstrate a personal and professional commitment to equality and diversity.
- You must adhere to the laws of the country in which you are practising.
- You must inform the NMC if you have been cautioned, charged or found guilty of a criminal offence.
- You must inform any employers you work for if your fitness to practise is impaired or is called into question.

Deal with problems

- You must give a constructive and honest response to anyone who complains about the care they have received.
- You must not allow someone's complaint to prejudice the care you provide for them.
- You must act immediately to put matters right if someone in your care has suffered harm for any reason.
- You must explain fully and promptly to the person affected what has happened and the likely effects.
- You must cooperate with internal and external investigations.

Be impartial

- You must not abuse your privileged position for your own ends.
- You must ensure that your professional judgement is not influenced by any commercial considerations.

Uphold the reputation of your profession

- You must not use your professional status to promote causes that are not related to health.
- You must cooperate with the media only when you can confidently protect the confidential information and dignity of those in your care.
- You must uphold the reputation of your profession at all times.

Information about indemnity insurance

The NMC recommends that a registered nurse, midwife or specialist community public health nurse, in advising, treating and caring for persons/clients, has professional indemnity insurance. This is in the interests of clients, persons and registrants in the event of claims of professional negligence.

Whilst employers have vicarious liability for the negligent acts and/or omissions of their employees, such cover does not normally extend to activities undertaken outside the registrant's employment. Independent practice would not be covered by vicarious liability. It is the individual registrant's responsibility to establish their insurance status and take appropriate action.

In situations where an employer does not have vicarious liability, the NMC recommends that registrants obtain adequate professional indemnity insurance. If unable to secure professional indemnity insurance, a registrant will need to demonstrate that all their clients/persons are fully informed of this fact and the implications this might have in the event of a claim for professional negligence.

(Nursing & Midwifery Council, 2008)

The capable practitioner

The capable practitioner is a framework and list of the practitioner capabilities required to implement the national service framework for mental health as devised by the Sainsbury centre.

This framework divides *capability* for modern mental health practice into five areas:

- Ethical practice. It makes assumptions about the values and attitudes needed to practice.

- Knowledge. It is the foundation of effective practice.
- Process of care. It describes the capabilities required to work effectively in partnership with users, carers, families, team members and other agencies.
- Interventions. These are capabilities specific to evidence-based, bio-psycho-social approaches to mental health care.
- Application. The above-mentioned capabilities are then used in *application* to specific service settings, for example, assertive outreach and crisis resolution, each requiring specialist capabilities. The specialist mental health settings are:

1. Primary Care
2. Community-Based Care Coordination (CMHTs)
3. Crisis Resolution and Early Intervention
4. Acute In-person Care
5. Assertive Outreach
6. Continuing Care, Day Services, Rehabilitation and Residential Care, and Vocational and Work Programmes
7. Services for people with complex and special needs (forensic, dual diagnosis) and people with personality disorders.

The national service framework for mental health

This national service framework sets out standards in five areas; each standard is supported by the evidence and knowledge base, by service models and by examples of good practice. Local milestones are proposed; timescales need to be agreed with NHS executive regional offices and social care regions, and progress will be monitored.

- Standard one addresses mental health promotion and combats the discrimination and social exclusion associated with mental health problems.
- Standards two and three cover primary care and access to services for anyone who may have a mental health problem.
- Standards four and five encompass the care of people with severe mental illness.
- Standard six relates to individuals who care for people with mental health problems.
- Standard seven draws together the action necessary to achieve the target to reduce suicides as set out in *Saving Lives: Our Healthier Nation*.

Standard one

Health and social services should:
- promote mental health for all, working with individuals and communities
- combat discrimination against individuals and groups with mental health problems, and promote their social inclusion.

Standards two and three: Primary care and access to services

Aim

To deliver better primary mental health care, and to ensure consistent advice and help for people with mental health needs, including primary care services for individuals with severe mental illness.

A Framework for Capable Practice

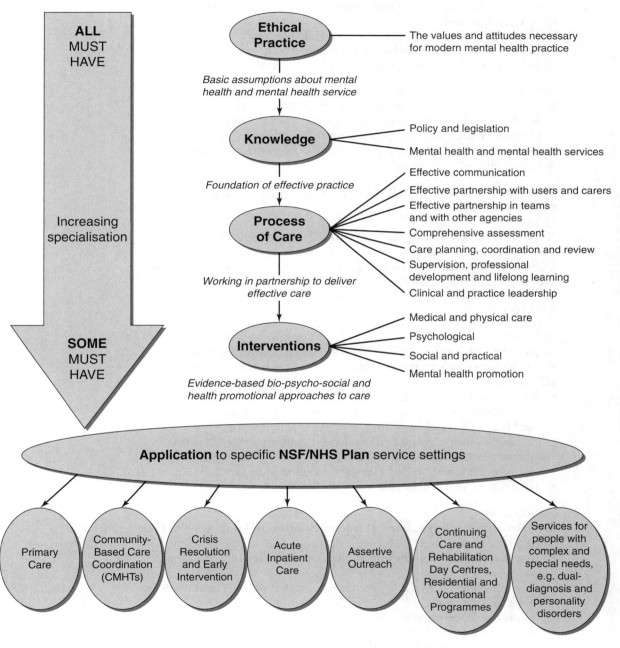

ALL MUST HAVE

Increasing specialisation

SOME MUST HAVE

Ethical Practice — The values and attitudes necessary for modern mental health practice

Basic assumptions about mental health and mental health service

Knowledge — Policy and legislation — Mental health and mental health services

Foundation of effective practice

Process of Care — Effective communication — Effective partnership with users and carers — Effective partnership in teams and with other agencies — Comprehensive assessment — Care planning, coordination and review — Supervision, professional development and lifelong learning — Clinical and practice leadership

Working in partnership to deliver effective care

Interventions — Medical and physical care — Psychological — Social and practical — Mental health promotion

Evidence-based bio-psycho-social and health promotional approaches to care

Application to specific **NSF/NHS Plan** service settings

- Primary Care
- Community-Based Care Coordination (CMHTs)
- Crisis Resolution and Early Intervention
- Acute Inpatient Care
- Assertive Outreach
- Continuing Care and Rehabilitation Day Centres, Residential and Vocational Programmes
- Services for people with complex and special needs, e.g. dual-diagnosis and personality disorders

Standard two
Any service user who contacts their primary health care team with a common mental health problem should:
• have their mental health needs identified and assessed
• be offered effective treatments, including referral to specialist services for further assessment, treatment and care if they require it.

Standard three
Any individual with a common mental health problem should:
• be able to make contact round the clock with the local services necessary to meet their needs and receive adequate care
• be able to use *NHS Direct*, as it develops, for first-level advice and referral on to specialist helplines or to local services.

Standards four and five: Effective services for people with severe mental illness

Aim
To ensure that each person with severe mental illness receives the range of mental health services they need; that crises are anticipated or prevented where possible; that each person receives prompt and effective help if a crisis does occur; and that each person has timely access to an appropriate and safe mental health place or hospital bed, including a secure bed, as close to home as possible.

Standard four
All mental health service users on Care Programme Approach should:
• receive care which optimises engagement, anticipates or prevents a crisis, and reduces risk
• have a copy of a written care plan which:
    – includes the action to be taken in a crisis by service users, their carer, and their care coordinator
    – advises their General Practitioner (GP) how they should respond if the service user needs additional help
    – is regularly reviewed by their care coordinator
• be able to access services 24 hours a day, 365 days a year.

Standard five
Each service user who is assessed as requiring a period of care away from their home should have:
• timely access to an appropriate hospital bed or alternative bed or place, which is:
    – in the least restrictive environment consistent with the need to protect them and the public
    – as close to home as possible
• a copy of a written after-care plan agreed on discharge which sets out the care and rehabilitation to be provided, identifies the care coordinator and specifies the action to be taken in a crisis.

Standard six: Caring about carers
Aim
To ensure health and social services assess the needs of carers who provide regular and substantial care for those with severe mental illness, and provide care to meet their needs.

Standard six
All individuals who provide regular and substantial care for a person on CPA should:
• have an assessment of their caring, physical and mental health needs, repeated on at least an annual basis
• have their own written care plan which is given to them and implemented in discussion with them.

Standard seven
Local health and social care communities should prevent suicides by:
• promoting mental health for all, working with individuals and communities (Standard one)
• delivering high-quality primary mental health care (Standard two)
• ensuring that anyone with a mental health problem can contact local services via the primary care team, a helpline or an A & E department (Standard three)
• ensuring that individuals with severe and enduring mental illness have a care plan which meets their specific needs, including access to services round the clock (Standard four)
• providing safe hospital accommodation for individuals who need it (Standard five)
• enabling individuals caring for someone with severe mental illness to receive the support which they need to continue to care (Standard six)
and in addition:
• support local prison staff in preventing suicides among prisoners
• ensure that staff are competent to assess the risk of suicide among individuals at greatest risk
• develop local systems for suicide audit to learn lessons and take any necessary action.

The 10 essential shared capabilities
There are 10 essential shared capabilities for mental health practice.
• Working in Partnership. Developing and maintaining constructive working relationships with service users, carers, families, colleagues, lay people and wider community networks. Working positively with any tensions created by conflicts of interest or aspiration that may arise between the partners in care.
• Respecting Diversity. Working in partnership with service users, carers, families and colleagues to provide care and interventions that not only make a positive difference but also do so in ways that respect and value diversity, including age, race, culture, disability, gender, spirituality and sexuality.

- Practising Ethically. Recognising the rights and aspirations of service users and their families, acknowledging power differentials and minimising them whenever possible. Providing treatment and care that is accountable to service users and carers within the boundaries prescribed by national (professional), legal and local codes of ethical practice.
- Challenging Inequality. Addressing the causes and consequences of stigma, discrimination, social inequality and exclusion on service users, carers and mental health services. Creating, developing or maintaining valued social roles for people in the communities they come from.
- Promoting Recovery. Working in partnership to provide care and treatment that enables service users and carers to tackle mental health problems with hope and optimism and to work towards a valued lifestyle within and beyond the limits of any mental health problem.
- Identifying People's Needs and Strengths. Working in partnership to gather information to agree health and social care needs in the context of the preferred lifestyle and aspirations of service users, their families, carers and friends.
- Providing Service User-Centred Care. Negotiating achievable and meaningful goals, primarily from the perspective of service users and their families. Influencing and seeking the means to achieve these goals and clarifying the responsibilities of the people who will provide any help that is needed, including systematically evaluating outcomes and achievements.
- Making a Difference. Facilitating access to and delivering the best quality, evidence-based, value-based health and social care interventions to meet the needs and aspirations of service users, their families and carers.
- Promoting Safety and Positive Risk Taking. Empowering the person to decide the level of risk they are prepared to take with their health and safety. This includes working with the tension between promoting safety and positive risk taking, including assessing and dealing with possible risks for service users, carers, family members and the wider public.
- Personal Development and Learning. Keeping up to date with changes in practice and participating in lifelong learning, personal and professional development for one's self and colleagues through supervision, appraisal and reflective practice.

NICE guidelines

NICE is an independent organisation responsible for providing national guidance on the promotion of good health and the prevention and treatment of ill health.

NICE produces guidance in three areas of health.
- Public health. Guidance on the promotion of good health and the prevention of ill health for those working in the NHS, local authorities and the wider public and voluntary sector.
- Health technologies. Guidance on the use of new and existing medicines, treatments and procedures within the NHS.
- Clinical practice. Guidance on the appropriate treatment and care of people with specific diseases and conditions within the NHS.

All of the conditions have a set of guidelines which are detailed in the relevant chapters.

Practice setting

A health care organisation's philosophy of mental health and mental illness – and its approach towards treatment – shapes the expectations of both the nurse and the service user. Administrative policies may either foster or limit the full use of the mental health nurse's practice abilities and expertise.

Personal initiative

The level at which a mental health nurse performs is influenced by her willingness to act as an agent of change, a thorough knowledge of personal strengths and weaknesses and realisation of her clinical competence.

Theoretical basis of mental health nursing

Like other nursing specialties, mental health nursing is theory based. Theoretical concepts gathered from numerous models of behaviour contribute to mental health nursing. (See *Theoretical models of behaviour*, pages 16 and 17.)

Nurse–service user relationship

The first step in caring for a service user with a mental health disorder is to establish a therapeutic relationship. Like other helping relationships, a therapeutic nurse–service user relationship is marked by caring, sensitivity, genuineness and empathy. Through your words and actions, you must convey that you respect the service user and that his feelings, thoughts and needs are important to you.

The relationship also is goal oriented, purposeful, time limited and focused on the service user's needs and growth. It evolves naturally through four distinct phases. (See *Phases of the nurse–service user relationship*, page 18.)

Power to the service user

An effective nurse–service user relationship empowers the service user. It allows you to plan, implement and evaluate care along *with* him – not just for him.

Can they trust you?

To establish an effective relationship, you must gain the service user's trust. A service user who feels safe and respected is more likely to provide accurate assessment information and to comply with treatment. To promote trust, always show sensitivity and display a positive regard towards the service user.

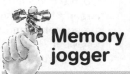

Memory jogger

To encourage your service user to trust you, think of the mnemonic TRUST.

T Try expression

R Reflection

U Use silence

S Set limits

T Time with the client

Theoretical models of behaviour

Learning about the various models of human behaviour gives you a better understanding of mental health disorders. These models are summarised below.

Remember, though, that human behaviour isn't fully understood, so no model or theory is considered right or wrong or better or worse than any other. Commonly, mental health and mental health nurses use an eclectic approach, drawing on several theoretical models.

Psychoanalytical model (Freud)

According to the psychoanalytical model, the personality consists of the:

- id, encompassing the primitive instincts and energies underlying all psychic activity
- ego, the conscious part of the personality, and the part that most immediately controls thought and behaviour
- superego, the conscience.

During childhood, development occurs in five psychosexual stages – oral, anal, phallic, latency and genital. Deviations in behaviour result from unsuccessful task accomplishment during earlier developmental stages. Freud also proposed that behaviour is motivated by anxiety, the cornerstone of psychopathology.

Understanding the psychosexual stages of childhood provides a framework for the nurse to understand adult behaviours. Also, the nurse can promote effective parenting by teaching parents about the child's needs during each psychosexual stage.

Interpersonal model (Sullivan, Peplau)

The interpersonal model holds that human development results from interpersonal relationships, and that behaviour is motivated by avoidance of anxiety and attainment of satisfaction.

Peplau drew on Sullivan's original theory to propose an interpersonal nursing theory, which advanced the practice of mental health nursing by defining it as an interpersonal process. She proposed that:

- nurses must promote the nurse–service user relationship to build trust and foster healthy behaviour
- therapeutic use of self promotes healing
- the therapeutic relationship is directed towards meeting the service user's needs.

Social model (Caplan, Szasz)

The social model proposes that the entire sociocultural environment influences mental health. Deviant behaviour is defined by the culture in which a person lives. Undesirable or abnormal behaviour in one society may be considered normal in another. In addition, social conditions and interactions predispose people to mental illness.

Existential model (Frankl, Perls, May)

The existential model centres on a person's present experiences rather than past ones. It holds that alienation from the self causes deviant behaviour, and that people can make free choices about which behaviours to display.

Based on the existential model of behaviour, nursing developed the concept that the nurse works to restore the service user to a state of 'full life' from a state of 'self-alienation'.

Theoretical models of behaviour *(continued)*

Nursing model (Rogers, Orem, Sister Roy, Peplau)

The nursing model emphasises the person as a biopsychosocial being. This holistic approach focuses on caring rather than curing, and promotes collaboration between the nurse and the service user. It establishes the nursing process as the basis for providing care.

According to the nursing model, the service user's needs direct the therapeutic relationship and the service user's reactions to nursing interventions guide future interventions.

Medical model

The medical model holds that disease is the cause of deviant behaviour. It focuses on the diagnosis and treatment of the disease. Application of the medical model to mental illness has led to identification of neurochemicals as possible causes of deviant behaviour. The medical model also accepts socioenvironmental influences as potential causes of deviant behaviour.

Communication models (Berne, Bandler, Grindler)

Communication theory proposes that all human behaviour is a form of communication and that the meaning of behaviour depends on the clarity of communication between the sender and the receiver. Unclear communication produces anxiety, which results in behaviour deviations.

The communication pattern used with individuals, families and social and work groups identifies the causes of the behavioural deviation. When communication improves, so does behaviour.

Nurses draw on the communication model when they teach service users effective communication techniques.

Behavioural model (Skinner, Wolpe, Eysenck)

According to the behavioural model, all behaviour – including mental illness – is learned. Unlike other models, which focus on the service user's emotions, behavioural theory focuses on the service user's actions.

Behaviourists believe that the behaviour that's rewarded will persist. Desired behaviours can be learned through rewards and negative behaviours eliminated through punishment. Thus, people can learn to behave in socially desirable ways.

Humanistic model (Maslow)

In the humanistic model, understanding human behaviour requires familiarity with a hierarchy that has six levels of need:

- Level 1: physiological survival (food, oxygen and rest)
- Level 2: safety, security and self-preservation
- Level 3: love and belonging (developing fulfilling relationships)
- Level 4: esteem and recognition (feeling like a worthwhile, contributing member of society, appreciating one's own uniqueness)
- Level 5: self-actualisation (self-fulfillment)
- Level 6: truth, harmony, beauty and spirituality.

Nursing draws from the humanistic model by striving to meet service users' lower-level needs before higher-level ones. By performing a needs assessment, the nurse determines appropriate intervention strategies to help service users meet their needs.

Phases of the nurse–service user relationship

The phases of a helping relationship include the preinteraction, orientation, working and termination phases.

Preinteraction phase

During the preinteraction phase – which may last a few seconds or several weeks – the nurse assesses the service user for unresolved problems. The service user may not be actively involved at this point.

Orientation (introductory) phase

The orientation (getting-to-know-you) phase sets the tone for the relationship. Introductions are made and each person's roles are defined. Trust begins to develop.

Usually, the nurse initiates this phase, setting the limits of the relationship as a professional one and establishing the focus for conversation based on assessment data.

Then the nurse and the service user may make an agreement, write a contract or discuss and establish goals. Be aware that some service users may be resistant during this phase, testing your true intent or denying they have a problem.

Working (exploration) phase

During the working phase, the nurse and the service user explore and evaluate problems and work towards achieving set goals. The nurse may take on the role of counsellor and facilitator, with the service user participating actively. The service user is free to examine problems and tries to gain insight or find solutions.

Termination (resolution) phase

During the termination phase, the nurse reviews and summarises the service user's progress. Together, the nurse and the service user determine if goals have been met – and, if not, why not.

Then the nurse formally ends the relationship, being sure to acknowledge the service user's feelings about termination. Be aware that the service user may feel hurt or angry at the nurse's 'abandonment'.

Effective communication

Although effective communication is important in all types of service user care, it's particularly crucial in mental health nursing. Communication involves both sending and receiving messages. It can be verbal or nonverbal. Usually, people send verbal and nonverbal messages simultaneously.

Verbal communication

In mental health nursing, verbal communication usually takes place through the spoken word but sometimes involves written communication (as when providing written instructions on taking self-administered medications).

Obliterating obstacles

Various factors can influence verbal communication, including the service user's past experiences, feelings, cultural or religious background and

> **Advice from the experts**
>
> ## Factors that influence verbal communication
>
> Various factors can prevent effective communication between the nurse and the individual. Be sure to consider the service user's:
>
> - native language
> - culture or nationality
> - sexual orientation or gender
> - age and developmental considerations
> - roles and responsibilities
> - social background or status
> - space and territoriality
> - physical, mental and emotional state
> - values
> - environment.

sociocultural status. To overcome these potential obstacles, you must learn about – and show sensitivity to – your service user's experiences, beliefs and background. (See *Factors that influence verbal communication*.)

Cutting through the fog

Communicating with mentally ill service users can be particularly challenging if their underlying disorder involves delusions, paranoia, hallucinations, dementia or thought disorders. Dealing with these problems may require special skills. (See *Reducing communication barriers*, page 20.)

¿Habla usted inglés?

If the service user doesn't speak English well, you may need to find an interpreter.

If his speech is impaired, consider using communication aids, such as a pad and felt-tipped pen, a dry erase board, sign language or flash cards with common words or phrases.

Service user patterns

Be sure to listen intently as the service user speaks. This will allow you not only to hear and analyse what he says but also to interpret his communication pattern.

Nonverbal communication

Nonverbal communication (body language) includes eye contact, facial expression, posture, gait, gestures, touch, physical appearance or attributes, dress or grooming, affect and even silence. In fact, most communication is nonverbal.

Advice from the experts

Reducing communication barriers

Acknowledging and reducing communication barriers can promote a more effective relationship with mental health service users.

Language difficulties or differences

Use words appropriate for the service user's educational level. Avoid medical terms that he's unlikely to understand.

Be aware of words that may have more than one meaning. To some service users, for instance, the word 'bad' may also be slang for 'good'.

If the person speaks a foreign language or uses an ethnic dialect, obtain an interpreter to help you communicate. However, remember that a third person's presence may make the person less willing to share his feelings.

Impaired hearing

If the person can't hear you clearly, he may misinterpret your questions or responses. Check whether he's wearing a hearing aid. If so, is it turned on? If not, can he read lips? If possible, face him and speak clearly and slowly, using common words. Keep your questions short, simple and direct.

If the person has a severe hearing impairment, he may have to communicate in writing, or you may need to collect information from his family or friends.

If the person is elderly, speak in low-pitched tones. With aging, the ability to hear high-pitched tones deteriorates first.

Inappropriate responses

Avoid appearing to discount the service user's feelings, as by changing the subject abruptly. Otherwise, the person may get the impression that you're disinterested, anxious or annoyed or that you're judging him.

Thought disorders

If the service user's thought patterns are incoherent or irrelevant, he may be unable to interpret messages correctly, focus on the interview or provide appropriate responses. When assessing him, ask simple questions about concrete topics, and clarify his responses. Encourage him to express himself clearly.

Paranoid thinking

Approach a paranoid person in a nonthreatening way. Avoid touching him, which he may misinterpret as an attempt to harm him. Also, keep in mind that a paranoid person may not mean the things he says.

Hallucinations

A hallucinating person can't hear or respond appropriately. Show concern but don't reinforce his hallucinatory perceptions.

Be as specific as possible when giving commands. For instance, if he says he's hearing voices, tell him to stop listening to the voices and listen to you instead.

Delusions

A deluded person defends irrational beliefs or ideas despite factual evidence to the contrary. Some delusions may be so bizarre that you'll recognise them immediately. Others may be hard to identify.

Don't condemn or agree with delusional beliefs, and don't dismiss a statement because you think it's delusional. Instead, gently emphasise reality without arguing.

Delirium

A delirious person experiences disorientation, hallucinations and confusion. Misinterpretation and inappropriate responses commonly result. Talk to him directly, ask simple questions and offer frequent reassurances.

Dementia

A person with dementia (irreversible deterioration of mental capacity) may experience changes in memory and thought patterns. His language may become distorted or slurred.

When interviewing him, minimise distractions. Use simple, concise language. Avoid making statements that could be easily misinterpreted.

Body talk

Besides analysing the service user's body language, you'll need to be aware of your own. Make sure your gestures, expressions and posture convey the proper messages – friendliness, openness and acceptance of the service user.

Using silence

Think of silence as a strategic communication tool. You can use it, for instance, to give the service user time to talk, think and gain insight into problems.

Remember, though, that strategic silence requires practice and timing. If you use it too much or at the wrong times, you could give the impression of disinterest or judgement.

Listening attentively

Always listen attentively. Facing the service user, acknowledge him and maintain eye contact. Stay relaxed, with your legs and arms uncrossed. You may lean forwards slightly so you don't seem stiff and distant.

When the service user speaks, convey acceptance. Don't interrupt or argue, but do provide verbal feedback as appropriate.

Checking for congruence

Ideally, the service user's nonverbal and verbal messages should match. Look for congruence (matching) between his verbal and nonverbal communication. Do his gestures and facial expression reinforce – or contradict – his words?

Therapeutic communication

Besides serving as the foundation for an effective nurse–service user relationship, therapeutic communication is the primary intervention in mental health nursing. Therapeutic communication reduces stress, encourages insight and supports problem solving.

Blunderin' and bunglin'

In contrast, nontherapeutic communication may create stumbling blocks in the relationship. (See *Nontherapeutic ways of communicating*, page 22.)

Therapeutic communication techniques

Therapeutic communication techniques include open-ended questions, validating, clarifying, sharing impressions, restating, focusing, suggestive collaboration and offering information.

Using open-ended questions

To initiate conversation, use open-ended or general questions. This encourages the service user to talk about any subject that comes to mind. For instance, you would ask, 'What would you like to talk about today?'

Advice from the experts

Nontherapeutic ways of communicating

Nontherapeutic techniques work against establishing an effective nurse–service user relationship. Avoid the following pitfalls when interacting with people.

Attacking or defending

- Getting angry with the person
- Arguing with him
- Challenging him or his beliefs
- Being defensive

Casting judgement

- Judging the person
- Criticising him
- Giving approval or disapproval

Interrogating

- Asking him why
- Asking excessive, inappropriate or leading questions
- Probing sensitive areas or making the person feel uncomfortable

Minimising

- Stereotyping the person
- Not listening to him
- Not perceiving him as human
- Not taking his beliefs seriously
- Failing to maintain eye contact
- Changing the subject inappropriately
- Working on a task while he's talking to you

- Letting your mind wander during a conversation
- Using clichés

Playing Ann Landers

- Giving advice
- Offering false reassurance

Pressuring

- Trying to talk the person into accepting treatment

Running off at the mouth

- Talking on and on
- Not letting the person respond
- Repeating a point you just made
- Interpreting or speculating on the dynamics of person problems
- Making inappropriate comments

Rushing

- Responding to the person before he finishes speaking
- Finishing his sentences for him

Taking sides

- Joining attacks led by the person
- Participating in criticism of staff members

Conversational cul-de-sacs

In contrast, closed-ended questions limit the range of responses, eliciting merely a 'Yes' or 'No'.

Validating

Validating – reviewing and rephrasing key service user statements – helps ensure that you've correctly understood what the service user has said.

Validating also encourages the service user to elaborate. Say, for example, the service user says he's angry at the way his friend treated him. To validate, you might reply, 'You're telling me you're feeling angry because of how your friend treated you yesterday. Is that right?'

Clarifying
Asking the service user to clarify a confusing or vague message shows your desire to understand what he's saying. It can also elicit precise information crucial to his treatment or recovery. You can use clarification to hone your understanding of the service user's expression of time, reality or sequence.

Sharing impressions
When you share impressions, you're describing the service user's feelings and then seeking corrective feedback from him. As an example, you might say, 'Tell me if my perception of what you're saying is correct.'

Share – Don't challenge
Like validating and clarifying, sharing impressions lets the service user clarify misperceptions or misunderstanding and gives you a better understanding of his true feelings. Just make sure your sharing doesn't change into challenging or confronting.

Restating
Restating involves summarising the service user's message in your own words and then allowing him to respond. It shows you're paying attention and want to hear more, and encourages him to expand on what he has said.

Say what?
Say, for example, the service user tells you his treatments 'make me want to scream'. You might respond, 'So what you're saying is that your treatments really upset you.'

Don't get carried away. Too much restating could make him feel you're mocking him.

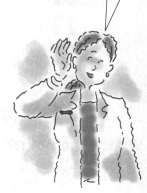

Ask the service user to clarify any confusing or vague information he provides.

Focusing
Focusing lets you redirect the service user's attention towards something specific – especially if he's vague or rambling. If you would like him to clarify or elaborate on something he said earlier, you would say, 'Let's go back to what we were just talking about.'

Suggestive collaboration
When used correctly, suggestive collaboration gives the service user a chance to explore the pros and cons of a suggested approach. For example, you might suggest, 'Perhaps we can meet with your parents to discuss the matter.' Use suggestive collaboration carefully, though, or you could end up 'directing' the service user.

Offering information
Offering information involves explaining the components or purpose of an activity or procedure. You're offering information any time you provide

teaching – such as when explaining why you're giving the service user a certain drug.

This technique promotes health teaching and establishes trust. Be sure to keep your statements simple and direct, and avoid giving advice.

> Making too many suggestions could make the service user feel you're directing him in a movie.

Assessment

Like other types of nursing, mental health nursing follows the nursing process steps. Mental health assessment is the scientific process of identifying a service user's psychosocial problems, strengths and concerns. Besides serving as the basis for treating mental health service users, mental health assessment has broad nursing applications.

Testing – one, two, three

The information you gather during assessment will permit caregivers to analyse the service user's mental, emotional and behavioural status. During assessment, you also may need to administer appropriate mental status tests.

Mental health nursing interview

A systematic mental health interview gathers broad information that helps you to:

 assess the service user's psychological functioning

identify the underlying or precipitating cause of his current problem

 understand his coping methods and their effect on his psychosocial growth

formulate the care plan

 gauge his progress and the effectiveness of treatments.

What's the point?

Sometimes the service user doesn't understand the purpose of the interview (or, for that matter, subsequent therapy). Help him identify the benefits of dealing with problems openly.

General guidelines

Follow the general guidelines below when conducting the service user interview.

Ensure privacy

Choose a quiet, calm, private setting. Interruptions and distractions threaten confidentiality and may interfere with effective listening. If necessary, reassure the service user that he's safe.

Just the two of us

Tell the service user you respect his need for privacy. Ask him privately who should be present at the interview. An adolescent, for instance, may refuse to discuss sexual activity in front of parents.

Show support and sensitivity

You're likely to encounter mental health service users who are angry and argumentative. Others will be too withdrawn even to say why they're seeking help.

To make the service user feel comfortable enough to discuss his problems, you must listen carefully and objectively, and respond with sensitivity. (See *Interview do's and don'ts*.)

Use reliable information sources

A mentally ill service user may not be a reliable source of information. If he can't provide answers to important questions or seems unreliable, ask for permission to interview family members or friends.

Advice from the experts

Interview do's and don'ts

When interviewing people with mental health problems, follow these guidelines.

Do set clear goals

The assessment interview isn't meant to be a random discussion. Make sure you have clearly set goals – such as obtaining information, screening for abnormalities or investigating for an identified mental health condition (depression, paranoia or suicidal thoughts, for instance).

Do heed unspoken signals

Listen carefully for indications of anxiety or distress. What topics does the person ignore or pass over vaguely? You may find important clues in his method of self-expression and in the subjects he avoids.

Do check yourself

Monitor your own reactions. The mental health person may provoke an emotional response strong enough to interfere with your professional judgement. For instance, a depressed person may make you depressed, a hostile one may provoke your anger and an anxious one may cause you to feel anxiety. A violent, psychotic person who has lost touch with reality may induce fear.

Don't rush

Don't rush through the interview. Remember that building a trusting therapeutic relationship takes time.

Don't make assumptions

Don't make assumptions about how past events affected the person emotionally. Try to discover what each event meant to him.

If he says one of his parents died, for instance, don't assume that the death provoked sadness. A death by itself doesn't cause sadness, guilt or anger. What matters is how the person perceives the loss.

Don't judge the person

Don't let personal values cloud your professional judgement. For example, when assessing the person's appearance, judge attire on its appropriateness and cleanliness, not on whether it suits your taste.

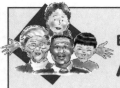

Bridging the gap

Abnormal – or just unfamiliar?

When dealing with a service user from an unfamiliar culture, you may need to consult an outside resource before drawing conclusions about his psychological state.

Say, for instance, the indivdiual blames bad luck on a power called 'juju'. In our culture, he may be considered delusional. However, in Nigeria, he would be considered normal.

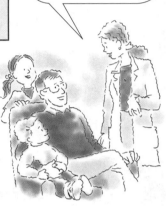

I'd like to ask you a few questions that Mrs. Clark couldn't answer.

Check and double-check

If he can answer your questions but his responses are questionable, verify them with family members, friends or health care personnel. Check hospital records from previous admissions, if possible, and compare his past behaviour, symptoms and circumstances with the current situation.

Consider the service user's culture

Be aware that service users come from diverse cultures. Some cultures frown on discussing intimate details with strangers, even nurses.

Gather cultural information early in the interview, and tailor your questions accordingly. (See *Abnormal – or just unfamiliar?*)

Beginning the interview

When meeting the service user for the first time, introduce yourself and explain the purpose of the interview. Ask how he would like you to address him.

Listening post

Sit at a comfortable distance from the service user and give him your undivided attention. Maintain a professional but friendly attitude. Speak in a calm, nonthreatening tone to encourage him to be candid.

Biographic data

Determine the service user's age, sex, ethnic origin, primary language, birthplace, religion and marital status. Use this information to validate his medical record.

Socioeconomic data

Gather information about your service user's educational level, housing conditions, income, current employment status and family – all of which may provide clues to his current problem.

Assessing his economic and personal situation helps you determine their impact on his current psychological status. Be aware that a service user experiencing economic or personal hardships is more likely to show symptoms of distress during an illness.

Bridging the gap

Culture and conduct

When conducting the service user interview, remember that behaviours considered appropriate in mainstream United Kingdom culture may be frowned on in other cultures – and vice versa. For example, a Brazilian from a low socioeconomic class may avoid direct eye contact with health care professionals as a way of showing respect.

Shame and stigma

Be aware, too, that many cultures view mental illness as a stigma. The family of a mentally ill person may keep that person hidden and refuse to answer questions about him.

Spiritual balance

A service user's cultural beliefs may affect his treatment decisions. For example, in certain black and African cultures, mental illness may be attributed to a person's level of spiritual balance.

Cultural beliefs

Find out about the service user's cultural beliefs. Beliefs can affect his response to illness, his adaptation to hospital care and even his behaviour during the interview. (See *Culture and conduct*.)

Chief complaint

When possible, fully explore the service user's chief complaint. Be sure to ask him:

 when his symptoms began

 whether they have an abrupt or gradual onset

 how severe they are

 how long they last

 how they affect his level of functioning.

For a recurrent problem, ask what prompted him to seek help at this time.

Can I quote you on that?

When documenting the service user's chief complaint, quote him directly.

You sure there's no problem?

Be aware that some service users don't have any overriding concern. Others insist nothing is wrong. In fact, service users enmeshed in a medical problem may fail to recognise their own depression or anxiety. Carefully observe such service users for signs of disturbed mental health.

Awareness check

When eliciting the chief complaint, keep in mind that the service user may not verbalise it directly. Instead, you, another nurse, family members or friends may note that he's having trouble coping or exhibiting unusual behaviour.

In this case, determine if he's aware of the problem. Document his response verbatim, enclosing his words in quotation marks.

Great expectations

Ask what the service user expects to accomplish through treatment. For instance, someone with low self-esteem may seek a better self-image. A schizophrenic may want to be rid of hallucinations.

Personal history

During this part of the interview, begin a more in-depth discussion of the development of the service user's personality. Stay alert for signs of stumbling blocks during the maturation process.

Ego function

Assess the service user's ego function. How does he cope with stress? Does he respond with violence or does he become withdrawn?

What's his usual coping pattern? Does he use denial to cope with stress? Can he control impulses and demonstrate good judgement? How strong is his sense of identity?

Areas of strength

Look for indications of the service user's talents, accomplishments, adaptability and capacity to find emotional support.

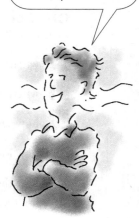

Go ahead. Ask me about my talents and accomplishments.

Mental health history

Discuss past mental health or psychological disturbances, such as episodes of delusions, violence, attempted suicides, drug or alcohol abuse or depression. Has the service user undergone mental health treatment before? If so, did it help?

Reluctant responders

Although the service user may be reluctant to respond to these questions, the answers could suggest early signs or symptoms of depression, dementia, suicide risk, psychosis or adverse reactions to drug therapy.

Psychosocial history

Taking the service user's psychosocial history helps you evaluate mental and social status and function. Ask about his beliefs, relationships, lifestyle, coping skills, diet, sleeping patterns and use of alcohol, tobacco or drugs.

Explore his social functioning by having him describe his work, school, religious practices, community life, hobbies and sexual activity. Also ask about his social network and support systems.

Upheaval index

Discuss life changes and how they've affected him. Explore how he coped with such changes as a recent marriage, divorce, illness, job loss or death of a loved one. How did he feel when these changes occurred?

Family history

To gain insight into environmental influences on the service user's development, ask about family customs, child-rearing practices and emotional support received during childhood.

How does he react when disclosing his family history? For example, if he talks about his parents' divorce, can you detect hints of hostility or unresolved grief?

> Find out how the person coped with a recent marriage, divorce or other major life change.

It's all relative

Ask about relatives' emotional health. Does the service user have a family history of substance abuse, alcoholism, suicide, psychological disorders, mental health hospitalisation, child abuse or violence?

Then ask about physical disorders. A family history of diabetes mellitus or thyroid disorders, for instance, may indicate that the service user's problem has an organic basis.

Medication history

Certain drugs may cause or contribute to signs or symptoms of mental illness. Have the service user list all the medications he takes, including over-the-counter drugs and nutritional and herbal supplements. Check for possible drug interactions.

> Review the person's medication history for therapeutic drug effects and adverse reactions.

Compliance check

If the service user is taking an antipsychotic, antidepressant, anxiolytic or antimanic drug, find out if he uses it as prescribed. Ask if his symptoms have improved since he started drug therapy and whether he has experienced adverse reactions.

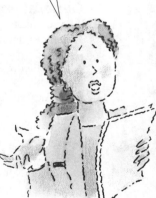

Physical illnesses

Find out if the service user has a history of medical conditions that could cause disorientation, distorted thought processes, depression or other signs or symptoms of mental illness. Such conditions include:
- kidney failure
- liver failure
- infection
- thyroid disease
- metabolic disorders
- increased intracranial pressure.

Mental status evaluation

Commonly included as part of the mental health interview, the mental status examination (MSE) is a tool for assessing psychological dysfunction and identifying causes of psychopathology. The MSE examines the service user's level of consciousness (LOC), general appearance, behaviour, speech, mood and affect, intellectual performance, judgement, insight, perception and thought content.

Master of the MSE?

Understanding the components of the MSE will help you accurately interpret the psychiatrist's findings and plan appropriate nursing interventions. Nursing responsibilities may include conducting all or a portion of the MSE.

Level of consciousness

Begin by assessing the service user's LOC – a basic brain function. Identify the intensity of stimulation needed to arouse him. Does he respond when spoken to in a normal conversational tone – or only to a loud voice? Does it take a light touch, vigorous shaking or painful stimulation to rouse him?

Stimulus response

Assess the service user's response to stimulation, including the degree and quality of movement, speech content and coherence, and level of eye opening and eye contact. Note and document his actions after the stimulus is removed.

An impaired LOC may indicate a brain tumour or abscess, haematoma, hydrocephalus, electrolyte or acid–base imbalance or toxicity caused by liver or kidney failure, alcohol or drugs. Refer the service user with an altered LOC for a more complete medical examination.

Oh dear. Kidney failure can cause an altered LOC.

General appearance

The service user's appearance may reflect his emotional and mental state. When evaluating his appearance, consider these questions:

 Is he dressed and groomed appropriately for age, sex and situation?

 Are his skin, hair, nails and teeth clean?

 Is his manner of dress appropriate?

If a female service user uses cosmetics, are they applied appropriately?

A dishevelled appearance may indicate self-neglect or a preoccupation with other activities. A pale, emaciated, sad appearance may signal depression.

Touchy subjects

Measure the service user's weight and height. Assess colouring, skin condition and body build. Check for obvious physical impairments and unpleasant odours.

Slouches, slumps and substances

Observe the service user's posture. Is he erect or does he slouch? Is his head lowered? Does he walk normally? Is his gait brisk, slow, shuffling or unsteady?

A slumped posture may mean depression, fatigue or suspiciousness. An uneven or unsteady gait could suggest physical abnormalities or the influence of drugs or alcohol.

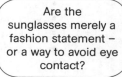

Are the sunglasses merely a fashion statement – or a way to avoid eye contact?

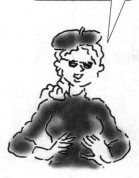

Facial facts

Note his facial expression. Does he look alert or stare blankly? Does he appear happy, sad or angry? Does he maintain or avoid direct eye contact? Does he stare at you for long periods?

Reality check

Find out if the service user's perceptions about his health match your observations. Note any discrepancies.

Behaviour

Evaluate the service user's demeanour and attitude. When entering the room, does he appear sad, joyful or expressionless? Does he acknowledge your initial greeting and introduction? Does he keep an appropriate distance between himself and others?

How does he respond to your questions? Is he cooperative, friendly, hostile or indifferent?

Gestures

Assess the service user's gestures. Are they appropriate? Disconnected gestures may indicate he's hallucinating. A service user who experiences auditory hallucinations, for instance, may speak to someone who isn't there and tilt his head to listen.

Mannerisms

Evaluate the service user's mannerisms. Does he have distinctive ones, such as tics or tremors? Does he bite his nails, fidget or pace? Does he gaze directly at you, at the floor or around the room?

Also note such unusual mannerisms as speaking to someone who isn't present.

Attitudes

Is the service user cooperative? Are his answers to your questions revealing – or overly revealing? Or is he mistrustful, hostile or embarrassed?

Activity level

Is the service user restless, calm, tense or rigid? Inability to sit still may indicate anxiety. Pressured, rapid speech and a heightened activity level may indicate the manic phase of bipolar disorder.

Speech

As the service user speaks, observe the content and quality of his speech. Be sure to note:
• illogical choice of topics
• irrelevant or illogical replies to questions

- speech defects, such as stuttering
- excessively fast or slow speech
- sudden interruptions
- excessive volume or barely audible speech
- altered vocal tone and modulation
- slurring
- excessive number of words (overproductive speech)
- minimal, monosyllabic responses (underproductive speech).

Sign language

If the service user communicates only with gestures, determine whether this is an isolated behaviour or part of a pattern of diminished responsiveness.

Time warp?

Notice how much time elapses before the service user reacts to your questions.

Where's the logic?

Note speech characteristics that may indicate altered thought processes, including:
- illogical or irrelevant replies to questions
- minimal or monosyllabic responses
- convoluted or excessively detailed speech
- repetitious speech patterns
- flight of ideas
- sudden silence for no obvious reason.

Mood and affect

Mood refers to a pervasive feeling or state of mind. Usually, a service user projects a prevailing mood – although this mood may change over the course of a day. For example, depressed service users may smile occasionally but will revert to their prevailing mood of sadness.

Affect, on the other hand, refers to expression of mood. Variations in affect are called range of emotion.

Feelings, wo-wo-wo, feelings

To assess mood and affect, enquire about the service user's current feelings. Ask him to describe these feelings in concrete terms, and have him suggest possible reasons for these feelings.

Observe for manifestations of mood and affect. Does the service user seem excited or depressed? Is he crying, sweating, breathing heavily or trembling?

Mood control

Can the service user keep mood changes under control? Mood swings may indicate a physiological disorder, stress, dehydration, electrolyte imbalances, medication effects or recreational drug or alcohol use.

Look for indications of mood in facial expression and posture. Also note inconsistencies between body language and mood. For instance, does the service user smile when discussing a situation that should provoke sadness or anger?

Flighty or flat?

Indications of a mood disorder include:
- lability of affect – rapid, dramatic fluctuation in the range of emotions
- flat affect – an unresponsive range of emotion, which may signify schizophrenia or Parkinson's disease
- inappropriate affect – inconsistency between affect and mood, as when the service user smiles when discussing an anger-provoking situation.

Intellectual performance

An emotionally distressed service user may be unable to reason abstractly, make judgements or solve problems. To develop a picture of the service user's intellectual abilities, use the series of simple tests described below (which also screen for organic mental syndrome).

If test results suggest organic mental syndrome, follow up with or refer the service user for additional physical, neurobehavioural and psychological testing.

Orientation

Evaluate the service user's orientation to time, place and person. Ask him to state his name and the time, date, place and circumstance.

Note confusion or disorientation. Look for signs that he's experiencing delusions, hallucinations, obsessions, compulsions, fantasies or daydreams.

Immediate recall

Test the service user's immediate recall by saying, 'I want you to remember three words: apple, house and umbrella'. Then ask, 'What are the three words I want you to remember?'

Delayed recall

Next, assess delayed recall by asking him to repeat the same words after an interval of 5–10 minutes.

Recent memory

To test recent memory, ask about an event that happened within the past few hours or days – for instance, 'When were you admitted to the hospital?' (You should know the correct response or be able to validate it with a family member.)

Memory masquerade

Keep in mind that a service user may make up plausible answers to mask memory deficits.

Remote memory

Assess the service user's ability to remember events in the distant past, such as where he was born or where he attended high school. Recent memory loss with intact remote memory may indicate an organic mental disorder.

Attention level

Assess the service user's attention span and ability to concentrate on a task for an appropriate length of time. (If you find that he has a short attention span, remember to provide simple, written health care instructions.)

Comprehension

Assess the service user's ability to understand the material, retain it and repeat the content. For instance, you might ask him to read part of a news article and explain it.

Concept formation

Test the service user's ability to think abstractly by asking him the meaning of a common proverb such as 'People in glass houses shouldn't throw stones'.

Aspire for the abstract

If he interprets this proverb to mean that you shouldn't criticise others when you could be criticised for doing the same thing, he's showing abstract thinking. People usually develop abstract thinking ability by about age 12.

Confoundingly concrete

But if he interprets the glass house proverb to mean that glass is breakable, he's showing concrete thinking. Concrete answers to abstract questions may indicate mental retardation, severe anxiety, organic mental syndrome or schizophrenia. Schizophrenics also may give elaborate or bizarre answers. Inability to give any answer may indicate low intellectual ability or brain damage.

General knowledge

To determine the service user's store of common knowledge, ask questions appropriate to his age and learning level, such as 'Who's the Prime Minister?'

Judgement

Assess the service user's ability to evaluate choices and draw appropriate conclusions. You can do this by asking questions that emerge naturally during conversation, as in 'What would you do if you ran out of medication?'

A response indicating good judgement would be 'I'd get my prescription renewed', or 'I'd call the doctor'. An inappropriate response to a hypothetical situation may indicate impaired judgement.

Insight

To assess the service user's insight, you might ask, 'What do you think is causing your anxiety?' or 'Have you noticed a recent change in yourself?'

Does his response indicate that he sees himself realistically? Is he aware of his illness and circumstances?

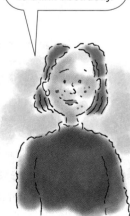

I'm only 12, but I'm old enough to think abstractly.

Degrees of insight

Expect service users to show varying degrees of insight. An alcoholic, for instance, may admit to having a drinking problem but blame it on his work schedule. Severe lack of insight may indicate a psychotic state.

Perception

Perception refers to interpretation of reality as well as use of the senses. Assess the service user's sensory perception and coordination by having him copy a simple drawing.

All in the interpretation

Experts have been placing increasing importance on interpretation of reality in psychological disorders. Psychoanalysts have long believed that depression results from internal, unresolved conflicts that are activated by a real or perceived loss. More recently, proponents of the cognitive theory have proposed that depression arises from distorted perceptions.

Sensory perception disorders

Some service users experience *hallucinations*, in which they perceive nonexistent external stimuli, or *illusions*, in which they misinterpret external stimuli. Tactile, olfactory and gustatory hallucinations usually indicate organic disorders.

Constant visual and auditory hallucinations may give rise to bizarre behaviour. Disorders associated with hallucinations include schizophrenia and acute organic mental syndrome after withdrawal from alcohol or barbiturate addiction.

Just an illusion?

Not all visual and auditory hallucinations are associated with psychological disorders. Heat mirages, visions of a recently deceased loved one, illusions evoked by environmental effects or those occurring just before falling asleep don't necessarily indicate abnormalities. Service users also may experience mild and transitory hallucinations.

Suspect the service user is hallucinating if she says she sees me and my germ buddies rowing gondolas.

Thought content

Assess the service user's thought content and pattern throughout the examination. Are his thoughts clear and well connected to reality? Do they progress in a logical sequence?

Also check for indications of abnormal beliefs and morbid thoughts or preoccupations.

Delusions

Usually associated with schizophrenia, delusions are false beliefs with no firm basis in reality. Grandiose and persecutory delusions are most common. Other types include somatic, nihilistic and control delusions.

Check the references

Ideas of reference (misinterpreting others' acts in a highly personal way) are closely related to delusions, although they don't represent the same level of ego disintegration.

Obsessions and compulsions

Some service users suffer intense obsessions, or preoccupations, that interfere with daily living – such as constantly thinking about hygiene. They also may have compulsions – obsessions that are acted out, such as constantly washing one's hands. Most compulsive service users must exert great effort to control their compulsions.

Morbid thoughts and preoccupations

Assess the service user for:

 suicidal, self-destructive, violent or superstitious thoughts

recurring dreams

 distorted perceptions of reality

feelings of worthlessness.

Sex drive

Changes in sex drive provide valuable information for psychological assessment. However, you may have to sharpen your interview skills to assess such changes, as many service users are uncomfortable discussing sexuality.

Language control

Introduce the subject of sex tactfully but directly. You might say, 'I'm going to ask you a few questions about your sexual activity because it's an important part of almost everyone's life.' Avoid language that assumes a heterosexual orientation.

Competence

Does the service user understand reality and the consequences of his actions? Does he understand the implications of his illness, its treatment and the consequences of avoiding treatment?

Be careful about competence

Use extreme caution when assessing for changes in competence. Unless the service user's behaviour strongly indicates otherwise, assume he's competent.

Remember that legally, only a judge has the power or right to declare a person incompetent to take decisions regarding personal health and safety or financial matters.

Defence mechanisms

In a stressful situation, a person may adopt defence, or coping, mechanisms – behaviours that operate on an unconscious level to protect the ego and reduce stress.

Name that defence mechanism

Examples of defence mechanisms include denial, regression, displacement, projection, reaction formation and fantasy.

Assess service users for excessive reliance on particular defence mechanisms. Be aware that most service users aren't aware they're using defence mechanisms. (For common defence mechanisms you may encounter, see *Defining defence mechanisms*.)

Defining defence mechanisms

People use defence, or coping, mechanisms to relieve anxiety. The definitions below will help you determine whether the person is using one or more of these mechanisms.

Acting out

Acting out refers to repeating certain actions to ward off anxiety without weighing the possible consequences of those actions.

Compensation

Also called substitution, compensation involves trying to make up for feelings of inadequacy or frustration in one area by excelling or overindulging in another.

Denial

A person in denial protects himself from reality – especially the unpleasant aspects of life – by refusing to perceive, acknowledge or face it.

Displacement

In displacement, the person redirects his impulses (commonly anger) from the real target (because that target is too dangerous) to a safer but innocent person. An example is the person who yells at the nurse after becoming angry at his mother for not calling him.

Fantasy

Fantasy refers to creation of unrealistic or improbable images as a way of escaping from daily pressures and responsibilities or to relieve boredom. For instance, a person may daydream excessively, watch TV for hours on end or imagine being highly successful when he feels unsuccessful. Doing these things makes him feel better for a brief period.

Identification

In identification, the person unconsciously adopts the personality characteristics, attitudes, values and behaviour of someone else (such as a hero he emulates and admires) as a way to allay anxiety. He may identify with a group to become more accepted by them.

Intellectualisation

Also called isolation, intellectualisation refers to hiding one's emotional responses or problems under a façade of big words and pretending there's no problem.

Introjection

A person introjects when he adopts someone else's values and standards without exploring whether they fit him.

(continued)

Defining defence mechanisms (continued)

Projection

In projection, the person attributes to others his own unacceptable thoughts, feelings and impulses.

Rationalisation

Rationalisation occurs when a person substitutes acceptable reasons for the real or actual reasons that are motivating his behaviour. The rationalising person makes excuses for shortcomings and avoids self-condemnation, disappointments and criticism.

Reaction formation

In reaction formation, the person behaves the opposite of the way he feels. For instance, love turns into hate and hate into love.

Regression

Under stress, a person may regress by returning to the behaviours he used in an earlier, more comfortable time in his life.

Repression

Repression refers to unconsciously blocking out painful or unacceptable thoughts and feelings, leaving them to operate in the subconscious.

Sublimation

In sublimation, a person transforms unacceptable needs into acceptable ambitions and actions. For instance, he may channel his sex drive into sports and hobbies.

Undoing

In undoing, the person tries to undo the harm he feels he has done to others. A person who says something bad about a friend may try to undo the harm by saying nice things about her or by being nice to her and apologising.

Withdrawal

Withdrawal refers to growing emotionally uninvolved by pulling back and being passive.

Potential for self-destructive behaviour

Next, assess the service user for self-destructive behaviour. Remember that a mentally healthy person may intentionally take death-defying risks such as engaging in dangerous sports. However, a self-destructive person takes risks that are death seeking, not death defying.

A thirst for pain

Not all self-destructive behaviour is suicidal in intent. Some service users engage in such behaviour because it helps them feel alive. Service users who have lost touch with reality may cut or mutilate body parts to focus on physical pain, which may be less overwhelming than emotional distress.

Death wish

Assess service users for suicidal tendencies, particularly if they have signs and symptoms of depression. Although not all such service users want to die, depressed service users have a higher suicide rate than others.

Schizophrenic service users also may attempt suicide, responding to voices that command them to kill themselves. Unfortunately, recognising suicide potential in these service users can be difficult.

Recognising and responding to suicidal service users

Assess your person for the following indications of suicidal ideation (thoughts of suicide):

- withdrawal from others (social isolation)
- signs and symptoms of depression – crying, sadness, fatigue, helplessness, poor concentration, reduced interest in sex and other pleasurable activities, constipation and weight loss
- overwhelming anxiety (the most common trigger for a suicide attempt)
- saying farewell to friends and family
- putting affairs in order
- giving away possessions
- conveying covert suicide messages and death wishes
- making obvious suicidal statements, such as 'I'd be better off dead'.

Responding to a suicide threat

If you believe the person intends to attempt suicide, assess the seriousness of his intent and the immediacy of the risk. Consider a person with a chosen method who plans to commit suicide in the next 48–72 hours a high risk.

Tell the person you're concerned, and urge him to avoid self-destructive behaviour until the staff has an opportunity to help him. Then consult with the treatment team about arranging for mental health hospitalisation or a safe equivalent such as having someone watch him at home.

Safety precautions

If you believe the person is at high risk for suicide, initiate the following safety precautions:

- Provide a safe environment. Check for and correct any conditions that pose a danger. Look for exposed pipes, windows without safety glass and access to the roof or open balconies.
- Remove dangerous objects – belts, razors, suspenders, light cords, glass, knives, scissors, nail files and clippers.
- Be alert when the person shaves, takes medication or uses the bathroom.
- Make the service user's specific restrictions clear to staff members.
- Plan for observation of the service user.
- Clarify day staff and night staff responsibilities.

Stay close

Helping the person build emotional ties to others is the ultimate means of preventing suicide. Besides observing the service user, maintain personal contact with him. Encourage continuity of care and consistency of primary nurses.

When to keep secrets

A person may ask you to keep his suicidal thoughts confidential. Remember that such requests are ambivalent – a suicidal person typically wants to escape the pain of life, but he also wants to live. A part of him wants you to tell other staff members about his suicidal thoughts so that he can be kept alive.

Tell the person you can't keep secrets that endanger his life or conflict with his treatment. You have a duty to keep him safe and ensure the best care.

If you note signs of hopelessness, perform a direct suicide assessment. (See *Recognising and responding to suicidal service users*.)

Crisis control

If the service user is in a suicidal crisis, take immediate steps to protect him from harm. After treatment, the service user will be able to think more clearly – and hopefully, find reasons for living.

Sizing up mental health assessment tests

Besides the Beck Depression Inventory, Minnesota Multiphasic Personality Inventory and other widely used tests, some persons may undergo the tests below.

- Mini–mental status examination: measures orientation, registration, recall, calculation, language and graphomotor function
- Cognitive Capacity Screening Examination: measures orientation, memory, calculation and language.
- Cognitive Assessment Scale: measures orientation, general knowledge, mental ability and psychomotor function
- Global Deterioration Scale: assesses and stages primary degenerative dementia based on orientation, memory and neurological function

- Functional Dementia Scale: measures orientation, affect and ability to perform activities of daily living.
- Eating attitudes test: detects patterns that suggest an eating disorder
- Michigan alcoholism screening test: 24-item, timed test in which a score of 5 or higher classifies the person as alcoholic
- CAGE questionnaire: four-question tool in which two or three positive responses indicate alcoholism
- Cocaine addiction severity test and cocaine assessment profile: used when cocaine use is suspected

Personality and projective tests

Personality and projective tests can provide insight into the service user's personality, mood and psychopathology. These tests include the Beck Depression Inventory, draw-a-person test, Minnesota Multiphasic Personality Inventory (MMPI), sentence completion test and thematic apperception test.

Other assessment tests may be given to aid diagnosis. (See *Sizing up mental health assessment tests*.)

I wonder what a psychologist would make of my draw-a-person test.

Beck Depression Inventory

The Beck Depression Inventory helps diagnose depression and determine its severity. Besides providing objective evidence of the need for treatment, it can be used to monitor the service user's response during treatment.

This self-administered, self-scored test asks service users how often they experience symptoms of depression, such as poor concentration, suicidal thoughts, guilt feelings and crying. Questions focus both on cognitive symptoms (such as impaired decision-making) and physical symptoms (such as appetite loss).

Postscript on scoring

Be aware that elderly and physically ill service users commonly score high on questions regarding physical symptoms. Their scores may stem from the effects of aging or physical illness as well as depression.

Draw-a-person test

In the draw-a-person test, the service user draws a human figure of each sex. The psychologist interprets the drawing, and systematically correlates his interpretation with the diagnosis. This test also can be used to estimate a child's developmental level.

MMPI

Consisting of 566 items, the MMPI is a structured paper-and-pencil test that assesses personality traits and ego function in adolescents and adults. Most service users who read English can complete it with little or no help.

The psychologist translates the service user's answers into a psychological profile and combines the profile with data gathered from the interview.

Patterns, pointers and potential

Results of the MMPI provide information about the service user's coping strategies, defences, strengths, gender identification and self-esteem. The test pattern may strongly suggest a diagnostic category, point to a suicide risk or indicate a potential for violence. If the results show a risk of suicide or violence, monitor the service user's behaviour.

If results show frequent physical complaints (indicating possible hypochondria), evaluate the service user's physical status. If his complaints lack medical confirmation, help him explore how these symptoms may signal emotional distress.

Sentence completion test

In the sentence completion test, the service user completes a series of sentences. A sentence might begin with 'When I get angry, I ....' The response may reveal the service user's fantasies, fears, aspirations or anxieties, among other things.

Thematic apperception test

In the thematic apperception test, a service user is shown a series of pictures depicting ambiguous situations and asked to tell a story describing each picture. The psychologist evaluates the stories systematically to gain insight into the service user's personality, especially regarding interpersonal relationships and conflicts. (See *Rorschach test: Do you see what I see?*)

Physical examination

Because some mental health problems may stem from organic causes or medical treatment, mental health service users usually undergo a physical examination. Observe service users for key signs and symptoms, and examine them through inspection, palpation, percussion and auscultation.

Diagnosis

After completing a thorough service user assessment, choose appropriate nursing diagnoses based on subjective and objective assessment findings.

Rorschach test: Do you see what I see?

The illustration below depicts 2 of 10 inkblots shown to service users in the Rorschach test. After looking at each inkblot, service users describe their impressions. Then the psychiatrist analyses the responses to aid personality evaluation.

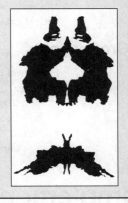

Planning

Planning involves setting and prioritising goals, formulating nursing interventions and developing a care plan based on the nursing diagnoses chosen. Effective planning must:
- focus on specific service user needs
- consider the service user's strengths and weaknesses
- encourage the service user to help set achievable goals and participate in his own care
- include feasible interventions
- fall within the scope of applicable nursing practice acts.

> The care plan isn't a mere formality. It helps ensure continuity of care.

Care plan

The care plan serves as a written guide for – and documentation of – the service user's care. It also helps ensure continuity of care delivered by all health care team members. The plan should be revised and updated as needed.

Setting goals

When formulating the plan, set one or more goals for each applicable nursing diagnosis. Appropriate goals help guide the selection of nursing interventions and serve as criteria for evaluating care. Goals may be short or long term, with short-term goals taking priority over long-term ones.

Groovy goals

Each goal must:
- relate directly to the nursing diagnosis
- be measurable and realistic
- be stated as a desired service user outcome of nursing care
- reflect the desires of the service user and his family
- be stated in a way that the service user and his family can understand.

Implementation

Implementation begins when the care plan is completed, and ends when established goals are achieved. During the implementation step, you work with the service user and his family to accomplish the interventions and move towards the outcomes specified in the plan. For implementation to be effective, members of the multidisciplinary team must collaborate closely.

Reassess the service user regularly to ensure that planned interventions continue to be appropriate. Periodic reassessment helps ensure a flexible, individualised and effective care plan.

Treatments

The diverse needs of mental health service users are mirrored by the wide range of treatments available today. Important mental health treatments include drug therapy, counselling, detoxification programmes and electroconvulsive therapy (ECT).

Drug therapy

Drugs used to treat mental health disorders include antidepressants, anxiolytic agents and antipsychotics. These drugs often require changes in dosage and careful monitoring.

Counselling and other therapies

Types of counselling include psychotherapy, behaviour therapy and milieu therapy.

Psychotherapy

Psychological treatment of mental and emotional disorders involves a range of approaches – from in-depth psychoanalysis to 1-day crisis counselling. Successful treatment usually involves two or more forms of therapy.

Regardless of the approach, most types of psychotherapy aim to change a service user's attitudes, feelings or behaviour. (See *Types of psychotherapy*, page 44.)

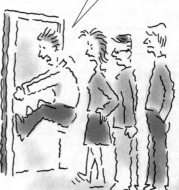

Okay, Rule #1: keep the unit doors unlocked.

Behaviour therapy

Behaviour therapy assumes that problematic behaviours are learned and, through special training, can be unlearned and replaced by acceptable behaviours. Unlike psychotherapy, behaviour therapy doesn't try to uncover the reasons for these behaviours. In fact, it tends to de-emphasise the service user's thoughts and feelings about them. (See *Drawing a bead on behaviour therapy*, pages 44 and 45.)

Milieu therapy

Milieu therapy uses the service user's environment as a tool for overcoming mental and emotional disorders. In essence, the service user's surroundings become a therapeutic community.

Milieu therapy may take place in a hospital or a community setting. The service user participates in planning, implementing and evaluating his care. Along with staff and other service users, he shares responsibility for establishing group rules and policies.

Out of uniform

Staff provide individual, group and occupational therapy. They usually wear street clothes, not uniforms. They keep units unlocked and run activities in a community room, which serves as the centre for meetings, recreation and meals.

Types of psychotherapy

The therapist may act as a neutral observer or active participant. The success of therapy depends largely on service user–therapist compatibility, treatment goals and the service user's commitment to therapy.

Individual therapy

Individual therapy involves a series of counselling sessions, which may be short or long term. After working with the person to establish appropriate goals, the therapist mediates the service user's disturbed behaviour patterns to promote personality growth and development.

Group therapy

Guided by a psychotherapist, a group of people (ideally 4–10) experiencing similar emotional problems meets to discuss their concerns. The duration of group therapy may vary from a few weeks for acute conditions requiring hospitalisation to several years for chronic conditions. Group therapy can be especially useful in treating addictions.

Cognitive therapy

According to cognitive theory, depression stems from low self-esteem and a belief that the future is bleak and hopeless. The goal of cognitive therapy is to identify and change the service user's negative generalisations and expectations – and thereby reduce depression, distress and other emotional problems.

The therapist assigns homework, such as making lists of pleasurable activities and reducing automatic negative thoughts and conclusions.

Family therapy

Family therapy aims to alter relationships within the family and change the problematic behaviour of one or more members. Useful in treating childhood or adolescent adjustment disorders, marital discord and abusive situations, family therapy may be short or long term.

Crisis intervention

Crisis intervention seeks to help service users develop adequate coping skills to resolve an immediate problem. The crisis may be developmental (such as a marriage or the death of a family member) or situational (such as a natural disaster or an illness).

Therapy focuses on helping the person resume the precrisis functional level. It usually involves just the person and the therapist but sometimes includes family members. It may consist of one session or of multiple sessions over several months.

Drawing a bead on behaviour therapy

Suitable for adults or children, behaviour therapy can be used either with an individual or with groups of persons who have similar problems.

The behavioural approach relies on therapies designed to change behavioural patterns. Commonly used therapies include assertiveness training, aversion therapy, desensitisation, flooding, positive conditioning, response prevention, thought stopping, thought switching and token economy.

Assertiveness training

Assertiveness training uses positive reinforcement, shaping and modelling to reduce anxiety. It teaches the person ways to express feelings, ideas and wishes without feeling guilty or demeaning others.

You can help the person by providing examples of appropriate behaviour and suggesting situations in which he can be more assertive.

Aversion therapy

In aversion therapy, a painful stimulus is applied to create an aversion to the obsession underlying the person's undesirable behaviour.

Desensitisation

The treatment of choice for phobias, desensitisation slowly exposes the person to something he fears.

Drawing a bead on behaviour therapy (continued)

Because phobias reflect unresolved conflicts, desensitisation works best if used with other treatments. The person learns to use deep breathing or another relaxation technique when confronted with a staged series of anxiety-producing situations.

During desensitisation, provide the person with reassurance and review relaxation techniques. Monitor his response to each anxiety-producing situation, and emphasise that he need not proceed to the next one until he feels ready.

Flooding

Also called implosion therapy, flooding can bring rapid relief from phobias such as travel phobias. Like desensitisation, it involves direct exposure to an anxiety-producing situation. However, instead of using relaxation techniques, it assumes that anxiety and panic can't persist and that confrontation helps the person overcome fear.

During flooding, monitor the person for signs of excitation. If he faints or has another extreme reaction, remove him from the anxiety-producing situation and assess for signs and symptoms of psychological trauma.

Positive conditioning

Building on the principle of desensitisation, positive conditioning attempts to gradually instill a positive or neutral attitude towards a phobia. This technique introduces a pleasurable stimulus such as music. The therapist encourages the person to heighten the pleasurable stimulus by associating it with other pleasurable experiences. Next, the therapist introduces the phobic stimulus along with the pleasurable one. Gradually, the person develops a positive response to the phobia.

If your person is undergoing positive conditioning, reinforce relaxation techniques and provide encouragement.

Response prevention

Response prevention seeks to prevent compulsive behaviour through distraction, persuasion or redirection of activity. To be effective, it may require that the person enter a hospital and his family get involved in treatment.

Thought stopping

Thought stopping helps the person break the habit of fear-inducing anticipatory thoughts. He's taught to stop such thoughts by saying 'stop' and then focusing his attention on achieving calmness and muscle relaxation.

Thought switching

In thought switching, the person learns to replace fear-inducing self-instructions with competent self-instructions. The therapist teaches the person to substitute positive thoughts for fear-inducing ones until the positive thoughts become strong enough to overcome the fear-inducing ones.

Token economy

Using token economy, the therapist rewards acceptable behaviour by giving out tokens, which the person uses to 'buy' a privilege or object. The therapist also may withhold or rescind tokens as punishment or to avert undesirable behaviour.

During this treatment, monitor the person's behaviour and provide or withhold rewards consistently and promptly.

Detoxification

Designed to help service users achieve abstinence, detoxification programmes offer a relatively safe alternative to self-withdrawal after prolonged dependence on alcohol or drugs. Performed in out-service user centres or in special units, these programmes provide symptomatic treatment as well as counselling or psychotherapy on an individual, group or family basis.

Treating service users undergoing detoxification requires skill, compassion and commitment. Because substance abusers typically have low self-esteem and try to manipulate people, you'll need to control your natural feelings of anger and frustration.

Electroconvulsive therapy

Although ECT was misused for decades, it has made a recent comeback. Today it's recognised as a legitimate treatment for depression. Nonetheless, it's still the most controversial treatment in psychiatry.

The Royal College of Psychiatrists has specific guidelines for ECT and recommends its use only in treating severe, debilitating mental disorders. Further standards for treatment are set out by Electroconvulsive Therapy Accreditation Service (ECTAS). Written and informed consent to treatment is required from the service user.

Candidates

Candidates for ECT may include:
- severely depressed service users for whom psychotherapy and medication have proven ineffective
- service users at immediate risk for suicide (because ECT produces much faster results than antidepressants)
- service users with certain schizophrenic syndromes.

Procedure

During an ECT treatment, the service user receives a short-acting general anaesthetic, along with medications, which paralyses the muscles temporarily. He's connected to devices that monitor his brain wave activity and heart rhythm.

Sleeping through a seizure

Then a tiny electric current is applied to the brain for 1 second or less, through electrodes placed above the temples. The current produces a seizure, which lasts 30 seconds to 1 minute or slightly longer.

When the service user wakes up 10–15 minutes later, he may experience a brief period of confusion, headache or muscle stiffness. These symptoms typically ease within 20–60 minutes.

A typical course of treatment involves a total of 6–12 ECT treatments, with 2 or 3 treatments given weekly.

Can't explain it

Most experts agree that when properly used, ECT can be an effective treatment for severe depression. However, no one is certain why the treatment works. The prevailing theory is that ECT acts by temporarily altering some of the brain's electrochemical processes.

Evaluation

Through evaluation, you obtain additional assessment data relating to the goals specified in the care plan. These data help you determine whether goals have been met totally or partially, or remain unmet.

Technically, evaluation is the final step in the nursing process. In reality, it occurs throughout the nursing process. You'll monitor the service user's progress based on established and measurable expected outcomes for each goal.

Documentation

Complete, accurate and timely documentation is crucial to the continuity of service user care and has many legal implications. The medical record is a legal and business record with many uses. It provides legal proof of the nature and quality of care that the service user received. A factual, consistent, timely and complete medical record defends you against allegations of negligence, improper treatment and omissions in care.

Legal duty

Health care professionals have a legal duty to maintain the medical record in sufficient detail. Inadequate documentation of care may result in liability or denial of reimbursement by third-party payers.

Care – or no care?

The old saying 'If it isn't documented, it hasn't been done' still holds true. Documentation of care has become synonymous with care itself, and failure to document implies failure to provide care.

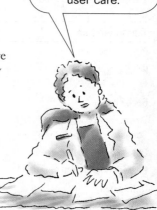

Documentation provides legal proof of the nature and quality of service user care.

Multidisciplinary care

The multidisciplinary care team may include many professionals of varying backgrounds and expertise – all of them focused on promoting the service user's psychological well-being. (See *Who's who on the multidisciplinary care team*, page 48.)

Trends and concerns in mental health care

The steady decline in funding for mental health programmes has markedly reduced mental health services and limited the training of new mental health professionals. There is a review of the roles that mental health professionals undertake and a move to develop new types of workers. The New Ways of Working builds on previous guidance and promotes a model where 'distributed responsibility' is shared amongst team members and no longer delegated by a single professional such as the consultant.

This cultural shift in services will mean that people with the most experience and skills will work face to face with people who have the most complex needs. More experienced staff will then support other staff to take on less complex or more routine work. All qualified staff will be able to extend

Who's who on the multidisciplinary care team

Professionals from varying disciplines and backgrounds may be involved in the care of mental health service users. The chart below identifies the education and responsibilities of each member of the multidisciplinary team.

Team member	Responsibilities
Psychiatrist	Diagnosis and treatment of mental disorders
Psychologist	Diagnosis of mental disorders, psychological testing and psychological treatments such as psychotherapy
Social worker	Diagnosis of mental disorders, and psychosocial therapies such as family and couple therapies, also linked with community resources
Counsellor	Counselling
Occupational therapist	Functional independence in tasks of living
Recreational therapist	Leisure-related activities
Nutritionist	Nutritional therapy, education and maintaining balanced diet
Speech therapist	Communication disorders
Expressive therapist (visual, musical, dance)	Expressive therapy through art, music or dance
Pastoral counsellor	Determination of spiritual and faith assets of each person in the healing process
Vocational counsellor	Evaluation of abilities, interests, talents and personality characteristics so that they can develop realistic academic and career goals
Clinical specialist	Provision of individual, family and group psychotherapy in inpatient, outpatient and community health settings and in private practice
Advanced practice nurse	Provision of mental health consultation to other nurses, service users and families within their speciality area

the boundaries of what they do (i.e. nonmedical prescription) and there will be more chances for new roles such as support time and recovery workers (STR), primary care mental health workers and assistant practitioners to take their places within teams.

Deinstitutionalisation

The push to deinstitutionalise mentally ill service users began several decades ago. The goal was to provide mental health services for these service users in the community.

Unfortunately, deinstitutionalisation has increased the number of both homeless and incarcerated persons with mental illness.

Shame and stigma

Despite more public education programmes and greater awareness of mental illness, the mentally ill continue to suffer stigmatisation and bias.

Drugs and dual diagnoses

The proliferation of street drugs poses a further challenge to mental health treatment. Some illicit drugs can cause permanent brain damage or lead to addiction with just one or two uses.

In addition, the number of service users with a dual diagnosis of chronic mental illness and substance abuse or dependence has been rising. These service users need challenging, long-term treatment, and many don't respond to conventional treatment protocols.

> Many service users suffer from both mental illness and substance abuse.

Legal Issues

Legal issues help shape the role of the mental health nurse. Mental health nurses are held to the same standards of reasonable and prudent behaviour expected of other professionals with the same education in similar circumstances. They must provide care that meets professional standards established by the NMC. In addition, they must know and abide by statutory provisions concerning service user admissions into mental health care.

The Mental Health Act 1983 as amended by the Mental Health Act 2007

Changes in 2007

The legislation governing the compulsory treatment of certain people who have a mental disorder is the Mental Health Act Amended 2007 (the 2007 Act). The 2007 Act does not replace the 1983 Act; it makes amendments to it as outlined below. It is also being used to introduce 'deprivation of liberty safeguards' by amending the Mental Capacity Act 2005 (MCA), and to extend the rights of victims by amending the Domestic Violence, Crime and Victims Act 2004.

The 2007 Act is largely concerned with the circumstances in which a person with a mental disorder can be detained for treatment for that disorder without his or her consent. It also sets out the processes that must be followed and the safeguards for people, to ensure that they are not inappropriately detained or treated without their consent. The main purpose of the legislation is to ensure that people with serious mental disorders which threaten their health or safety or the safety of the public can be treated irrespective of their consent where it is necessary to prevent them from harming themselves or others.

The changes in relation to the MCA are in response to the 2004 European Court of Human Rights (ECHR) judgement involving an autistic man who was kept at Bournewood Hospital by doctors against the wishes of his carers. The ECHR found that admission to and retention in hospital of HL under the common law of necessity amounted to a breach of ECHR Article 5(1) (deprivation of liberty) and Article 5(4) (right to have lawfulness of detention reviewed by a court).

The 9 key changes to the Mental Health Act 1983 are:
* Single definition of Mental Disorder Changes to: 'any disorder or disability of the mind.'
* This wide definition now applies to all sections of the MHA.
* The four categories of mental disorder (mental illness, mental impairment, severe mental impairment and psychopathic disorder) have disappeared.
* Appropriate Medical Treatment Introduces a new 'appropriate treatment' test.
* As a result, it will not be possible for patients to be compulsorily detained or their detention continued unless 'medical treatment' which is appropriate to the patient's mental disorder and all other circumstances of the case' (Code of Practice 2007) is available to that patient.
* 'Medical treatment' includes psychological treatment, nursing, habilitation and rehabilitation as well as medicine.

Age Appropriate Services It requires hospital managers to ensure that people aged under 18 admitted to hospital for a mental disorder are accommodated in an environment that is suitable for their age (subject to their needs).

Broadening Professional Groups It is broadening the group of practitioners who can take on the functions previously performed by the approved social worker (ASW) and the responsible medical officer (RMO). These roles are now undertaken by approved mental health professionals (AMHP) and responsible clinicians (RC) respectively.

Nearest Relative It gives people the right to make an application to displace their nearest relative and enables county courts to displace a nearest relative where there are reasonable grounds for doing so. The provisions for determining the nearest relative have been amended to include civil partners amongst the list of relatives.

The Independent Mental Health Advocate It places a duty on the appropriate national authority to make arrangements for help to be provided by independent mental health advocates

Patients and ECT It introduces new safeguards for people.

Supervised Community Treatment Supervised Community treatment orders (SCTO). It introduces SCTO for people following a period of detention in hospital. It is expected that this will allow a small number of people with a mental disorder to live in the community whilst subject to certain conditions under the 1983 Act as amended, to ensure they continue with the medical treatment that they need.
* Mental Health Review Tribunal (MHRT) Introduces earlier referrals by Hospital Managers of detained patients who have not used their rights of appeal to the MHRT.
* The annual referral to the MHRT for those under 16 has been raised to those under 18.
* The existing multiple regional tribunals are to be replaced with two tribunals, one for England and one for Wales.

The changes to the MCA provide for procedures to authorise the deprivation of liberty of a person in a hospital or care home who lacks capacity to consent. The MCA principles of supporting a person to take a decision when possible, and acting at all times in the person's best interests and in the least restrictive manner, will apply to all decision-making in operating the procedures. The main points covering the most commonly used sections of the Mental Health Act 2007 are described below.

Definitions

Mental Illness is defined as 'any disorder or disability of the mind'.

Four categories of mental disorder are specified as follows:

- Mental illness. Not defined.
- Severe mental impairment. 'A state of arrested or incomplete development of mind, which includes severe impairment of intelligence and social functioning and is associated with abnormally aggressive or seriously irresponsible conduct on the part of the person concerned'.
- Mental impairment. A state defined in the same way as severe mental impairment except that the phrase 'severe impairment' is replaced by 'significant impairment'.
- Psychopathic disorder. 'A persistent disorder or disability of mind (whether or not including significant impairment of intelligence) that results in abnormally aggressive or seriously irresponsible conduct on the part of the person concerned'.

Note: some forms of mental disorder fall outside the scope of these four categories, for example, a state of arrested or incomplete development of mind, which includes severe or significant impairment of intelligence and social functioning, but is not associated with abnormally aggressive or seriously irresponsible conduct.

Some sections of the Act apply to people suffering from mental disorder, while others apply only to people suffering from one of the four specified categories of mental disorder.

Persons involved in criminal proceedings (part III)

Hospital order (section 37)

Duration of order: up to 6 months, renewable for a further 6 months, and then for 1 year at a time.

Procedure: a hospital order can be made by the Crown Court, or Magistrates' Court in the case of an offender convicted of an offence that it could punish with a prison sentence (such offences include manslaughter but not murder). The Magistrates' Court can make a hospital order without recording a conviction, if an offender is suffering from mental illness or severe mental impairment, and magistrates are satisfied that she or he committed the act as charged. The court can make a hospital order on evidence from two doctors that:

(a) the offender is suffering from a disorder or disability of the mind of a nature or degree that makes detention for medical treatment appropriate

Detention under the Mental Health Act 2007

Compulsory admission to hospital or guardianship for persons not involved in criminal proceedings (part II)

Admission for assessment (section 2)

Duration of detention: 28 days maximum.

Application for admission: by an AMHP (Approved Mental Health Professional) or the person's nearest relative. The applicant must have seen the person within the previous 14 days.

Procedure: two doctors must confirm that:

(a) the person is suffering from a mental disorder of a nature or degree that warrants detention in hospital for assessment (or assessment followed by medical treatment) or at least a limited period
(b) she or he ought to be detained in the interests of her or his own health or safety, or with a view to the protection of others.

Discharge: by any of the following:

- RC.
- Hospital managers.
- The nearest relative, who must give 72 hours notice. The RC can prevent her or him discharging a person by making a report to the hospital managers.
- Mental Health Review Tribunal (MHRT). The person can apply to a tribunal within the first 14 days of detention the Health, Education and Social Care Chamber of the First-tier Tribunal.

Admission for assessment in cases of emergency (section 4)

Duration of detention: 72 hours maximum.

Application for admission: by an AMHP or the nearest relative. The applicant must have seen the person within the previous 24 hours.

Procedure: one doctor must confirm that:

(a) it is of 'urgent necessity' for the person to be admitted and detained under section 2
(b) waiting for a second doctor to confirm the need for an admission under section 2 would cause 'undesirable delay'.

Note: The person must be admitted within 24 hours of the medical examination or application, whichever is the earlier, or the application under section 4 is null and void.

Admission for treatment (section 3)

Duration of detention: up to 6 months, renewable for a further 6 months, and then for 1 year at a time.

Application for admission: by the nearest relative, or an AMHP in cases where the nearest relative does not object, or is displaced by the county court, or it is not 'reasonably practicable' to consult her or him.

Procedure: two doctors must confirm that:

(a) the person is suffering from a disorder or disability of the mind of a nature or degree that makes it appropriate for her or him to receive medical treatment in hospital
(b) if the person is suffering from a psychopathic disorder or mental impairment, such treatment is likely to 'alleviate or prevent a deterioration' of her or his condition
(c) it is necessary for her or his own health or safety, or for the protection of others that she or he receives such treatment and it cannot be provided unless she or he is detained under this section.

Renewal: under section 20, the RC can renew a section 3 detention if the original criteria still apply and treatment is likely to 'alleviate or prevent a deterioration' of the person's condition. In cases where the person is suffering from mental illness or severe mental impairment, but treatment is not likely to alleviate or prevent a deterioration of her or his condition, detention may still be renewed, if she or he is unlikely to be able to care for her or himself, to obtain the care she or he needs or to guard her or himself against serious exploitation.

Discharge: by any of the following:

- RC.
- Hospital managers.
- The nearest relative, who must give 72 hours notice. If the RC prevents the nearest relative discharging the person, by making a report to the hospital managers, the nearest relative can apply to an MHRT within 28 days.
- A person can apply to a tribunal once during the first 6 months of his detention, once during the

Detention under the Mental Health Act 2007 *(continued)*

second 6 months and then once during each period of 1 year. If the person does not apply in the first 6 months of detention, her or his case will be referred, automatically, to the MHRT. After that, the case is automatically referred when a period of 3 years has passed since a tribunal last considered it (1 year, if the person is under 16).

Compulsory detention of informal persons already in hospital (section 5)

A doctor in charge of an informal person's treatment (including inpatients being treated for a physical problem) can detain a person for up to 72 hours by reporting to hospital managers that an application for compulsory admission 'ought to be made'. A suitably qualified nurse (a nurse trained to work with mental illness or learning disabilities) can detain an informal person who is receiving treatment for mental disorder for up to 6 hours, or until a doctor with authority to detain her or him arrives, whichever is earlier.

Guardianship (sections 7–10)

Duration of guardianship order: up to 6 months, renewable for a further 6 months, and then for 1 year at a time.

Application for reception into guardianship: by an AMHP or the nearest relative.

Procedure: two doctors must confirm that:

(a) the person is suffering from a disorder or disability of the mind of a nature or degree that warrants reception into guardianship
(b) it is necessary in the interests of the person's welfare or for the protection of others.

Note: The person must be over 16. The guardian must be a local social services authority, or person approved by the social services authority, for the area in which she or he (the guardian) lives.

Effect: under section 8, a guardian has the following powers:

* to require a person to live at a place specified by the guardian

* to require a person to attend places specified by the guardian for occupation, training or medical treatment (although the guardian cannot force the person to undergo treatment)
* to ensure that a doctor, a social worker or another person specified by the guardian can see the person at home.

Discharge: by any of the following:

* RC.
* Local social services authority.
* Nearest relative.
* MHRT. The person can apply to a tribunal once during the first 6 months of guardianship, once during the second 6 months and then once during each period of 1 year.

Mentally disordered persons found in public places (section 136)

Duration of detention: 72 hours maximum.

Procedure: if it appears to a police officer that a person in a public place is 'suffering from mental disorder' and is 'in immediate need of care or control', she or he can take that person to a 'place of safety', which is usually a hospital, but can be a police station. Detention under section 136 lasts for a maximum of 72 hours, so that the person can be examined by a doctor and interviewed by an AMHP and 'any necessary arrangements' made for her or his treatment or care.

Warrant to search for and remove persons (section 135)

Duration of detention: 72 hours maximum.

Procedure: if there is reasonable cause to suspect that a person is suffering from mental disorder and:

(a) is being ill-treated or neglected or not kept under proper control
(b) is unable to care for herself or himself and lives alone, a magistrate can issue a warrant authorising a police officer (with a doctor and an AMHP) to enter any premises where the person is believed to be and move her or him to a place of safety.

(b) taking into account all the relevant circumstances, including the past history and character of the offender and alternative methods of dealing with her or him, a hospital order is the most suitable option.

Discharge: by any of the following:
- RC.
- Hospital managers.
- MHRT. The person can apply to a tribunal once in the period between 6 and 12 months after a hospital order is made, and then once during each period of 1 year. A person's case is automatically referred to a tribunal when a period of 3 years has passed since a tribunal last considered it (1 year if the person is under 16).

Restriction order (section 41)

Duration of order: may be specified by the court or without a limit of time.

Procedure: the Crown Court that has made a hospital order under section 37 can also impose a restriction order if:

(a) this is necessary to protect the public from 'serious harm'
(b) at least one of the doctors who made recommendations for the hospital order gave her or his evidence orally.

A Magistrates' Court cannot make a restriction order, but can commit an offender to a Crown Court so that a section 41 order can be imposed. Persons on restriction orders are usually known as restricted persons.

Discharge: by any of the following:
- The Home Secretary.
- MHRT. A person can apply to a tribunal once in the period between 6 and 12 months after a restriction order is made, and then once during each period of 1 year. The person's case is automatically referred to a tribunal when a period of 3 years has passed since a tribunal last considered it (1 year, if the person is under 16).

Transfer to hospital from prison (section 47)

Duration of detention: up to 6 months, renewable for a further 6 months, and then for 1 year at a time. If the Home Secretary imposes a restriction direction (section 49), it continues in force until the earliest date on which the person would have been released from prison with remission.

Procedure: the Home Secretary orders the transfer, if satisfied by evidence from two doctors that:
- an offender has any disorder or disability of the mind of a nature or degree that makes detention for medical treatment appropriate

Discharge: if no restriction direction has been imposed, the person can be discharged by any of the following:
- RC.
- Hospital managers.
- MHRT. The person can apply to a tribunal once during the first 6 months of transfer, once during the second 6 months, and then once during each

period of 1 year. The Home Secretary must refer her or his case to a tribunal if the MHRT has not considered it in the previous 3 years (1 year if the person is under 16).

Until the end of her or his prison sentence (allowing for remission), a person under a restriction direction can only be discharged by the Home Secretary. She or he can apply to a tribunal once during the first 6 months of transfer, once during the second 6 months and then once during each period of 1 year, but an MHRT can only recommend to the Home Secretary that the person be discharged. The Home Secretary may order a return to prison instead. At the end of the prison sentence (allowing for remission), the restriction direction ceases to have effect and the above provisions apply.

Remand to hospital for medical report (section 35)

Duration of remand: up to 28 days, renewable for further periods of 28 days to a maximum of 12 weeks in total.

Procedure: the Crown Court or Magistrates' Court remands the accused person to hospital on evidence from one doctor that:

(a) there is 'reason to suspect' that she or he is suffering from a disorder or disability of the mind
(b) it would be 'impracticable' for a report on her or his mental condition to be made if she or he were remanded on bail.

Remand to hospital for treatment (section 36)

Duration of remand: up to 28 days, renewable for further periods of 28 days to a maximum of 12 weeks in total.

Procedure: the Crown Court remands the accused person to hospital for treatment, on evidence from two doctors that she or he is suffering from mental illness or severe impairment, of a nature or degree that makes detention for treatment appropriate.

Interim hospital order (section 38)

Duration of order: 12 weeks, renewable for 28 days at a time, to a maximum of 6 months in total.

Procedure: the Crown Court or Magistrates' Court makes an interim hospital order on evidence from two doctors that:

(a) a convicted offender is suffering from a disorder or disability of the mind
(b) there is reason to suppose that it is appropriate for the order to be made.

Note: A hospital order or prison sentence may subsequently be imposed on an offender who has been subject to an interim hospital order.

Hospital and limitation direction (section 45A)

Duration of direction: the same as for a transfer direction under section 47, together with a restriction direction under section 49. The offender may be transferred to prison at any time during her or his sentence, by warrant of the Home Secretary, on the recommendation of her or his RC or MHRT.

Procedure: if the Crown Court, having considered making a hospital order (section 37), instead imposes a fixed-term sentence of imprisonment, it may direct the immediate admission of the offender to hospital, if it is satisfied by evidence from two doctors that:

(a) she or he suffers from a psychopathic disorder of a nature or degree that makes medical treatment appropriate
(b) such treatment is 'likely to alleviate or prevent a deterioration of her or his condition'.

Discharge: before the end of the prison sentence, the offender can only be discharged by the Home Secretary, on recommendation of the RC or MHRT. She or he may order a return to prison instead. At the end of the prison sentence (allowing for remission), the limitation direction ceases to have effect, and the offender is treated as if she or he were on a hospital order (section 37).

Consent to treatment (part IV)

Part IV of the Mental Health Act applies to:
• treatments for mental disorder
• all formal persons except those who are detained under sections 4, 5, 35, 135 and 136, subject to guardianship or conditionally discharged. These persons have the right to refuse treatment, as have informal persons, except in emergencies.

Part IV states that:

(a) any treatment can be given without the person's consent, unless the Mental Health Act or DoH regulations specify otherwise
(b) under section 57, psychosurgery and treatments specified in DoH regulations as giving rise to special concern can only be given if:

1. the person consents
2. a multidisciplinary panel appointed by the Mental Health Act Commission confirms that her or his consent is valid
3. the doctor on the multidisciplinary panel certifies that the treatment should be given. Before doing so, she or he must consult two people, one a nurse and the other neither a nurse nor a doctor, who have been concerned with the person's treatment.

Note: As the treatments specified in section 57 give rise to particular concern, this section applies to all formal and informal persons.

(c) under section 58, certain treatments can only be given if:

1. the person consents or
2. an independent doctor appointed by the Mental Health Act Commission confirms that treatment should be given. Before doing so, she or he must consult two people, one a nurse and the other neither a nurse nor a doctor, who have been concerned with the person's treatment.

Section 58 applies to treatments named in DoH regulations (including electroconvulsive therapy). Medication can be given without the person's consent for 3 months. After that, it is subject to the safeguards laid down in section 58.

Note: Under section 62, any treatment for mental disorder can be given without consent in specific emergencies, subject to restrictions when a treatment is irreversible or hazardous.

Quick quiz

1. The popular system that is used to classify and diagnose mental disorders was established by the:
- A. American Nurses Association.
- B. American Psychiatric Association.
- C. state boards of nursing.
- D. American Medical Association.

Answer: B. The American Psychiatric Association established the currently used system of classifying and diagnosing mental disorders. The latest version, published in *Diagnostic and Statistical Manual of Mental Disorders*, Fourth Edition, Text Revision (*DSM-IV-TR*), emphasises observable data and de-emphasises subjective and theoretical impressions.

2. The mental status examination (MSE) investigates all of the following except the service user's:
- A. LOC.
- B. mood, affect and perceptions.
- C. medication effects.
- D. activities of daily living.

Answer: C. The MSE examines the service user's LOC, general appearance, behaviour, speech, mood and affect, perceptions, intellectual performance, judgement, insight and thought content.

3. Over the course of a day, a service user may exhibit changes in:
- A. orientation.
- B. mood.
- C. affect.
- D. consciousness.

Answer: B. Mood refers to the pervading feeling or state of mind. The service user's prevailing mood may change over the course of a day.

4. Which test assesses a service user's orientation and recall?
- A. Beck Depression Inventory
- B. Thematic apperception test
- C. Mini–mental status examination
- D. Millon Clinical Multiaxial Inventory-III

Answer: C. The mini–mental status examination assesses the service user's orientation, registration, recall, calculation, language and graphomotor function.

5.   A preoccupation that's acted out is called:
     A.   an obsession.
     B.   a compulsion.
     C.   a delusion.
     D.   a hallucination.

Answer: B. A compulsion is a repetitive behaviour that the service user feels compelled to perform in response to an obsession.

Scoring

☆☆☆   If you answered all five items correctly, superb! Your mental health sagacity is spectacular!

☆☆   If you answered three or four items correctly, well done! You're obviously all psyched up about mental health disorders.

☆   If you answered fewer than three items correctly, don't despair! You have plenty of time to digest the *DSM-IV-TR*!

Just the facts

In this chapter, you'll learn:

♦ theories of growth and development

♦ characteristics of mentally healthy young people

♦ signs and symptoms of mental illness in children and adolescents

♦ treatment options for children and adolescents with mental illness.

A look at disorders of children and adolescents

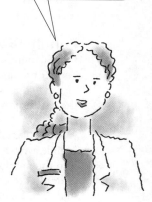

Some mental health problems may start in early childhood.

Because children and adolescents are in a state of rapid change and growth, a wide range of behaviour is considered normal. Nonetheless, many children and adolescents experience emotional and mental distress that's more severe than the normal ups and downs of growing up. Although some get better over time, others have serious and persistent problems that affect their daily activities – problems that require professional help.

Not long ago, most clinicians believed depression and certain other mental illnesses began only after childhood. Now we know these problems can start in early childhood and can affect the way a child develops. Unfortunately, it can be hard to tell whether a child or adolescent has a mental illness or is demonstrating normal – if extreme – behaviour for his age and developmental stage.

Illness inventory

This chapter discusses some of the most common mental illnesses affecting youths:

• attention deficit hyperactivity disorder (ADHD)

• oppositional defiant disorder (ODD)

- conduct disorder
- depression
- Tourette's syndrome (TS).

Surprising stats

About 1 in 10 children and adolescents in the United Kingdom suffers from mental illness severe enough to cause impairment. However, fewer than one in five receive treatment – even though many of these disorders can be treated effectively with psychotherapy and drug therapy.

Risk factors

Mental illnesses occur in children and adolescents of all social classes and backgrounds. Certain factors put a child at greater risk. They include:
- low birth weight
- physical problems
- family history of mental or addictive disorders
- multigenerational poverty
- separation from caregivers
- abuse and neglect.

Psychosocial consequences

A child or adolescent with mental illness has many challenges to overcome. Despite greater public awareness and understanding of mental disorders, these illnesses still carry a stigma that can affect a person for life. A child who behaves oddly may frighten or offend other children, making him a social outcast.

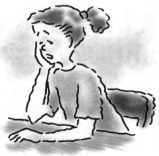

Family discord

Family members may lack adequate knowledge of mental illness and may feel guilty or embarrassed at having a disturbed child. If they don't understand or can't cope with his behaviour, they may become frustrated. Ultimately, the frustration may escalate to verbal or physical abuse of the child.

Placement issues

A child whose behaviour disrupts the family or who can't be integrated into the family unit may require temporary or permanent placement in a structured facility. The placement decision may be influenced by social, financial, religious and cultural considerations.

Educational issues

Although most children and adolescents with mental illness can attend regular schools, those with severe disorders may be better off in special classes or special educational facilities. However, these classes may be out of reach financially for some families.

Childhood development

To understand childhood disruptions and the mental health problems that can result, you must be familiar with the patterns of normal child development. A child moves from infancy through childhood to adolescence in an orderly manner. As the child grows, the personality develops.

I could write a book about child development! Just call me Sigmunda Freud!

Nature plus nurture

Personality formation is influenced by genetic and environmental factors. Sigmund Freud, Erik Erikson and Jean Piaget proposed developmental theories to describe the progressive stages of childhood and adolescence. (See *Theories of growth and development*, page 62.)

When you're familiar with theories of growth and development, you can apply them to clinical situations, determining a child's developmental level and assessing his accomplishment of the tasks defined for each stage.

Recognising the typical characteristics of mentally healthy young people also helps you compare a child's or adolescent's behaviour against the norm. (See *Characteristics of mentally healthy young people*, page 63.)

Communicating with children and adolescents

When caring for a child or an adolescent with a mental illness, your first task is to establish rapport. To do this, you must show empathy and understanding.

Keep in mind that the child may be frightened at first. To break the ice, initiate conversation by asking about toys, hobbies, pets and other subjects he's interested in.

Communing with kids

To further enhance communication, follow these guidelines:
- Keep verbal communication brief and use simple language.
- Ask direct questions when seeking specific information.
- Use body language to reinforce what you've said and help the child express ideas and feelings.
- Give feedback when appropriate, based on the child's developmental stage.
- Talk about reality by focusing on the 'here and now'.
- Speak quietly but firmly when reinforcing behavioural limits.
- Avoid arguments.
- Make your expectations clear.
- Role-model effective ways of communicating.

Theories of growth and development

As children grow, they develop intellectually, emotionally, sexually, socially and spiritually. They learn to think abstractly and logically, to use language and to explore the world around them. Several theorists, including Sigmund Freud, Erik Erikson and Jean Piaget, explain how this growth occurs.

Freud: Psychosexual development

Freud theorised that the human mind consists of three major entities – id, ego and superego. The id seeks instant gratification. The ego orients the person to reality, intercepting impulses from the id. The superego (conscience) develops during childhood – the product of rewards and punishments bestowed on the individual.

According to Freud, a child must master each developmental stage before he can move on to the next one.

- **Oral phase (birth to age 1):** The infant is totally dependent and narcissistic and starts to become aware of the self as an individual. Ego development begins.
- **Anal phase (ages 1–3):** The child learns to postpone immediate gratification and to manipulate surroundings. Episodes of negativity, rebellion and conflict may occur. The superego begins to develop.
- **Phallic phase (ages 3–6):** The child becomes aware of gender and develops cooperation and socialisation skills.
- **Latency period (ages 6–12):** As the child identifies with peers, parents become less important. Intellectual curiosity increases.
- **Adolescence (ages 12 and older):** The child establishes close relationships with the opposite sex and devotes energy towards work, achievement and interpersonal relationships. He moves away from emotional ties with family members.

Erikson: Psychosocial development

Erikson's theory of human development indicates that major personality changes occur throughout the life cycle. Passage from one stage to another depends on successfully gaining the skills of the preceding stage. Unlike many other theorists, Erikson suggests that new experiences may provide opportunities to cope with deficits in earlier stages.

- **Trust vs. mistrust (birth to age 1):** The infant derives a sense of security from gratification of needs.
- **Autonomy vs. shame and doubt (ages 1–3):** The child begins to view the self as a person apart from the parents.
- **Initiative vs. guilt (ages 3–6):** The child starts to behave assertively as he's guided to explore and investigate the world.
- **Industry vs. inferiority (ages 6–12):** Accomplishment occurs and a sense of responsibility develops as the child masters tasks and social skills.
- **Identity vs. role diffusion (ages 12–18):** The adolescent develops a sense of personal and role identity.

Piaget: Cognitive development

Piaget's cognitive theory of development describes successive stages of mental activity that occur during childhood. By successfully encountering new experiences, the child adapts and progresses to the next stage.

- **Sensorimotor stage (birth to age 2):** The infant's world focuses on the self. He experiences and understands the world through the senses and motor movements.
- **Preoperational stage (ages 2–7):** The child develops language and egocentric thought, and begins symbolic play.
- **Concrete operations stage (ages 7–11):** The child develops the concepts of time, space, categories, numbers and reversibility.
- **Formal operations stage (ages 12–15):** The adolescent begins to think abstractly and logically and starts to envision options and possibilities.

Characteristics of mentally healthy young people

When assessing a child for possible mental health disorders, you'll need a basis for comparison. A mentally healthy child or adolescent:

- trusts parents and appropriate caregivers
- views the world as a safe place where needs will be met
- has an age-appropriate sense of reality
- perceives the personal environment realistically

- demonstrates a positive sense of self
- handles age-appropriate stress and frustration effectively
- shows age-appropriate coping skills
- demonstrates mastery of developmental tasks
- communicates or expresses himself
- has useful and satisfying relationships.

Assessment

To assess a child or adolescent for a mental illness, you should evaluate the family as well. Begin by collecting biographic data, including the ages of all family members, from the parents. Gather information about the family's health, school, housing, economic situation and religious, ethnic and cultural background.

Document your description of the parents, including any marital problems.

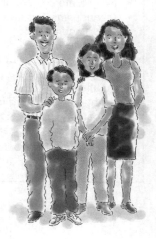

How do Mum and Dad feel?

Next, ask the parents what their concerns are. Ask them how they view their child's problem and what they think might have caused it. Evaluate each parent's attitude towards the child and his condition. Then obtain the child's developmental history from the parents. Find out which, if any, services and agencies are involved in the family's or child's care.

Then begin your interview of the child, including an assessment of his mental status. (See *Assessing the mental status of a child or adolescent*, page 64.)

Diagnosis

A child with signs or symptoms of mental illness should be evaluated by a medical doctor. Based on findings, the doctor may recommend further evaluation by a specialist in child behavioural problems, such as a psychiatrist, psychologist or social worker.

Specialist, speak

When evaluating the child, the specialist considers the child's developmental level, social and physical environment and reports from parents and teachers. He tries to rule out other possible causes for the child's signs and symptoms.

Advice from the experts

Assessing the mental status of a child or adolescent

When evaluating the mental status of a child or adolescent, be sure to assess:

- physical appearance (including whether the person looks his age)
- hygiene and grooming
- attention level and behaviour during the interview
- understanding of his role in the interview
- speech or language development
- intellectual functioning
- judgement
- insight into self and the situation
- mannerisms, tics and other involuntary movements
- mood and affect
- anxiety level
- obvious obsessive or compulsive behaviours
- frustration tolerance
- impulsiveness
- acting out or oppositional behaviour
- verbal or physical aggression
- thought disorders, hallucinations or delusions.

Especially for adolescents

If the service user is an adolescent, also evaluate for:

- depression
- communication problems
- difficulty expressing feelings
- low self-esteem
- unmet needs for attention and affection
- emotional closeness to peers
- relationship difficulties
- overachievement or underachievement
- noncompliance with family or school rules
- ineffective support system
- limited coping or problem-solving skills
- limited social skills
- impulsive behaviour
- procrastination
- lack of leisure skills
- academic or employment problems
- discomfort with sexual feelings or inappropriate sexual behaviours
- money problems
- drug and alcohol use.

If appropriate, the specialist makes a diagnosis according to criteria established by the American Psychiatric Association (APA). As for adults, mental illness in children and adolescents are classified and diagnosed according to the APA's *Diagnostic and Statistical Manual of Mental Disorders*, Fourth Edition, Text Revision (*DSM-IV-TR*).

Attention deficit hyperactivity disorder

A neurobiological disorder, ADHD is marked by developmentally inappropriate inattention, impulsiveness and, in some cases, hyperactivity. Unless identified and treated properly, ADHD may progress to conduct disorder, academic and job failure, depression, relationship problems and substance abuse.

Most children with ADHD experience signs and symptoms by age 4. A few aren't diagnosed until they enter school.

Are you still paying attention?

ADHD affects roughly 3–5% of school-age children in the United Kingdom.

Boyz to men

ADHD affects at least twice as many boys as girls. The child's behaviour may cause problems at school, in the home and in the community, and may influence his emotional development and social skills.

Until recently, experts thought children outgrew ADHD by adolescence. We now know that many symptoms continue into adulthood, causing frustrated dreams and emotional pain. In fact, the disorder affects approximately 2–4% of adults.

Causes

No known biological basis for ADHD exists. Research shows that the disorder tends to run in families, suggesting a genetic influence. For example, when one identical twin has the disorder, the other is likely to have it, too.

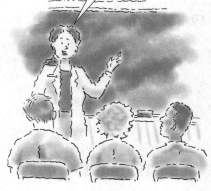

On average, one child in every classroom has attention deficit hyperactivity disorder.

It may be relative

Typically, a child with ADHD has at least one close relative who also has the disorder. At least one-third of men who had ADHD in their youth have children with the disorder.

Risk factors

Some scientists believe the following conditions may predispose a child to ADHD:

- drug exposure *in utero*
- birth complications, such as toxaemia, hypoxia or head trauma
- low birth weight
- preexisting neurological conditions, such as cerebral palsy or epilepsy
- lead poisoning
- multiple stressful events
- child abuse.

Signs and symptoms

Signs and symptoms of ADHD fall into three categories:

 inattention

 impulsiveness

 hyperactivity.

'What a bore'

Commonly, these behaviours intensify when the child is bored, in an unstructured situation, or required to concentrate or focus on a task for an extended period.

Inattention

Children with ADHD have a short attention span, don't seem to listen and have a hard time keeping their minds on any one thing. They get bored easily, tiring of tasks after just a few minutes.

Head in the clouds

Although children with ADHD may give effortless attention to the things they enjoy, they have difficulty focusing deliberate, conscious attention on organising and completing a task or learning something new. Inattention causes them to lose things, be forgetful and make careless mistakes.

Follow-through failure

Children with ADHD don't follow through on instructions, fail to finish tasks and have trouble organising tasks. Easily distracted, they're reluctant to engage in tasks that call for sustained mental effort. (See *ADHD and psychosis: A possible link?*)

Impulsiveness

Children with ADHD have trouble curbing their immediate reactions. They act before they think. They interrupt others – for instance, blurting out inappropriate remarks or answering a question before the person has finished asking it.

Take a number!

Waiting their turn and waiting for things they want are also challenging for these children. When upset, they may grab another child's toy or strike out physically.

Hyperactivity

Children with ADHD are always in motion and can't seem to sit still. They try to do several things at once.

In school, they fidget or squirm in their seat, roam around the room or talk excessively. They have trouble engaging in quiet activities and may find it impossible to sit through a class. Some tap their pencils incessantly, wiggle their feet or touch everything.

Diagnosis

The child should undergo a complete medical evaluation, with emphasis on a neurological examination, hearing and vision. A psychiatric evaluation should be performed to assess intellectual ability, academic achievement and potential learning disorder problems. Sometimes, speech and language evaluations are necessary.

The diagnosis of ADHD hinges on specific features. Characteristic behaviours must appear before age 7, continue for at least 6 months and be more frequent or severe than in other children of the same age.

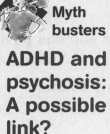

Myth busters

ADHD and psychosis: A possible link?

Myths and misinformation can cause needless worry in parents of children with attention deficit hyperactivity disorder (ADHD). One myth involves the reputed link between ADHD and psychosis.

Myth: Children with ADHD can easily become psychotic.

Reality: Children with ADHD may seem disorganised because of their impulsiveness and distractibility. However, few have psychotic symptoms, such as delusions, hallucinations or thought disorders.

An angel at home?

Also, the behaviours must create a real handicap in at least two areas of the child's life, such as school, home or social settings. A child who's overly active at school but functions well elsewhere wouldn't be diagnosed with ADHD. (See *Diagnostic criteria: Attention deficit hyperactivity disorder*.)

Treatment

Treatment focuses on coordinating the child's psychological and physiological needs. Psychotherapy can reduce ADHD symptoms and teach the child ways to modify behaviour. Such drugs as Atemoxetine help to ease inattention, impulsiveness and hyperactivity. (See *Pharmacological options for treating ADHD*, pages 68 and 69.)

Diagnostic criteria: Attention deficit hyperactivity disorder

The *Diagnostic and Statistical Manual of Mental Disorders*, Fourth Edition, Text Revision groups a selection of symptoms into inattention and hyperactivity-impulsivity categories. To qualify for the diagnosis of attention deficit hyperactivity disorder, the person must have at least six symptoms from the inattention group or at least six from the hyperactivity-impulsivity group. Symptoms must have persisted for at least 6 months to a degree that's maladaptive and inconsistent with the person's developmental level.

Symptoms of inattention

The person manifesting *inattention:*

- often fails to pay close attention to details or makes careless mistakes in school, work or other activities
- often has trouble sustaining attention in tasks or play activities
- often seems not to listen when spoken to directly
- often fails to follow through on instructions or to finish schoolwork, chores or workplace duties (not because of oppositional behaviour or failure to understand instructions)
- often has trouble organising tasks and activities
- often avoids, dislikes or is reluctant to engage in tasks that require sustained mental effort (such as schoolwork or homework)
- often loses things necessary for tasks or activities (toys, school assignments, pencils, books, tools)
- often becomes distracted by extraneous stimuli
- often demonstrates forgetfulness in daily activities.

Symptoms of hyperactivity-impulsivity

The person manifesting *hyperactivity:*

- often fidgets with his hands or feet or squirms in his seat
- often leaves his seat in the classroom or in other situations in which remaining seated is expected
- often runs about or climbs excessively in inappropriate situations
- often has trouble playing or engaging in leisure activities quietly
- often is described as 'on the go' or 'driven by a motor'
- often talks excessively.

The person manifesting *impulsivity:*

- often blurts out answers before questions have been completed
- often has difficulty awaiting his turn
- often interrupts or intrudes on others in conversations or games.

Additional features

- Some symptoms causing impairment appear before age 7.
- Impairment from the symptoms is present in two or more settings (at school and at home).
- Clinically significant impairment in social, academic or occupational functioning is clearly evident.

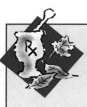

Meds matters

Pharmacological options for treating ADHD

Three central nervous system stimulants have been used effectively to control symptoms of attention deficit hyperactivity disorder (ADHD) in both children and adults – dextroamphetamine (Dexedrine), methylphenidate (Ritalin) and pemoline (Cylert). For many people, these drugs dramatically reduce hyperactivity and improvetheir ability to focus, learn and work.

Drug	Adverse reactions		Contraindications
Dextroamphetamine	• Anorexia • Weight loss or decrease in expected weight gain • Diarrhoea • Insomnia • Hyperactivity	• Restlessness • Headache • Mild blood pressure elevation • Dizziness • Mild depression • Skin rash	• Use of monoamine oxidase inhibitor therapy within previous 14 days (may cause a hypertensive crisis) • Tartrazine allergy
Methylphenidate	• Anorexia • Nausea • Weight loss or decrease in expected weight gain • Temporary growth delay • Stomachache • Abdominal pain	• Lethargy • Headache • Insomnia • Transient motor tics • Mild blood pressure elevation • Social withdrawal • Rebound hyperactivity or irritability • Nervous habits	• Tourette's syndrome • Diabetes mellitus • Kidney disease • Cardiovascular disease
Atomoxetine	• Anorexia • Dry mouth • Nausea • Vomiting • Abdominal pain • Constipation • Dyspepsia • Flatulence • Palpitation • Tachycardia • Increased blood pressure • Postural hypotension • Hot flushes • Sleep disturbacne • Dizziness • Headache • Fatigue	• Depression • Anxiety • Irritability • Tremor • Rigours • Urinary retension • Enuresis • Prostatis • Sexual dysfunction • Menstrual disturbances • Mydriasis • Conjunctivitis • Dermatitis • Pruritus • Rash • Sweating • Weight changes	

Nursing interventions

- Give first dose on awakening, followed by second dose in 4–6 hours.
- Discuss concurrent use of prescription and over-the-counter (OTC) drugs with child's primary health care provider.
- Monitor growth and development regularly.
- Monitor sleep patterns.
- Be aware that stimulant drugs have the potential for abuse.

- Give with meals to minimise anorexia.
- Administer at least 6 hours before bedtime.
- Monitor growth and development regularly. Weigh the child two to three times weekly.
- Monitor growth parameters.
- Monitor vital signs.
- Monitor for tics.
- Monitor for depression.
- Be aware that stimulant drugs have the potential for abuse.

- Give either single dose in the morning or in two divided doses with last dose no later than early evening
- Monitor vital signs
- Seek prompt medical attention in case of severs abdominal pain, unexplained nausea, malaise, darkening of urine or jaundice.
- Inform parents of heightened risk of suicidal ideation and to report clinical worsening, suicidal thoughts or behaviour, irritability, agitation or depression.
- Monitor growth.

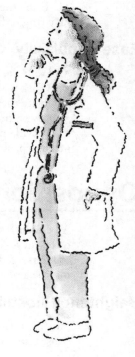

The child also may benefit from an individualised educational plan, with special services that support his strengths and minimise problems stemming from his vulnerabilities.

Nursing interventions

These interventions may be appropriate for a child with ADHD:
- Develop a trusting and accepting relationship with the child.
- Encourage him to talk about problems, difficulties and feelings.
- Assess his risk of injury related to hyperactivity and gross motor behaviours.
- Maintain a safe, calm environment that minimises stimulation and distractions and helps the child remain in control.

Cultivate better conduct

- Help the child determine acceptable and unacceptable behaviours. Discuss with him disruptive behaviours, patterns of losing control and consequences of disruptive behaviours.
- Teach him how to make choices and select appropriate ways of behaving.
- Monitor his activities and help him set limits, stay calm and take opportunities to control undesirable behaviours.

Subdue the frenzy

- Schedule frequent breaks to help him control impulsiveness and minimise hyperactive behaviours.
- Teach the parents that hunger, thirst, fatigue and other physical problems may trigger hyperactivity.

Ease impulsivity

- Help the child learn how to take his turn, wait in line and follow rules.
- Work with him to divide tasks into doable steps so that he's more likely to complete them successfully.
- Give him opportunities to participate in activities with peers.
- Provide positive feedback for improvement as he starts to take steps to manage problematic behaviours.

Oppositional defiant disorder

All children sometimes talk back, argue, disobey and defy their parents or teachers – especially when they're hungry, tired or stressed. In fact, for toddlers aged 2 or 3 and for young adolescents, such oppositional behaviour may be a normal part of development.

Heightened hostility

Hostile, uncooperative behaviour in a child may signal ODD if it's more consistent and severe than that of other children of the same age and

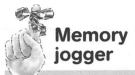

Memory jogger

The word PEPS can help you recall the major treatment components for attention deficit hyperactivity disorder.

P Psychotherapy

E Education

P Pharmacology

S Strengths

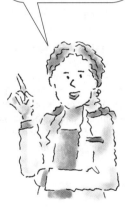

Maintain a safe, calm environment for a child with ADHD.

developmental level – and if such behaviour affects the child's social, family and academic life.

A child with ODD is consistently negative, disobedient, argumentative and hostile. He behaves in a provocative manner deliberately meant to annoy and upset authority figures.

Defiant, disobedient and hostile – could I have ODD?

No end to the argument

During an argument, a child with ODD doesn't back down, even if he stands to lose privileges. To him, the important thing is the struggle, which overshadows the reality of the situation. If anyone objects to his behaviour, he views it as stimulation to continue the argument. ODD may be a precursor to conduct disorder (discussed below).

A lot of ODD

Roughly 5–15% of school-age children have ODD. Onset occurs between ages 3 and 19.

Before puberty, ODD is more common in boys. After puberty, it affects both genders equally.

Causes

No known biological basis for ODD exists.

Risk factors

Various biological, psychosocial and environmental risk factors may play a role. These factors include:
- parental rejection
- inconsistent, unsupervised child rearing
- inconsistent or punitive discipline or limit setting
- parental modelling of defiant interactions with others
- family conflict
- marital discord between the child's parents
- disrupted child care with a succession of different caregivers.

Signs and symptoms

Signs and symptoms of ODD usually occur in more than one setting, although they may be more noticeable at home or at school. They include:
- persistent or consistent pattern of defiant, disobedient, hostile behaviour
- disobeying directly by not following rules
- disobeying indirectly by procrastinating and being sneaky
- refusing to cooperate
- being touchy and easily annoyed
- frequent bouts of anger and resentment
- persistent fighting
- excessive arguing
- stubbornness

- testing of behavioural limits
- temper tantrums
- deliberate attempts to upset or annoy people
- vindictiveness
- blaming others for his own misbehaviour
- violating others' rights.

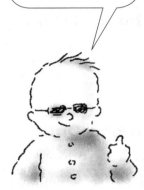

I'm not supposed to wear my shades indoors, but I'm feeling defiant.

Diagnosis

A child with suspected ODD should undergo a complete psychiatric evaluation. The family should be assessed, too, with particular attention to family interactions and communication patterns. (See *Diagnostic criteria: Oppositional defiant disorder*.)

Treatment

Treatment of ODD focuses on meeting the child's and family's psychological and psychosocial needs – and preventing ODD from progressing to conduct disorder. The child may benefit from individual psychotherapy, with an emphasis on anger management.

Teach the parents well

Parents may benefit from training programmes that teach them how to manage the child's behaviour. Together, the parents and the child may

---

Diagnostic criteria: Oppositional defiant disorder

Oppositional defiant disorder is diagnosed when the person meets the criteria in the *Diagnostic and Statistical Manual of Mental Disorders*, Fourth Edition, Text Revision.

Negative behaviour pattern

The person demonstrates a pattern of negative, hostile and defiant behaviour lasting at least 6 months, during which at least four of these criteria are present:

- often loses his temper
- often argues with adults
- often defies or refuses to comply with adults' requests or rules
- often annoys people deliberately
- often blames others for his mistakes or misbehaviour
- often is touchy or easily annoyed by others
- often is angry and resentful
- often is spiteful or vindictive.

These behaviours must occur more frequently than is typically seen in people of the same age and developmental level. Also, the behaviour disturbance must cause clinically significant impairment in social, academic or occupational functioning.

Additional criteria

- The behaviours don't occur exclusively during the course of a mood or psychotic disorder.
- The person doesn't meet the criteria for conduct disorder or (in a person aged 18 or older) antisocial personality disorder.

undergo family psychotherapy to improve communication. (See *Family therapy for ODD*.)

Usually, drug therapy is reserved for children who also have symptoms of anxiety or depression.

Nursing interventions

These nursing interventions may be appropriate for a child with ODD:
• Convey acceptance to help establish a trusting relationship.
• Discuss with the child the limits and consequences of oppositional behaviour.

Negate the negativity

• Help him address negative feelings – especially anger and resentment. Determine appropriate strategies for handling these feelings.
• Assist him in addressing situations and issues that trigger negative thoughts and feelings.
• Discuss strategies he can use to control negative situations.

Stop the plotting

• Help the child learn to accept responsibility for his own behaviour rather than blaming others, becoming defensive and plotting revenge.
• Teach him how to express anger appropriately and control his temper.
• Identify his use of passive-aggressive behaviour, evaluate its effect on others and devise strategies to eliminate it.

Role-play and reinforce

• Teach the child problem-solving and communication skills. Provide role-playing opportunities so that he can become comfortable and self-confident when using these new skills.
• Reinforce the child's acceptable behaviour and positive behaviour changes.
• Work with the child and his family to address conflict, clear expectations and improvement in communication skills.

Conduct disorder

Aggressive behaviour is the hallmark of conduct disorder. A child with this disorder fights, bullies, intimidates and assaults others physically or sexually. Typically, he has poor relationships with peers and adults. He violates others' rights and society's rules.

Future jailbird?

A child with conduct disorder rarely performs at the level predicted by IQ or age. His behaviour interferes with his school or work performance. He may be expelled from school and have problems with the law.

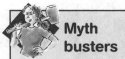

Myth busters

Family therapy for ODD

In some circles, it's assumed that the family of a child with oppositional defiant disorder (ODD) should stay out of the child's therapy. However, this isn't necessarily true.

Myth: Family therapy generally isn't helpful for a child who has ODD.

Reality: Family therapy provides a useful means for discussing family problems and resolving conflict. It gives family members the chance to learn and build on communication and coping skills.

Myth busters

Just a rambunctious kid?

All children misbehave now and then. In fact, misbehaviour is so common in children that some people think it's normal. But misbehaviour that's persistent and pronounced is *not* normal.

Myth: A child with conduct disorder is just a rambunctious kid involved in normal mischief.

Reality: Conduct disorder is a serious mental health problem. A child with this disorder engages in dangerous antisocial behaviour, which may lead to involvement with the juvenile justice system or even incarceration.

> AARGH! This is one type of behaviour you certainly shouldn't role-model!

If the child is removed from the home, he may have difficulty staying in an adoptive or foster family or a group home, further complicating his development.

(Mostly) boys behaving badly

Among children aged 9–17, the prevalence of conduct disorder is approximately 1–4%. Although the disorder occurs in both males and females, it's more common in males.

Conduct disorder has an onset before age 18. Children with early onset (before age 10) are predominantly male, have a worse prognosis and are more likely to develop antisocial personality disorder as adults. In fact, 25–50% of highly antisocial children become antisocial adults. (See *Just a rambunctious kid?*)

Consequences

Besides adult antisocial personality disorder, a child with conduct disorder is at high risk for:
- sexually transmitted diseases
- rape
- teenage pregnancy
- injuries
- substance abuse
- depression
- suicidal thoughts, suicide attempts and suicide itself.

Causes

The cause of conduct disorder isn't fully known. Studies of twins and adopted children suggest the disorder has both biological (including genetic) and psychosocial components.

A dash of ADHD

Studies show that roughly 30–50% of clinical populations with conduct disorder also have ADHD.

Social risk factors

Various social factors may predispose a child to conduct disorder. All of these factors can lead to lack of attachment to the parents or family unit – and eventually, to lack of regard for societal rules. They include:
- early maternal rejection
- separation from parents, with no adequate alternative caregiver available
- early institutionalisation
- family neglect, abuse or violence
- frequent verbal abuse from parents, teachers or other authority figures
- parental psychiatric illness, substance abuse or marital discord
- large family size, crowding and poverty.

Other risk factors

Certain physical factors and other conditions also increase the risk of conduct disorder. These include:
- neurological damage caused by low birth weight or birth complications
- underarousal of the autonomic nervous system
- learning impairments
- insensitivity to physical pain and punishment.

Signs and symptoms

Signs and symptoms of conduct disorder include:
- fighting with family members and peers
- speaking to others in a nasty manner
- being cruel to animals
- vandalising or destroying property
- cheating in school
- skipping classes
- smoking cigarettes
- using drugs or alcohol
- stealing or shoplifting
- engaging in precocious sexual activity
- abusing others sexually.

Diagnosis

Understanding the deviant behaviours of a child with conduct disorder may require a complete team approach – including medical and psychiatric evaluations, feedback from parents, a school consultant's recommendations, a case manager's plan and a probation officer's report. A team approach is important because antisocial behaviours tend to go under-reported. (See *Diagnostic criteria: Conduct disorder*, page 76.)

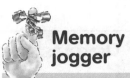

Memory jogger

To remember the signs and symptoms of conduct disorder, simply think of the term itself.

C   Cheats

O   Obnoxious

N   Nasty in speech and behaviour

D   Drug and alcohol use

U   Unpredictable behaviour

C   Cruel to people or animals

T   Truant

D   Destroys property

I   Intimidates

S   Steals

O   Onset of antisocial personality disorder

R   Rages

D   Disrespectful

E   Esteem low

R   Reckless or risky behaviour

Diagnostic criteria: Conduct disorder

A person is diagnosed with conduct disorder if he meets the criteria in the *Diagnostic and Statistical Manual of Mental Disorders*, Fourth Edition, Text Revision. At least three of the criteria from any of the categories below must have been present in the past year, and at least one criterion must have been present within the past 6 months:

Aggression to people and animals

The person exhibiting conduct disorder:

- often bullies, threatens or intimidates others
- often initiates physical fights
- has used a weapon that can cause serious physical harm to others (for instance, a bat, brick, broken bottle, knife or gun)
- has been physically cruel to people
- has been physically cruel to animals
- has stolen while confronting a victim (as in mugging, purse snatching, extortion or armed robbery)
- has forced someone into sexual activity.

Destruction of property

The person has:

- deliberately set a fire with the intention of causing serious damage
- deliberately destroyed others' property (other than by setting a fire).

Deceitfulness or theft

The person:

- has broken into someone else's house, car or building
- often lies to obtain goods or favours or to avoid obligations (in other words, 'cons' others)
- has stolen items of nontrivial value, without confronting a victim (such as by shoplifting [without breaking and entering] or by committing forgery).

Serious violations of rules

The person:

- often stays out at night despite parental prohibitions, starting before age 13
- has run away from home overnight at least twice while living in the parent's or surrogate parent's home (or once without returning for a lengthy period)
- often skips school, beginning before age 13.

Additional criteria

- The behaviour disturbance must cause clinically significant impairment in social, academic or occupational functioning.
- The person is age 18 or older and doesn't meet the criteria for antisocial personality disorder.

Other features

- Conduct disorder is considered *mild* if the person exhibits few if any conduct problems beyond those required to make the diagnosis and if the conduct problems cause only minor harm to others.
- The disorder is considered *moderate* if the conduct problems and their effects on others are intermediate between 'mild' and 'severe'.
- The condition is considered severe if the person has many conduct problems beyond those needed to make the diagnosis, or if the conduct problems cause considerable harm to others.

Anything else going on?

Educational assessments must be reviewed to determine if the child also has cognitive deficits, learning disabilities or problems in intellectual functioning. A neurological examination may be needed if he has a history of head trauma or seizures.

Treatment

Treatment focuses on coordinating the child's psychological, physiological and educational needs. Psychotherapy can help him learn problem-solving skills, decrease disruptive symptoms and modify behaviour. Drugs may be prescribed to treat neurological difficulties. Educational strategies focus on encouraging and helping the child continue with school.

ID them early

Early identification of at-risk children is important, because many risk factors for conduct disorder emerge in the first years of life. Studies show that children who behave aggressively at age 3 continue to do so at ages 11–13.

Tough love

Parents of a high-risk child should be taught how to deal with the child's demands. They may need to learn to reinforce appropriate behaviours and to use harsh punishment for inappropriate behaviours. At the same time, they should be encouraged to find ways to bond more strongly with him.

Here come da judge!

Ultimately, some children with conduct disorder enter the juvenile justice system. Juvenile justice interventions provide structured rules and a means for monitoring and controlling the child's behaviour.

Nursing interventions

These nursing interventions may be appropriate for a child or adolescent with conduct disorder:
• Work to establish a trusting relationship with the child. Be sure to convey that you accept him.
• Provide clear behavioural guidelines, including consequences for disruptive and manipulative behaviour.
• Talk to him about making acceptable choices.
• Teach him effective problem-solving skills, and have him demonstrate them in return.
• Help him identify personal needs and the best strategies for meeting them.

Avert abuse

• Identify abusive communication, such as threats, sarcasm and disparaging comments. Encourage the child to stop using them.
• Teach him how to express anger appropriately through constructive methods to release negative feelings and frustrations.
• Monitor him for anger as well as signs that he's internalising anger, as shown by depression or suicidal ideation.

Rein in revenge

- Work on helping the child accept responsibility for behaviour rather than blaming others, becoming defensive and wanting revenge.
- Teach him effective coping skills and social skills.
- Use role-playing so that he can practise ways of handling stress and gain skill and confidence in managing difficult situations.

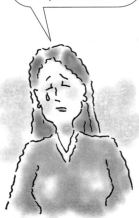

Depression puts me at risk for illnesses and lingering psychosocial problems.

Major depression

Everyone feels sad now and then. In fact, mood changes are normal. However, when a sad mood persists and causes difficulty eating, sleeping or concentrating, clinical depression may be present.

Ripple effect

Depression can have widespread effects on a child's adjustment and functioning. Depressed children may feel unloved, pessimistic or even hopeless about the future. They may think life isn't worth living. What's more, a depressed child is at increased risk for physical illness and psychosocial difficulties that persist long after the depressive episode resolves.

The blahs and the blues

Major depression (also called unipolar depression) is a syndrome of persistently sad or irritable mood accompanied by disturbances in sleep and appetite, lethargy and inability to experience pleasure. (See *Bipolar predisposition?*)

Two excruciatingly long weeks

Major depressive disorder is characterised by one or more major depressive episodes, defined as episodes of depressed mood lasting at least 2 weeks.

Myth busters

Bipolar predisposition?

Many people think children who experience depression are likely to develop bipolar disorder (manic-depression) later in life. On the whole, this isn't true.

Myth: Children who experience childhood depression are highly likely to develop bipolar disorder as adults.

Reality: Only a small percentage of children with depression develop bipolar disorder as adults. However, a family history of both bipolar disorder and childhood depression – not just depression alone – makes bipolar disorder more likely.

About one-half of depressed service users experience a single episode and recover completely. The rest have at least one recurrence.

Agonising episode

In children and adolescents, a major depressive episode lasts an average of 7–9 months. Depressed children and adolescents are sad and lose interest in activities that used to please them. They're often irritable, and their irritability may lead to aggressive behaviour. They have difficulty taking decisions and concentrating. They lack energy or motivation and may neglect their appearance and hygiene.

Many miserable kids

Roughly 2–3% of children and more than 8% of adolescents in the United Kingdom suffer from depression. What's more, depression now has an earlier onset than it did in past decades.

For all too many children, early-onset depression persists, recurs and continues into adulthood. In fact, depression in youth may predict more severe depressive illness in adult life.

Substances and suicide

Depressed adolescents are at increased risk for substance abuse and suicidal behaviour. Suicide attempts peak during the mid-adolescent years. The incidence of death from suicide increases steadily throughout the adolescent years. In fact, among adolescents, suicide is the third leading cause of death.

Causes

The multiple causes of depression are controversial and not completely understood. Current research suggests possible genetic, familial, biochemical, physical, psychological and social causes. In many service users, the history identifies a specific personal loss or severe stress that probably interacts with a person's predisposition to major depression.

Biological tip-offs

Among depressed service users, researchers have found imbalances in the major neurotransmitters – serotonin, norepinephrine, dopamine, acetylcholine and gamma-aminobutyric acid (GABA).

Also, computed tomography (CT) and positron emission tomography (PET) scans show abnormally slow activity in the prefrontal cortex and temporal lobes of depressed service users. This finding suggests faulty glucose metabolism in those areas.

Melancholy genes

Some scientists believe depression may be linked to genetic abnormalities involving chromosomes 4, 11, 18 and 21. Also, a family history of depression increases the risk of the disorder.

Medical miseries

Depression is also linked to certain medical conditions, namely:
- neurological problems, such as brain tumour, brain trauma, multiple sclerosis, Parkinson's disease and Huntington's disease
- cardiovascular disease
- acquired immunodeficiency syndrome
- electrolyte imbalances (especially calcium, magnesium, sodium and potassium)
- endocrine disorders, such as Addison's disease, Cushing's syndrome, thyroid disorders, diabetes mellitus and parathyroid disorders
- nutritional imbalances, such as deficiencies in B and C vitamins, iron, zinc and protein.

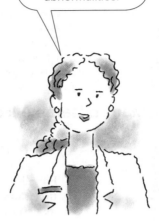

Depression may be linked to certain chromosomal abnormalities.

Risk factors

Common risk factors associated with major depression include:
- family history of depression
- excessive stress
- abuse or neglect
- physical or emotional trauma
- loss of a parent
- loss of a relationship
- other mental illnesses
- other chronic illnesses
- other developmental, learning or conduct disorders.

Signs and symptoms

Early diagnosis and treatment of depression is crucial for healthy emotional, social and behavioural development. Assess the child for such signs and symptoms as:
- persistent sadness
- irritable, cranky mood
- physical complaints, such as headache or stomachache
- crying for no apparent reason
- inability to concentrate or take decisions
- withdrawal from peers and social situations
- restlessness, fidgeting or frequent moving
- boredom with daily activities
- difficulty sleeping, or sleeping more than usual
- disorganisation with periods of agitation
- fatigue or lack of energy
- rejection of self or others
- not caring about self, others or activities
- sense of worthlessness
- verbal or physical fights with others
- thoughts of death, suicidal ideation, suicide attempts and high-risk behaviours

- struggling with normal developmental adjustments
- absence of expected weight increase for growth and developmental stage.

Under the radar

All too often, depression goes unrecognised by the child's family, doctor and teachers. Signs and symptoms may be mistaken for the normal mood swings typical of a particular developmental stage. Also, symptoms of depression may be expressed in varying ways depending on the child's developmental stage.

In addition, children and young adolescents may have trouble identifying and describing their emotional states. Instead of expressing how bad they feel, they may act out their feelings, which may be interpreted as misbehaviour.

Leery of labels

To complicate matters further, some health care professionals may be reluctant to label a young person mentally ill by assigning a diagnosis of depression.

Depression with a difference

Despite some similarities, childhood depression differs from adult depression in two key ways.

 Psychotic features are less common in children and adolescents.

 Anxiety symptoms (such as reluctance to meet people) and physical symptoms (such as aches and pains, stomachache and headache) are more common in depressed children and adolescents.

Diagnosis

The diagnosis of depression can be made from person self-reports, interviews and observations. A team approach is crucial. The team should include a medical and psychiatric evaluation, a school consultant's recommendations and feedback from parents. (See *Diagnostic criteria: Major depression*, page 82.)

Tool time

Certain tools may be useful in screening children and adolescents for major depression. Two such tools are:

 Children's Depression Inventory (CDI) for ages 7–17

 Beck Depression Inventory for adolescents.

A child who screens positive on one of these instruments should undergo a comprehensive diagnostic evaluation by a mental health professional. The evaluation should include interviews with the child, parents and, when possible, other informants (such as teachers and social services personnel).

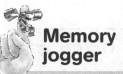

Memory jogger

To help remember the major signs and symptoms of depression in children and adolescents, think of SWAP.

S School problems

W Withdrawal

A Alterations in sleep, appetite and energy levels

P Physical health problems

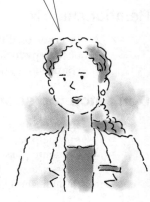

The child may be screened with the Children's Depression Inventory or the Beck Depression Inventory.

Diagnostic criteria: Major depression

A person is diagnosed with major depression if he meets these criteria for a single major depressive episode from the *Diagnostic and Statistical Manual of Mental Disorders*, Fourth Edition, Text Revision.

- At least five of the following symptoms must have been present during the same 2-week period and must represent a change from previous functioning. One of these symptoms must be either depressed mood or loss of interest in previously pleasurable activities:
  - depressed mood (irritable mood in children and adolescents) most of the day, nearly every day, as indicated by either a subjective account or observation by others
  - markedly diminished interest or pleasure in all, or almost all, activities most of the day, nearly every day
  - significant weight loss or gain when not dieting, or a decrease or increase in appetite nearly every day (in children, failure to make expected weight gains)
  - insomnia or excessive sleeping nearly every day
  - psychomotor agitation or retardation nearly every day
  - fatigue or loss of energy nearly every day

  - feelings of worthlessness or excessive or inappropriate guilt nearly every day
  - diminished ability to think or concentrate, or indecisiveness, nearly every day
  - recurrent thoughts of death, recurrent suicidal ideation without a specific plan, a suicide attempt or a specific plan for committing suicide.

Other criteria

- Symptoms cause clinically significant distress or impairment in social, occupational or other important areas of functioning.
- Symptoms don't stem from the direct physiological effects of a substance or a general medical condition.
- Symptoms aren't better accounted for by bereavement.
- Symptoms last longer than 2 months or are characterised by marked functional impairment, morbid preoccupation with worthlessness, suicidal ideation, psychotic symptoms or psychomotor retardation.

Treatment

Treatment of major depression may entail psychotherapy (particularly cognitive-behavioural therapy), medication or a combination. Targeted interventions may involve the home or school environment.

Relationship Rx

Interpersonal therapy may be another psychotherapy option. This type of therapy focuses on working through disturbed relationships that may contribute to depression.

Don't stop too soon

Continuing psychotherapy for several months after symptom remission may help service users and families strengthen the skills they learned during the acute phase of depression. It may also help them cope with depression after-effects, address environmental stressors and understand how the child's thoughts and behaviours could contribute to a relapse.

Pharmacotherapy

Although antidepressant drugs can be effective treatments for adults with depressive disorders, their use in children and adolescents is controversial. Many doctors have been reluctant to prescribe psychotropic medications for young people because, until fairly recently, little evidence was available about the safety and efficacy of these drugs in youth.

Prozac inclination

Although medication is never the primary intervention, recent studies in the United States show that selective serotonin reuptake inhibitors (SSRIs), such as fluoxetine (Prozac), are safe and effective for the short-term treatment of depression in young people. Prozac recently was approved for use in children aged 8 and older. (See *Pharmacological options for treating depression*, page 84.)

First in line

Medication may be considered a first-line treatment for children and adolescents who:

 have severe symptoms that would make effective psychotherapy difficult

 can't undergo psychotherapy

have psychosis or chronic or recurrent depressive episodes.

Rebuffing a relapse

After symptom remission, the doctor may recommend that the child continue drug therapy because of the high risk that depression will recur. As appropriate, antidepressant medication should be discontinued gradually over at least 6 weeks or longer.

Nursing interventions

These nursing interventions may be appropriate for a child or adolescent with major depression:
- Structure and maintain a safe, secure environment.
- Find ways to sustain the child's typical routine.
- Monitor him for dangerous or self-destructive behaviour.
- Work with him to address his needs.
- Provide appropriate times to eat, rest, sleep and play or relax.

Put it in writing

- Develop an agreement or contract with the child that he'll seek out staff if he feels desperate or suicidal.
- Teach him to talk things out rather than act things out.

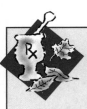

Meds matters

Pharmacological options for treating depression

A child or adolescent with major depressive disorder may receive a selective serotonin reuptake inhibitor (SSRI). The chart below details the adverse reactions, contraindications and nursing interventions for three SSRIs.

Drug	Adverse reactions		Contraindications	Nursing interventions
Fluoxetine	• Anorexia • Nausea • Appetite changes • Dry mouth • Headache • Nervousness • Fatigue	• Tremor • Dizziness • Seizures • Chest pain • Skin rash • Blurred vision • Flulike reaction	• Kidney problems • Liver problems • Diabetes mellitus • Suicidal ideation	• Give in the morning. • Supervise people at risk for suicide. • Monitor weekly for weight changes. • Monitor for safety because drug may cause dizziness.
Sertraline	• Anorexia • Nausea • Appetite changes • Dry mouth • Headache • Insomnia • Nervousness • Fatigue • Emotional lability • Tremor • Dizziness	• Seizures • Chest pain • Cough • Blood pressure changes • Tachycardia • Skin rash • Blurred vision • Flulike reaction • Liver problems	• Liver problems • Concurrent use of a monoamine oxidase inhibitor	• Tell people to take drug with food. • Supervise people at risk for suicide. • Monitor weekly for weight changes. • Monitor people with a history of seizure disorder.

Probe problems

- Discuss concerns and issues that upset or bother him.
- Help him talk about problems and stressors.
- Work on age-appropriate strategies for solving problems.
- Encourage him to express his feelings openly.
- If he has suffered a major loss, talk about the loss, what it means to him and how to grieve for it.

Get physical

- Provide physical outlets for energy and aggression release (such as sports, music or art) to help the child express feelings and develop healthy coping skills.
- Help him rethink negative statements about self and identify and build on current strengths.
- Have him identify supportive people and learn ways to talk to these people about his feelings and needs.

Do you have any concerns you'd like to discuss?

Tourette's syndrome

TS is a neurobehavioural disorder characterised by sudden, involuntary muscle movements (motor tics) and vocalisations (vocal tics). In some cases, the tics may include inappropriate words. Symptoms, which may range from mild to severe, usually appear before age 18.

Tic combination

Motor tics tend to affect the head, trunk or limbs. They sometimes change in severity, frequency and location. *Verbal* tics may involve a wide variety of sounds, such as clicks, yelps, barks and snorts.

Most TS sufferers gradually develop a combination of different motor and vocal tics. The tics may occur a few times or many times during the day.

Tics may grow less frequent and severe during adolescence or adulthood. In a few cases, they disappear completely after adolescence.

TS in toddlers

TS usually becomes apparent between ages 2 and 15. Roughly one-half of service users experience symptoms by age 7.

The disorder is more common in males than females. It affects from 0.1% to 1.0% of the general population.

Apart and alone

Many people with TS have associated behavioural problems, such as obsessions and compulsions, inattention, hyperactivity and impulsivity. Because of their odd behaviour, they tend to experience distress and difficulties in social situations, in school and on the job.

Causes

The cause of TS is unknown. Many researchers suspect the disorder is linked to abnormalities in neurotransmitters, because abnormal levels of dopamine, serotonin, GABA, norepinephrine and acetylcholine have been found in TS service users. Also, the basal ganglia and other brain regions show decreased metabolic activity.

TS has been linked to decreased metabolic activity in certain brain regions.

Genes and wombs

Predisposing factors for TS may include:

☝ genetic factors (in a few cases, TS may be inherited from both parents)

✌ pregnancy and prenatal problems, such as emotional problems, stress during pregnancy and severe nausea and vomiting during the first trimester of pregnancy.

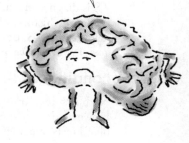

Signs and symptoms

Facial tics, such as eye blinking, typically are the first sign of TS. The tics commonly begin around age 7, although some children as young as age 2 have them. Over time, facial grimacing, neck or head jerking, neck stretching, foot stamping or body twisting and bending may occur.

What makes tics tick

Tics tend to worsen during stress, excitement, boredom or fatigue and to ease during relaxation, sleep and when the person is absorbed in an activity. Although some people can suppress the tics for a short time, tension eventually builds and the tic escapes.

Some people with TS periodically clear their throat, cough, sniff, grunt, snort, yelp, bark or shout. They may touch other people excessively or repeat actions obsessively and unnecessarily. A few engage in self-harming behaviours, such as lip and cheek biting and head banging.

Tics tend to ease during relaxation. I recommend bubble bath therapy.

Additional inklings

Other signs and symptoms of TS may include:
- coprolalia (swearing or using obscene language)
- copropraxia (making obscene gestures)
- low self-esteem
- feelings of shame
- obsessive thinking
- compulsive behaviours.

Waxing and waning

In most TS sufferers, symptoms wax and wane, periodically decreasing or increasing in frequency and intensity. Some service users may go weeks or even years with few or no symptoms.

Diagnosis

TS is diagnosed clinically from person observation and the evaluation of the family history, which may reveal a familial predisposition to TS. For a diagnosis of TS, tics must be present for at least 1 year. (See *Diagnostic criteria: Tourette's syndrome*, page 87.)

Copycat conditions

No blood tests or other laboratory tests can diagnose TS definitively. However, to rule out conditions that resemble TS, the person may undergo blood tests, magnetic resonance imaging and CT scans and EEG.

Diagnostic criteria: Tourette's syndrome

A person is diagnosed with Tourette's syndrome if he meets these criteria from the *Diagnostic and Statistical Manual of Mental Disorders,* Fourth Edition, Text Revision.

Motor and vocal tics

- Both multiple motor tics and one or more vocal tics must have been present during the illness, although not necessarily at the same time. (A tic is a sudden, rapid, recurrent, nonrhythmic, stereotyped motor movement or vocalisation.)
- The tics occur many times per day – usually in clusters – nearly every day or intermittently during a period exceeding 1 year. During this period, the person has never had a tic-free period lasting more than 3 consecutive months.
- Onset of the tics occurred before age 18.

Other criteria

The disturbance doesn't result from direct physiological effects of substances (such as stimulants) or a general medical condition (for instance, postviral encephalitis or Huntington's disease).

A complete neurological history and examination can determine if the child has additional neurological problems or movement disorders. A thorough psychiatric evaluation also is done, focusing on anxiety, mood, behaviour and age-appropriate developmental level.

Treatment

Treatment of TS may involve child and family psychotherapy and, possibly, medications. Psychotherapy promotes and maintains the child's self-esteem and helps the person and family learn about:
- the nature of the disorder and how to manage symptoms
- stress management strategies, with a focus on how to best handle distress or crisis
- strategies for coping with the stigma of the illness, especially peer teasing
- social skills and ways to manage disagreements, anger and conflict at school, at home and in the community.

Pharmacotherapy

Most TS service users don't require medication. However, some may take it when symptoms interfere with their functioning. Medications also may promote normal child development. Unfortunately, no one drug eliminates all symptoms or helps all TS service users.

Specific drug therapy may involve one of three types of drugs:

low-dose antipsychotic agents, such as pimozide, risperidone and (for severe tics) haloperidol

SSRIs, such as fluoxetine, for people who also have obsessive–compulsive disorder

clonidine, an antihypertensive drug. (See *Pharmacological options for treating Tourette's syndrome*, page 88.)

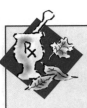

Meds matters

Pharmacological options for treating Tourette's syndrome

A child or adolescent with Tourette's syndrome may receive an antipsychotic drug to relieve tics and other symptoms. The chart below gives the adverse reactions, contraindications and nursing interventions for two antipsychotic agents.

Drug	Adverse reactions		Contraindications	Nursing interventions
Haloperidol	• Extrapyramidal reactions (Parkinsonian symptoms) • Tardive dyskinesia (with prolonged use) • Dry mouth • Anorexia • Nausea • Insomnia • Restlessness • Anxiety • Agitation	• Drowsiness • Depression • Fatigue • Headache • Dizziness • Seizures • Photosensitivity • Tachycardia • Blood pressure changes • Blurred vision • Urinary retention	• Seizure disorder • Severe depression • Urinary retention • Glaucoma • Severe cardiovascular disease	• Teach the person to take the drug with a full glass of water or with food or milk. • Assess for mental status changes. • Monitor closely for adverse reactions, especially Parkinsonian symptoms and tardive dyskinesia. As needed, obtain an order for benztropine (Cogentin) to relieve Parkinsonian symptoms. • Monitor for seizures. • Encourage adequate fluid intake. • Monitor for dental problems. • Caution the person about overexposure to the sun. Instruct him to wear sunglasses and use sunscreen.
Pimozide	• Extrapyramidal reactions (Parkinsonian symptoms) • Tardive dyskinesia (with prolonged use) • Dry mouth • Anorexia • Weight change • Nausea • Restlessness	• Insomnia • Agitation • Headache • Seizures • Photosensitivity • Blood pressure changes • Blurred vision • Urinary retention or frequency	• Seizure disorder • Kidney problems • Liver problems	• Obtain a baseline electrocardiogram before drug therapy begins. • Tell the person to take the drug with a full glass of water or with food or milk. • Know that dry mouth may worsen as the dosage increases. • Assess for mental status changes. • Monitor closely for adverse reactions, especially Parkinsonian symptoms and tardive dyskinesia. As needed, obtain an order for benztropine to relieve Parkinsonian symptoms. • Monitor for seizures. • Encourage adequate fluid intake. • Monitor for dental problems. • Caution the person about overexposure to the sun. Instruct him to wear sunglasses and use sunscreen. • Instruct the person to taper the dosage gradually rather than stopping the drug abruptly.

Dainty doses

Usually, these drugs are given to children in small doses, with the dosage increased gradually as appropriate.

Nursing interventions

These nursing interventions may be appropriate for a child or adolescent with TS:
- Develop a relationship with the child that fosters trust and acceptance.
- Teach him about the disorder and ways to manage symptoms.
- Help him address behaviours that contribute to irritability and frustration.

Bookworm therapy

- Explain to the child and family that stress tends to increase tic frequency, whereas quiet activities (such as reading) can diminish the intensity of tics. If appropriate, recommend relaxation and biofeedback therapy.
- Encourage the child to express feelings about the illness and the problems he experiences.
- Help him learn to cope with impulses, negativity and unacceptable behaviours.

Souped-up self-esteem

- Promote the child's strengths and self-esteem.
- Address ways for him to stay positive about himself.
- Work with family members to decrease their focus on the child's symptoms and to reduce critical comments.
- If he has difficulty in regular classes, help the family obtain information about special education options as appropriate. (See *Tourette's syndrome and special schooling?*.)

Quick quiz

1. What should the nurse teach the parents of a child who's receiving methylphenidate (Ritalin)?
   - A. Monitor the child's blood glucose level because the drug increases the diabetes risk.
   - B. Monitor the child's growth closely because the drug may interfere with growth and development.
   - C. Have the child undergo IQ testing because the drug may decrease intelligence.
   - D. Have the child's hearing tested because the drug can cause hearing loss.

Answer: B. The child's physical growth should be monitored because Ritalin may cause weight loss and temporary interference with growth and development.

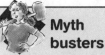

Myth busters

Tourette's syndrome and special schooling?

Some people have mistaken notions about the educational needs of children with Tourette's syndrome (TS).

Myth: Children who experience tics frequently must be hospitalised and removed from school because of their special needs and impaired school performance.

Reality: Most children with TS are treated on an outpatient basis and attend regular school. Only those with extremely severe tics and concomitant mental health problems may need a few days of hospitalisation for a comprehensive evaluation and medication therapy.

2. In a child with conduct disorder, aggressive behaviour is:
    A. caused by anxiety.
    B. masking low self-esteem.
    C. caused by temporary changes in relationships.
    D. caused by heredity.

Answer: B. A child with conduct disorder struggles with low self-esteem and a low tolerance for frustration – even though he may attempt to portray an aggressive image.

3. A child with depression has limited interaction with classmates. When working with him, the nurse should assign top priority to:
    A. developing his strengths and improving his self-esteem.
    B. addressing ways for him to learn to complete tasks.
    C. determining strategies to help him handle fear.
    D. developing his communication skills.

Answer: A. A depressed child needs assistance with learning how to feel good about himself.

4. Signs and symptoms of ODD include:
    A. anxiety.
    B. compulsive behaviour.
    C. testing of limits.
    D. hallucinations.

Answer: C. Children with ODD engage in persistent testing of behavioural limits, bully others to get what they want and try to win no matter what the consequences may be.

5. A child with Tourette's syndrome who has both motor and vocal tics is most likely to experience:
    A. academic difficulties.
    B. peer teasing.
    C. poor social skills.
    D. speech impediment.

Answer: B. Children with Tourette's syndrome who have motor and vocal tics are often ridiculed and teased by other children.

Scoring

✰✰✰   If you answered all five items correctly, congrats! Your commitment to understanding kids is commendable!

✰✰   If you answered three or four items correctly, pat yourself on the back! We're proud of your paediatric proficiency!

✰   If you answered fewer than three items correctly, don't get depressed! Review the chapter – only this time, stop fidgeting and pay more attention!

3 Disorders of the elderly

Just the facts

In this chapter, you'll learn:

♦ mental status changes of older adulthood

♦ care settings for older adults with psychiatric disorders

♦ diagnosis, treatment and nursing interventions for older adults with age-related cognitive decline (ARCD), Alzheimer's dementia and vascular dementia.

A look at psychiatric disorders in older adults: UK Data

People in the UK are living longer than ever before, with the vast majority surviving to at least age 65. Likewise the elderly population is increasing. A significant number of older adults are disabled – sometimes severely – by psychiatric disorders, such as depression, anxiety and dementia. As the life expectancy of people in the UK continues to rise, the number of older adults experiencing mental disorders will keep growing. Unfortunately, many health care professionals lack the training to identify these disorders, whose symptoms may mimic those of other medical conditions.

A depressing thought . . .

Almost one in four people aged 85 or older experiences severe symptoms of depression. Older adults have the highest suicide rate, accounting for 20% of suicides.

Beyond recognition?

Despite the substantial need for mental health services, older adults make little use of them. Some older adults deny that they have mental

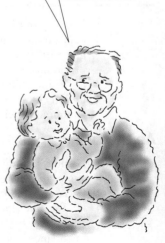

My granddaughter keeps me happy and alert, but some of my friends aren't so lucky

Barriers to treatment

Many older adults need – but don't get – treatment for psychiatric disorders. Here are some reasons for this unmet need:

- Many people (elderly and otherwise) believe that senility, depression and hopelessness are natural conditions of ageing that can't or don't need to be treated.
- Many older adults are reluctant to discuss psychological symptoms, dwelling instead on their physical problems.
- Some older adults prefer primary care – yet many primary care providers lack the training to diagnose and treat psychiatric disorders in the older adults.
- Treatment of mental disorders in older adults can be complex even for properly trained professionals.
- Some health care providers are reluctant to inform older people that they have a mental disorder.
- Health care delivery systems may impose time pressures or fail to reimburse the costs of treating mental disorders.

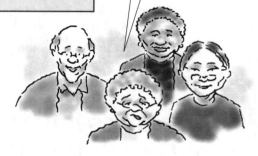

I don't see what they're so happy about. Being old is depressing!

disorders, and many health care providers fail to identify the characteristic signs and symptoms.

Even among older adults who acknowledge their mental disorders, only about one-half receive treatment from any health care provider, and only a fraction of those receive specialty mental health services. (See *Barriers to treatment*.)

Mental status changes of older adulthood

Throughout life, a person continues to develop and change. The brain continuously interacts with and responds to multiple influences. At any given time, the expression of mental health or mental illness can be subtle or pronounced.

Vulnerability to the various types of mental disorders changes throughout life. In children, this vulnerability is taken for granted, but in older adults, it's commonly overlooked, and mental problems in older adults can go undetected.

As the brain ages . . .

During late adulthood, health changes may grow more pronounced and the ability to compensate for deficits may decrease. With age, the brain's capacity for certain mental tasks tends to diminish.

Yet other mental abilities normally remain intact. Well into late adulthood, cognitive skills training and problem-solving strategies can be used to enhance a person's ability to solve problems.

Myth busters

Shaking off 'old people' stereotypes

Does the brain grow brittle and inflexible with age, much the way bones do? Don't bet on it.

Myth: Older adults are slow thinking, inflexible and unproductive.

Reality: With normal ageing, intellectual functioning remains stable, as do the capacity for change and productive engagement with life. Research shows that people have the capacity for constructive change in later life – even in the face of mental illness, adversity and chronic mental health problems. Many older adults remain flexible in both behaviour and attitude and are able to grow intellectually and emotionally.

Neurobiological changes of normal ageing

Although many physiological functions decline with advancing age, extreme disability in older people – including disability from mental disorders – isn't inevitable.

Normal ageing brings certain changes in mental functioning. Most older adults experience a slight decline in intelligence, learning ability, short-term memory and reaction time. This decline grows more significant by about age 75. (See *Shaking off 'old people' stereotypes*.)

Physical changes of the brain

With age come certain physical changes in the brain. These include:
- 20% decrease in the brain's weight by age 90
- selective loss of 5–20% of neurons (brain cells)
- shrinking of neurons
- 15–20% decline in synapses (communication areas between two neurons) in the frontal lobes.

Cognitive changes

Cognition involves intelligence, language, learning and memory. With advancing years, cognitive capacity declines somewhat, but important functions are spared. Age-related cognitive changes vary significantly among individuals.

Cognitive research

Cognitive neuroscientists and cognitive ageing psychologists are conducting research to determine:
- what happens to the mind as we age
- how changes in cognitive behaviours (such as remembering and problem-solving) relate to brain function

> It says here that neurons shrink with age. Does that mean I don't have to diet?

Studying the ageing brain

Increasing evidence suggests that old brains aren't organised like young brains – and that the brain continuously changes and reorganises in response to the demands of ageing.

In one study, researchers found that young adults used the left frontal cortex to perform a verbal working memory task, whereas older adults used both the left and right hemispheres. Other studies also have found that older adults use more parts of their brain than young adults do when performing certain tasks.

Memory and manipulation

Cognitive researchers tested adults ranging from ages 20 to 90 on a variety of basic cognitive tasks. They examined how rapidly the subjects performed mental operations and explored the limits of their working memories (how much information they could simultaneously remember, manipulate and retrieve).

They also tested the subjects' memories for visual-spatial and verbal materials.

They found that age-related cognitive declines occurred in a continuous and gradual fashion, starting from age 20 and continuing at the same pace until age 90. These findings refute the conventional notion that memory problems begin in late adulthood.

Been there, done that

Although mental processing grows less efficient with age, world knowledge and experience usually remain intact. When researchers tested older adults' world knowledge, they found accumulated world knowledge intact even in subjects who showed decline in processing efficiency. In some subjects, accumulated world knowledge actually increased. This finding suggests that knowledge gained through experience remains stable with age.

• whether young brains are more specialised than older ones
• whether old brains are able to reorganise so that decreased functioning in one area is compensated for by another area.

Researchers are also investigating the ageing mind through brain-imaging techniques. (See *Studying the ageing brain*.)

Cognitive disorders

Marked by disruption of cognitive functioning, cognitive disorders manifest clinically as mental deficits in people who previously didn't show such deficits. A cognitive deficit is a prominent feature of many mental and physical disorders seen in older adults. This can pose a challenge to health care professionals trying to pinpoint the underlying problem.

A cognitive disorder can result from any condition that alters or destroys brain tissue and, in turn, impairs cerebral functioning.

Vocabulary, fluid intelligence and processing capacity

A person's vocabulary increases slightly until about age 75 and then starts to decline. Likewise, fluid intelligence – the ability to solve novel problems – also declines over time. Yet research shows that fluid intelligence can be enhanced through training in cognitive skills and problem-solving strategies.

Mental processing capacity – the ability to understand text, make inferences and pay attention – also decreases with age.

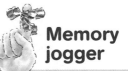

Memory jogger

To help remember the possible causes of cognitive disorders, think of the three Ds:

• Disease – primary brain disease
• Disturbance – the brain's response to a systemic disturbance, such as a medical condition
• Drugs – the brain's reaction to a toxic substance, as in substance abuse

Advice from the experts

Using pictures and words

Ageing doesn't seem to affect a person's ability to recognise pictures. So you can use pictures to help jog the memory of older adults with memory impairments. Here are some other ways to aid memory retention:

- Choose text instructions that explicitly represent material rather than those that force the person to make subtle inferences or draw conclusions.
- Avoid irrelevant details, which can be distracting and require more mental processing.

Cognitive processes minimally affected by ageing

Certain cognitive processes show little or no decline with age. They include:
- implicit memory (information that can't be brought to mind but that can affect behaviour)
- prospective memory (remembering things you need to do)
- highly practised expert skills, such as typing or playing bridge or chess
- picture recognition. (See *Using pictures and words*.)

Working memory and long-term memory

Studies show that working memory and long-term memory decline with ageing. *Working* memory is used for tasks such as keeping a phone number in mind just long enough to write it down as well as in planning, organising and rehearsing. *Long-term* memory is responsible for storing information on a relatively permanent basis.

Haven't I seen you somewhere before?

Researchers have found that ageing affects recall (the process of bringing an experience back into consciousness) more than it affects recognition (the ability to recognise someone or something through remembering).

Implications for teaching

Because age-related cognitive changes lead to slower learning, you'll need to repeat new information frequently when teaching older adults. Also, to reduce the memory load of new information, have older adults practise new skills and habits until these become automatic. When practised sufficiently, any skill becomes automatic – and isn't likely to be completely lost at a later time.

Remember, though, that older adults need much more practice than do younger adults to achieve such automatisation, although they may derive a much greater benefit.

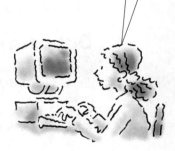

Highly practised skills like typing and playing bridge rarely decline with age.

Predictors of cognitive performance

One comprehensive research study found that high cognitive performance in older adults depends on four variables:

 educational level

 activity level

 peak pulmonary flow rate

self-efficacy (a person's judgement of his ability to reach a specific goal).

It's cool to stay in school

A person's educational level, indicated by years of schooling, was the strongest predictor of high cognitive functioning. This finding suggests that education affects brain function early in life and foreshadows sustained productive behaviour in later life.

Complaints of memory problems

Approximately 50–80% of older adults report subjective memory complaints. Interestingly, those who complain about memory problems perform better than those who don't complain. Such complaints are thought to reflect depression more than a decline in memory.

Depression in older adults

Late-life depression can have serious consequences, including increased illness and death from suicide. Depression typically results from such losses as:
• deaths of friends and loved ones
• loss of physical capacities
• loss of social status and self-esteem.

Bereavement and depression

Bereavement – the natural response to a loved one's death – causes sorrow, anxiety, crying, agitation, insomnia and appetite loss. Although these symptoms may coincide with major depression, they don't in themselves constitute mental illness.

Woeful widows

Nonetheless, bereavement is an important risk factor for depression. Roughly 10–20% of widows and widowers develop clinically significant depression during the first year of bereavement.

Without treatment, such depression tends to persist and become chronic, leading to further disability and health impairment (possibly including altered endocrine and immune function).

> Late adulthood can bring loss of loved ones, physical capacities, social status and self-esteem.

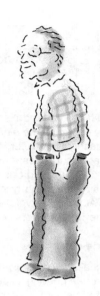

Bereavement red flags

Bereavement is common among older adults who survive family members and friends. Sometimes, though, bereavement can turn into a major depressive disorder. Suspect this is happening if your person experiences:

- frequent thoughts of death
- sense of worthlessness
- guilt about things other than the actions he took, or failed to take, at the time of the loved one's death
- pronounced slowing of psychomotor functions

- prolonged, marked functional impairment.

Not-so-harmless hallucinations

Some bereaved people hallucinate, thinking they've heard the dead person's voice or seen that person's face. Some report that they've seen their deceased spouses in a crowd or heard them call their name while drifting off to sleep. These hallucinations are common among bereaved people.

But a person who has other types of hallucinations may be suffering a serious mental disorder and needs help.

If bereavement symptoms last 2 months or more, the older adult is at risk for adjustment disorder or major depressive disorder. Even when it lasts less than 2 months, bereavement may warrant clinical attention because it's a highly stressful condition that increases the likelihood of mental and somatic (physical) disorders. (See *Bereavement red flags*.)

Traumatic grief

Bereavement-related depression commonly coexists with traumatic grief. Signs and symptoms of traumatic grief include those exhibited in pathological grief (extreme decline in functioning, harming oneself or others and changes in interpersonal relationships) and post-traumatic stress disorder (insomnia, an exaggerated startle response, angry outbursts and hypervigilance). Extremely disabling, these symptoms are associated with health and functional impairments as well as persistent thoughts of suicide. (See *Guiding people through grief*, page 98.)

Preventing depression

With early recognition of symptoms, depression and suicidal behaviour may be averted through grief counselling. Be aware that suicide prevention strategies are important for new residents of long-term facilities – one-half of those newly admitted are at increased risk for depression.

Assessment

Assessing and diagnosing psychiatric disorders in older adults can be challenging. For one thing, these disorders may present differently in older adults than in younger ones. Additionally, older adults are more likely to

Advice from the experts

Guiding people through grief

To help older adults work through their grief, you need to recognise the signs and symptoms of grief and its phases. Grief refers to a sequence of mood changes that occur in response to an actual or perceived loss, such as a loved one's death or a change in family role, residence or body image caused by illness or injury.

Acute grief typically lasts 1–2 years. Prolonged grieving may persist for up to 12 years.

Grieving stages

Usually, successful adaptation requires progressing through grieving stages. Discrete stages of grieving are listed below. But people don't necessarily move through the stages in an orderly way. They may experience several stages at once or may even regress.

- *Disequilibrium*. The person has feelings of shock and disbelief, followed by a numbed sensation. He may cry and feel anger and guilt.
- *Disorganisation*. Restlessness and the inability to organise and complete tasks are common. The person typically experiences loss of self-esteem; profound feelings of loneliness, fear and helplessness; preoccupation with the image of the lost person or object; feelings of unreality; and emotional distance from others.
- *Reorganisation*. The person establishes new goals and interpersonal relationships. He begins to test new behaviours and expand his sense of identity.

Pathological grief

The person who can't cope with change risks developing a maladaptive or pathological grief reaction. Stay alert for such warning signs as:

- prolonged, excessive activity with no sense of loss
- physical symptoms similar to those that the deceased person experienced
- psychosomatic illness
- progressive social isolation
- extreme hostility
- wooden or formal conduct
- activity detrimental to social or economic well-being
- manic episodes
- depression
- substance abuse or other self-destructive behaviour.

Coping with grief

To help your person cope with grief in a positive way, take the following steps:

- Explain the normal stages of grieving, emphasising that a wide range of feelings and behaviours may occur.
- Establish rapport and build trust.
- Convey a caring attitude to encourage the person to express his feelings.
- Discuss the person's loss and the concrete changes that have resulted.
- Encourage him to express sadness, guilt or anger. If he becomes angry with you, don't get defensive.
- Help him to determine what realistic changes he needs to make.
- Suggest that he use more adaptive ways of coping and make concrete plans for the future.
- Urge him to review and share both good and bad memories. Gradually help him shift his focus from sharing memories to coping with the present and planning for the future.

report physical symptoms of depression than psychological ones; however, such somatic complaints may not meet the full criteria for depressive disorders.

Masking and mimicking

Coexisting medical disorders are common in older adults and may mask or mimic psychopathology. What's more, some mental disorders may be confused with nonpathological types of ARCD.

History lessons

Obtaining an accurate person history is crucial. If the person's cognitive status is poor, you may need to gather history information from family members or caregivers.

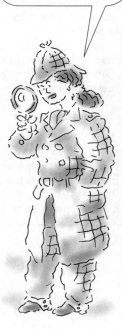

Shifting into detective mode can help you assess a mental disorder in an older adult.

Treatment

Depending on the cause of the psychiatric disorder, treatment may include medication, psychotherapy, support groups and sociocultural supports. Ideally, a multidisciplinary team approach is used, with the person (when able) and his family helping to set goals and make decisions about treatment options.

The team typically includes a nurse, doctor, psychologist, psychiatrist, physiotherapist, occupational therapist, social worker, and other professionals (such as a pharmacist or dietitian) as needed. For optimal results, make referrals early in the treatment process.

Keep it confidential

Everyone, including older adults, have a right to confidentiality in matters related to health care. You must obtain a signed informed consent from the person (or a family member, if the person lacks or has reduced mental capacity) before sharing information with other health care professionals or facilities. Never disclose the person's identity to the public.

Outpatient care

Outpatient care is usually provided by experienced mental health professionals, such as mental health nurses, psychiatrists, psychologists, psychotherapists and social workers. A multidisciplinary team approach helps to ensure comprehensive community care.

Care can be provided to individuals, couples, families or groups.

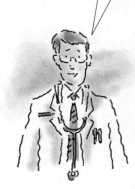

Some older adults see psychiatrists or other mental health professionals on an outpatient basis.

Support groups

Support groups give older adults a chance to discuss how their illnesses affect their lives and to help each other by sharing workable solutions. The support group usually consists of people (and family members) with a common problem. A mental health professional facilitates the group, monitoring and focusing the discussion.

Support groups commonly meet in community centres.

Care settings

Nurses must be prepared to meet older adults' mental health needs in such settings as general hospitals, outpatient clinics, short-term rehabilitation,

Providing psychiatric care for hospitalised older adults

Health care professionals who provide psychiatric care for older adults in general hospitals must be knowledgeable in all aspects of older adult health needs – not just the problem presenting at the time of admission.

Most acute-care hospital stays are short. You'll have little time to get to know the person and help him adjust to the environment, and you'll also need to perform an accurate assessment.

Touting teamwork

Many hospitals have established multidisciplinary liaison-psychiatric intervention teams to aid in rapid expert assessment and interventions. These teams can deescalate crisis situations, teach hospital staff specific interventions, counsel families and make referrals for postdischarge specialty care.

Dealing with behavioural problems

Behavioural problems in hospitalised older adults can lead to serious complications, so the staff must be trained to recognise these problems early.

Anxious, agitated older adults are at a much greater risk for falls. Nonetheless, physical restraints should be used only in emergency situations after other interventions have failed.

Be aware that the use of physical restraints and side rails in older adults may lead to pressure ulcers, infections, incontinence, functional impairment, cardiac stress, altered nutrition and agitation. Strangulation, accidental death and serious injuries also have been reported.

---

adult day care, long-term care facilities and in their own homes. (See *Providing psychiatric care for hospitalised older adults.*)

Home care

An older adult may be returning home after being discharged from the hospital, a rehabilitation centre or a group home. Or, he may simply need mental health nursing care to remain in the home.

Services provided in the home are expanding rapidly. Currently they include medication management, psychotherapy, detoxification and dementia care.

Deescalate and coordinate

When providing mental health care in a person's home, you'll need to be thoroughly familiar with:
• physical assessment techniques
• commonly prescribed medications (especially cardiac, hypertensive and psychiatric drugs) and their interactions
• crisis deescalation
• community services for older adults.

You may also need to serve as the care coordinator if the person is receiving simultaneous services from a community mental health clinic, primary care clinics, social care and voluntary agencies.

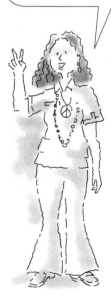

Peace and love, people! When caring for a person at home, you may have to deescalate a crisis.

Cutting down on crime

The older adult who is cared for at home may be vulnerable to crime and abuse. If you learn of crimes against the person you are caring for, threats of crime or other unusual situations, report these to the police. Remember, even if the person has a mental disorder, his descriptions of threatening situations may be reality based.

Long-term care facilities

Admission to a nursing home or other long-term care facility can cause situational depression. Help the person adjust to the change of environment and stay alert for signs of depression.

If the person was admitted for a short-term rehabilitation programme, remind him that his stay is only temporary and that his goal is to return home.

Some older adults with chronic mental health problems such as Alzheimer's disease may be placed in specialised units in long-term care facilities. These units provide a low-stimulus environment with trained staff who assist in activities of daily living (ADLs), nutrition and safety.

Hospital emergency departments

An older adult may be taken to a hospital emergency department (A&E) for a medical emergency, a suicide attempt or an episode of violent or threatening behaviour. An older adult with a history of acting-out behaviour should undergo a thorough physical assessment with baseline diagnostic tests, including electrocardiography, complete blood profile and urinalysis.

Intervention aims to:
- keep the person from harming himself or others
- provide rapid tranquilisation or sedation
- avoid overmedication and toxicity
- identify any underlying physical condition that may be contributing to their behaviour such as toxic confusional state.

The linking liaison

To address the problems of caring for the mentally ill in the A&E, some hospitals employ mental health liaison nurses. Working collaboratively with other staff, these nurses act as the links among crisis intervention, outreach and continuity-of-care staff. They can provide valuable information to the intervention team and expedite rapid referrals.

Inpatient care

Inpatient care is used to assess people for suspected dementia and to stabilise aggressive or suicidal people. Efforts focus on rapid evaluation to rule out physical illness, rapid mood stabilisation and discharge planning. Stays on these units typically are brief, reflecting the trend towards community-based health care.

Day hospitals

Mental health day hospitals provide intense, structured, multidisciplinary therapy for people who have more acute needs than outpatients do. Usually, people are driven to the day hospital site in the morning and return home later in the day.

Adult day care

In some locations, adult day care centres are available for older adults with chronic mental disorders. These programmes provide structured activities, personal care, recreation, socialisation, nutritional support and health care. They often include social services and carer support.

Adult day care offers respite for family members and other carers, allowing them to maintain their jobs. It also helps postpone or avoid institutionalising the older adult.

Community education programmes

In many communities, senior centres, hospitals and clinics sponsor public education programmes on mental illness. Depression and anxiety screening programmes encourage older adults and their families to learn more about mental health and help connect them with skilled practitioners for treatment.

Many community and mental health hospitals also offer free educational programmes on psychiatric issues, such as family dynamics, depression and anxiety. They may also include psychoeducation programmes, carer education and carer support groups.

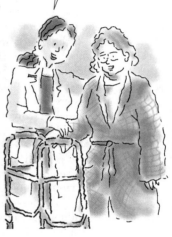

Teaching people how to cope with the real world is one of the things I love most about my job.

Drug therapy

If the person is receiving drugs to treat a mental illness, be aware of the increased possibility of side effects and drug interactions. Many older adults take concurrent multiple medications for coexisting illnesses – a practice called polypharmacy. This puts them at high risk for drug interactions, side effects and adverse reactions.

A slower metabolic rate in older adults increases the risk of drugs even further. Older adults are more vulnerable to adverse reactions, including tardive dyskinesia – a motor disorder causing involuntary jerky movements of the face, tongue, jaws, trunk and limbs. Also, some prescribed drugs may worsen a coexisting medical disorder. Be sure to adjust dosage and administration schedules appropriately.

Curbing prescriber chaos

To complicate matters, some older adults have multiple drug prescribers, who may not be aware that the person is seeing other practitioners.

To help ensure safe and effective drug administration, keep the person's medication list up to date and monitor him for side effects and drug interactions. As appropriate, use assessment scales to check for tardive

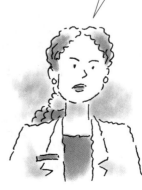

Polly Pharmacy? That was my college roommate's nickname.

dyskinesia and other drug side effects. (See *Dyskinesia Identification System: Condensed User Scale*, pages 104 and 105.)

Also, find out if the person is taking nonprescription medications or nutritional or herbal supplements. Some of these may pose dangers to older adults. (See *Using St. John's wort to treat depression*, page 106.)

Start low, titrate slow

Generally, dosages for older adults should start at 25% of the amount used for younger adults; then increased gradually as tolerated. The doctor may want to monitor blood or urine drug levels to ensure that the person isn't getting a toxic dose.

Because of lower dosages and slower administration schedules, however, an older adult may not achieve adequate blood drug levels to treat his condition effectively.

Compliance complaints

Compliance with drug treatment can be a challenge in older adults, especially those with moderate to severe cognitive deficits. Those with poor vision may misread instructions or mistake one drug for another. Those with cognitive impairment may not remember whether they have taken all of their doses.

Other challenges to compliance may include a poor doctor–patient relationship, inadequate teaching about the necessity or procedure for taking drugs, a large number of daily dosages and multiple drugs taken at the same time.

Administering psychotropic drugs

Psychotropic drugs (such as antidepressants, sedatives, tranquilisers or lithium) may cause oversedation in an older adult. Because of diminished kidney and liver functions, drugs take longer to be metabolised and excreted in older people.

As a result, the person may not respond to a psychotropic drug immediately. Misguided caregivers may then administer more of the medication, which can cause drug accumulation – with side effects that may range from a hangover feeling to near-coma.

Falls and withdrawal

Older people who receive psychotropic medications also are at high risk for falls – especially if they have other illnesses or mobility problems.

Problems also may arise if these medications are discontinued before surgery and then resumed a few days later. In people on benzodiazepines or certain other psychotropic medications, this administration schedule may lead to withdrawal symptoms.

For many older people, managing medications is a difficult juggling act.

Dyskinesia Identification System: Condensed User Scale

Name __Marjorie Jenkins__
__Stewart Memorial Hospital__
(facility)

Dyskinesia Identification System:
Condensed User Scale (DISCUS)

Current psychotropics/anticholinergic
and total mg/day

__Haldol, 0.5 mg P.O.__ ____1__ mg
_____ _____ mg
_____ _____ mg

Exam type (check one)
☑ 1. Baseline
☐ 2. Annual
☐ 3. Semi-annual
☐ 4. D/C — 1 month
☐ 5. D/C — 2 month
☐ 6. D/C — 3 month
☐ 7. Admission
☐ 8. Other

Cooperation (check one)
☐ 1. None
☑ 2. Partial
☐ 3. Full

Scoring

0 Not present (movements not observed, or some movements observed but not considered abnormal)

1 Minimal (abnormal movements difficult to detect, or movements easy to detect but occurring only once or twice in a short, nonrepetitive manner)

2 Mild (abnormal movements easy to detect and occurring infrequently)

3 Moderate (abnormal movements easy to detect and occurring frequently)

4 Severe (abnormal movements easy to detect and occurring almost continuously)

NA Not assessed (or not able to assess)

Assessment

DISCUS item and score (circle one score for each item)

Face	1.	Tics	0	1	2	3	4	NA	
	2.	Grimaces	⓪	1	2	3	4	NA	
Eyes	3.	Blinking	⓪	1	2	3	4	NA	
Oral	4.	Chewing/lip smacking	⓪	1	2	3	4	NA	
	5.	Puckering/sucking/ thrusting lower lip	⓪	1	2	3	4	NA	
Lingual	6.	Tongue thrusting/ tongue in cheek	⓪	1	2	3	4	NA	
	7.	Tonic tongue	⓪	1	2	3	4	NA	
	8.	Tongue tremor	⓪	1	2	3	4	NA	
	9.	Athetoid myokymic/ lateral tongue	⓪	1	2	3	4	NA	
Head/	10.	Retrocollis/torticollis	⓪	1	2	3	4	NA	
neck/ trunk	11.	Shoulder/hip torsion	⓪	1	2	3	4	NA	
Upper limb	12.	Athetoid/myokymic finger-wrist-arm	⓪	1	2	3	4	NA	
	13.	Pill rolling	⓪	1	2	3	4	NA	
Lower limb	14.	Ankle flexion/ foot tapping	⓪	1	2	3	4	NA	
	15.	Toe movement	⓪	1	2	3	4	NA	

Comments _____

15-item score ____1____

Rater's signature and title
__Angela Bavaro, RN__

Exam date __5/14/03__
Next exam date __12/14/03__

Evaluation

1. Greater than 90 days' neuroleptic exposure

	Yes	No
2. Scoring/intensity level met	Yes	No
3. Other diagnostic conditions?	Yes	No

(If yes specify) _____

4. Last exam date _____
Last total score _____
Last conclusion _____
Preparer's signature and title for items 1 to 4 (if different from doctor)

_____

5. Conclusion (circle one)

A. No tardive dyskinesia (TD); if scoring prerequisite met, list other diagnostic condition or explain in comments

B. Probable TD
C. Masked TD
D. Withdrawal TD
E. Persistent TD
F. Remitted TD
G. Other (specify in comments)

6. Comments _____
_____
_____

Doctor's signature _____
Date _____

Simplified diagnoses for tardive dyskinesia

Prerequisites

The three prerequisites for diagnosing tardive dyskinesia (TD) are as follows, although exceptions may occur.

1. A history of at least 3 months' total cumulative neuroleptic exposure. (Include amoxapine and metoclopramide in all categories below as well.)
2. Scoring/intensity level. Total score of 5 or more. Also be alert for any change from baseline or scores below 5 which have at least a moderate (3) or severe (4) movement on any item or at least two mild (2) movements on two items located in different body areas.
3. Other conditions are not responsible for the abnormal involuntary movements.

Diagnoses

The diagnosis is based on the current exam and its relation to the last exam. It can shift depending on whether movements are present or not, whether movements are present for 3 months or more (6 months for a semiannual assessment), and whether neuroleptic dosage changes occur and affect movements.

- No TD (Movements not present on this exam, or movements present but caused by some other condition. The last diagnosis must be No TD, Probable TD or Withdrawal TD.)
- Probable TD (Movements present on this exam for the first time, or for the first time in 3 months or more. The last diagnosis must be No TD or Probable TD.)
- Persistent TD (Movements present on this exam and have been present for 3 months or more with this exam or present at some point in the past. The last diagnosis can be any except No TD.)
- Masked TD (Movements not present on this exam, but this is due to a neuroleptic dosage increase or restart after an earlier exam when movements were present. Or movements not present due to the addition of a nonneuroleptic medication to treat TD. The last diagnosis must be Probable TD, Persistent TD, Withdrawal TD or Masked TD.)
- Remitted TD (Movements are not present on this exam, but persistent TD has been diagnosed and no neuroleptic dosage increase or restart has occurred.

The last diagnosis must be Persistent TD or Remitted TD. If movements reemerge, the diagnosis shifts back to Persistent TD.)
- Withdrawal TD (Movements are not present while person receives neuroleptics or at the last dosage level, but are seen within 8 weeks after neuroleptic reduction or discontinuation. The last diagnosis must be No TD or Withdrawal TD. If movements continue for 3 months or more after neuroleptic reduction or discontinuation, the diagnosis shifts to Persistent TD. If movements do not continue for 3 months or more after the reduction or discontinuation, the diagnosis shifts to No TD.)

Instructions

1. The rater completes the Assessment according to the standardised exam procedure. If the rater also completes the Evaluation items 1–4, he must also sign the preparer box. The form is given to the physician. Or the doctor may perform the assessment.
2. The physician completes the Evaluation section. The physician is responsible for the entire Evaluation section and its accuracy.
3. A doctor should examine any person who meets the three prerequisites or has movements not explained by other factors. He should obtain any neurological assessments or differential diagnostic tests that may be needed.
4. File form according to policy or procedure.

Other conditions (partial list)

1. Age
2. Blind
3. Cerebral palsy
4. Contact lenses
5. Dentures, no teeth
6. Down's syndrome
7. Drug intoxication (specify)
8. Encephalitis
9. Extrapyramidal adverse effects (specify)
10. Fahr's syndrome
11. Heavy metal intoxication (specify)
12. Huntington's disease
13. Hyperthyroidism
14. Hypoglycaemia
15. Hypoparathyroidism
16. Idiopathic torsion dystonia
17. Meige's syndrome
18. Parkinson's disease
19. Stereotypies
20. Sydenham's chorea
21. Tourette's syndrome
22. Wilson's disease
23. Other (specify)

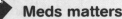

Meds matters

Using St. John's wort to treat depression

St. John's wort *(Hypericum perforatum)* is a wild-growing, yellow-flowered herb sometimes promoted for the treatment of mild to moderate depression and anxiety. It's available as a capsule, tea, tincture (alcoholic or nonalcoholic), oil extract for topical use and bulk dried leaves.

St. John's wort can be obtained without a prescription – but make sure the doctor approves its use before the person starts taking it. The doctor will want to monitor the person for beneficial and adverse effects. Make sure the person's other health care providers also know that he's using St. John's wort.

Cautionary notes

- Be aware that St. John's wort shouldn't be taken concomitantly with other antidepressants.
- Teach the person (or his family members) to watch for side effects of St. John's wort, including dry mouth, dizziness, GI symptoms, fatigue and confusion.
- Advise him to follow sun-exposure precautions to help prevent photosensitivity symptoms, such as dermatitis, severe burning and blisters.

Age-related cognitive decline

ARCD refers to an objectively identified decrease in cognitive functioning related to ageing that's within normal limits and not attributable to a specific mental disorder or neurological condition.

ARCD is characterised by deterioration in memory, learning, attention, concentration, thinking, language use and other mental functions. It usually emerges gradually.

Caught in the middle

Some older adults have greater memory and cognitive problems than others, but their symptoms aren't severe enough to qualify as Alzheimer's disease. Although some will progress to Alzheimer's disease, others won't. Clinicians refer to this middle category as mild cognitive impairment or mild neurocognitive disorder.

Causes

ARCD may stem from the natural slowing that occurs with age. Age differences are found in many cognitive tasks, even when the subjects have unlimited time to do them.

All in the timing

An older adult's slower mental processing (which may stem from decreased mental capacity) makes timing more critical in complex situations, such as when approaching a traffic junction on a main road at high speed. Practice can help improve cognitive speed in older adults, although to a lesser degree than in younger adults.

Working that memory

A faulty inhibitory mechanism in working memory (the type of memory that enables us to ignore irrelevancies) may underlie ARCD. Specifically, it may cause the older adult to heed irrelevant details and to interpret context incorrectly. (Studies show that older adults find irrelevant information more distracting than younger adults do.)

Risk factors

Risk factors for ARCD include advancing age, female gender, heart failure and a history of myocardial infarction.

> Tarot cards are fun, but you don't need them to know that some cognitive abilities decline with age.

Signs and symptoms

Typically, the person with ARCD complains that he can't remember appointments or solve complex problems. Other signs and symptoms may include:
- poor hygiene
- inappropriate dress
- weight loss
- indicators of depression, such as a stooped posture, shuffling gait, poor eye contact and abnormal movements.

Be sure to assess the person's alertness level and orientation to person, place and time. When evaluating memory, investigate remote, recent and immediate memory.

Detecting defensiveness

During the interview, note the person's responses and the effort required to answer your questions. Stay alert for hostility, resistance and defensiveness.

Diagnosis

Diagnosing ARCD requires a specialised professional evaluation. The person should undergo neuropsychological and cognitive testing to determine and measure the severity and rate of the cognitive decline, evaluate the functional expression of the disorder and assess functional capacities.

Mental status examination

Diagnosis rests on various evaluations that encompass elements of the mental status examination. Areas assessed in this examination may include:
- physical appearance, which may give clues to overall health and self-esteem
- remote, recent and immediate memory

> ## Diagnostic criteria: Age-related cognitive decline
>
> According to the *Diagnostic and Statistical Manual of Mental Disorders*, Fourth Edition, Text Revision, age-related cognitive decline (ARCD) or mild cognitive impairment (MCI) may be diagnosed when the focus of clinical attention is an objectively identified age-related decline in cognitive functioning that's within normal limits given the person's age. A person with ARCD may report difficulty remembering names or appointments or difficulty solving complex problems.
>
> This diagnosis should be considered only after other mental disorders and neurological conditions have been eliminated as the cause of the cognitive impairment.

- speech characteristics
- higher language skills
- calculation skills
- decision-making ability
- affective function, such as mood and anxiety level
- motor function, which may indicate depression, affective illness or behavioural disturbances
- social skills, which may suggest cognitive deficits or psychosocial impairment
- responses to questions, which may suggest cognitive or psychological impairment
- orientation, which may reflect cognitive deficits
- degree of contact with reality, which may indicate delusions, paranoia, hallucinations or illusions
- alertness level, which may indicate undetected medical disturbances.

Many physicians base the diagnosis of ARCD on the criteria in the *Diagnostic and Statistical Manual of Mental Disorders*, Fourth Edition, Text Revision (*DSM-IV-TR*). (See *Diagnostic criteria: Age-related cognitive decline*.)

Treatment

Various drugs, vitamins, herbs and dietary therapies are being investigated as treatments for cognitive decline. The person should be followed closely by his doctor because any new medical problems could further impair cognitive function.

Interdisciplinary management should include psychiatrists, social workers and other health care professionals. Treatment should encompass sociocultural supports and counselling.

Nursing interventions

These nursing interventions may be appropriate for a person with ARCD:

Cut through the confusion

- Reduce and eliminate factors that may worsen confusion, such as dehydration, malnutrition and difficulty sleeping. Carefully monitor fluid

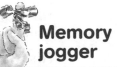

Memory jogger

Use the acronym PILE to help people with cognitive deficits maintain their maximal level of functioning.

P Promote 'here and now' interactions

I Interact briefly but frequently

L Link talk to meaningful topics

E Encourage self-expression

and electrolyte status, and replace as needed. Promote adequate fluid intake. Provide a well-balanced diet.

• Promote normal sleep–rest activities. Avoid giving sedative-hypnotic drugs when possible.

Optimise senses and stimuli

• Promote optimal vision and hearing by keeping rooms well lit, cleaning cerumen out of ears, promoting frequent eye and ear examinations and ensuring that hearing aids are in good working order and positioned properly in the ear.

• Reduce unnecessary stimulation and make the environment as stable as possible. Avoid changing rooms and moving furniture or possessions around.

Orient – always

• Provide frequent meaningful sensory input and reorientation. Place a large clock and calendar in every room. Provide outdoor activities or a bed by the window.

• Add orienting material to every conversation. Frequently tell the person your name and what you're going to do.

• Encourage the person to participate in therapeutic groups, such as those centred on reality orientation, remotivation, reminiscence, recreational therapy, pet therapy, music therapy and sensory training.

• Frequently assess his need for medications, appropriateness of dosage and side effects. Be especially aware of possible drug interactions.

Avert injury

• Check the person frequently because he may be prone to falls, wandering and self-poisoning.

• Take extra safety measures regarding bath water and food temperature to avoid accidental burns.

Dementia of the Alzheimer's type (late onset)

Alzheimer's-type dementia is marked by global, progressive impairment of cognitive functioning, memory and personality. The dementia is irreversible and progressive. The average duration of illness from symptom onset to death is 8–10 years.

No safety in these numbers

The most common cause of dementia among people aged 65 and older is Alzheimer's disease which affects an estimated 700,000 people in the UK. It's the sixth leading cause of death among white women aged 85 and older.

Myth busters

Debunking dementia myths

Misunderstandings about dementia can lead to unrealistic expectations.

Myth: Dementia is reversible if diagnosed early.

Reality: For most people, dementia takes a progressive, deteriorating, irreversible course.

Myth: Vascular dementia isn't as serious a health problem as Alzheimer's disease.

Reality: Marked disruption in cerebral blood flow with destruction of brain cells, vascular dementia reduces life expectancy to a greater degree than does Alzheimer's disease.

Myth: Dementia causes rapid loss of language skills.

Reality: Only the most severe forms of dementia result in aphasia and the inability to speak. As dementia progresses, though, most people struggle to name objects and express themselves.

As more people in the UK live longer, the incidence of Alzheimer's disease will continue to grow, unless a cure or effective prevention is discovered.

There goes the memory

Typically, memory loss is the earliest symptom of Alzheimer's disease. As the disease progresses, symptoms progressively interfere with the person's social and occupational functioning. (See *Debunking dementia myths.*)

Causes

No one knows exactly what causes Alzheimer's disease. Researchers suspect it's linked to specific biological factors, which are triggered by various environmental and genetic factors.

Biological factors in the brain

In people with Alzheimer's disease, brain-imaging techniques have found a significant loss of neurons and volume in the brain regions devoted to memory and higher mental functioning. Abnormalities found on biopsy include neurofibrillary tangles (twisted nerve cell fibres) and a build-up of beta amyloid (a sticky protein).

Neurofibrillary tangles

Neurofibrillary tangles are the damaged remains of microtubules – the support structures that permit nutrients to flow through neurons. A key component in neurofibrillary tangles is an abnormal form of the tau protein, which aids in assembling microtubules. The defective tau appears to block the actions of the normal version.

Tangles and freaky taus – two more things that are dangerous to my health!

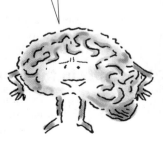

Beta amyloid

An insoluble protein, beta amyloid accumulates and forms sticky patches called neuritic plaques. In the brains of people with Alzheimer's disease, these patches are surrounded by the debris of dying neurons.

Amyloid overdose

High beta amyloid levels are associated with decreased levels of acetylcholine, a neurotransmitter crucial to memory and learning. Beta amyloid also may damage the brain's sodium, potassium and calcium channels, disrupting the electrical charges that allow messages to pass between neurons.

Oxidation and the inflammatory response

In trying to determine why beta amyloid is so toxic to nerve cells, some researchers are focusing on oxidation and the inflammatory processes. As beta amyloid breaks down, it releases oxygen-free radicals. These unstable chemicals bind to other molecules through the process of oxidation.

Oxidant overflow

When oxidants are overproduced, they can cause severe damage to cells and tissue. Oxidation is known to play a part in such diseases as coronary artery disease and cancer, and some experts believe that it may contribute to Alzheimer's disease.

Oxidation triggers the activity of immune factors to repair injury. But too many immune factors may trigger the inflammatory response, resulting in damage to cells. Inflammatory factors of interest to Alzheimer's disease researchers are the enzyme cyclooxygenase and its products, the prostaglandins.

Genetic factors

Certain genetic factors are thought to play a role in the beta amyloid build-up found in the brain of people with Alzheimer's disease. A major focus of research is apolipoprotein E (Apo E), which aids cholesterol transport and nerve cell repair. (See *Alzheimer's disease and apolipoprotein E*, page 112.)

Environmental factors

Researchers are exploring whether such environmental factors as infection, metals and toxins may trigger oxidation, inflammation and the Alzheimer's disease process (especially in people with genetic susceptibility).

Infection

According to one theory, a person with a genetic susceptibility to Alzheimer's disease may be vulnerable to the actions of certain viruses – particularly when the immune system is weakened. Although no specific virus has been definitively linked to Alzheimer's disease, researchers are focusing on herpesvirus 1 and *Chlamydia pneumoniae*.

Alzheimer's disease and apolipoprotein E

Apolipoprotein E (Apo E), a plasma protein involved in cholesterol transport, is a current focus of research on Alzheimer's disease. The Apo E gene comes in three major types – Apo E4, Apo E3 and Apo E2.

Apo E and beta amyloid

Studies show the greatest number of deposits of beta amyloid (a protein) in people with the Apo E4 gene. People with Apo E3 have fewer beta amyloid deposits, and those with Apo E2 have fewer still.

Because significant beta amyloid accumulations are characteristic of Alzheimer's disease, Apo E4 may be a major risk factor for late-onset Alzheimer's disease.

One copy or two?

Everyone inherits a copy of one type of the Apo E gene from each parent. According to some researchers, the number of Apo E4 copies inherited affects the risk of Alzheimer's disease:

- People with no copies of Apo E4 have a 9–20% chance of developing Alzheimer's disease by age 85.
- People with one copy of the gene have a 25–60% chance.
- People with two copies have a 50–90% chance.

No foregone conclusions

Nonetheless, Alzheimer's disease isn't inevitable even in people with two Apo E4 copies. In addition, most people with late-onset Alzheimer's disease don't even carry the Apo E4 gene.

Increasingly, researchers are speculating that many cases of Alzheimer's disease stem from a combination of genetic factors involved in beta amyloid production or degradation.

Metals

Some studies report excessive amounts of metal ions, such as zinc and copper, in the brains of people with Alzheimer's disease. These ions may change the chemical architecture of beta amyloid, making it more harmful. A mildly acidic environment seems to help these metals bind to beta amyloid. An acidic environment and higher zinc and copper levels commonly result from the inflammatory response to local injury.

Other factors

Researchers are studying other factors for their possible role in Alzheimer's disease. (See *Alzheimer's disease research round-up*, page 113.)

Signs and symptoms

Decreased intellectual function, personality changes, impaired judgement and changes in affect are common manifestations of Alzheimer's disease, which has three identifiable stages.

Stage 1

In stage 1, signs and symptoms typically include:
- agitated or apathetic mood
- attempts to cover up symptoms
- deterioration in personal appearance
- decline in recent memory

Alzheimer's disease research round-up

Besides biological, genetic and environmental factors, some researchers suspect other factors may cause or contribute to Alzheimer's disease. Recent studies have explored such wide-ranging possibilities as vitamin deficiencies, depression, head injury and lower educational level.

Vitamin B deficiencies

Some research suggests that deficiencies of vitamins B6, B12 and folate (which all help to protect nerves) may be a risk factor for Alzheimer's disease. These deficiencies may increase levels of homocysteine, an amino acid that may interfere with nerve cell repair. The weakened cells are then more susceptible to the harmful effects of oxidised beta amyloid (the insoluble protein that builds up in the brains of people with Alzheimer's disease).

Depression

Depression and dementia coexist in many older people. Some evidence suggests there may be common genetic factors in people who have both early depression and Alzheimer's disease.

Head injury

Some studies suggest a link between serious head injuries in early adulthood and later development of Alzheimer's disease. It's unclear whether such injuries cause Alzheimer's disease directly or simply accelerate the disease process in susceptible people.

Lower educational level

Several studies have shown a higher risk for Alzheimer's disease in people with less education and a lower risk in people who remain mentally active. Experts speculate that learning may stimulate more neurons to grow and thus create a larger reserve in the brain, so that it takes longer for brain cells to be destroyed.

- poor concentration
- depression
- disorientation to time
- sleep disturbances
- inability to retain new memories
- susceptibility to falls
- transitory delusions of persecution
- wandering.

Stage 2

In stage 2, expect to find:
- bowel and bladder incontinence
- confabulation (filling of memory gaps with fabrications that the person believes to be facts)
- continuous, repetitive behaviours
- decreasing ability to understand or use language
- disorientation to person, place and time
- failure to recognise family members
- inability to retain new information
- inability to perform ADLs without assistance
- increased appetite without weight gain
- socially unacceptable behaviour
- tantrums.

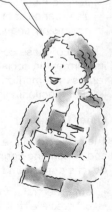

Signs and symptoms of Alzheimer's disease occur in three stages, matching the progression of the disease.

Stage 3

In stage 3, look for:

- severe decline in cognitive functioning
- compulsive touching and examination of objects
- decreased response to stimuli
- deterioration in motor ability
- emaciation
- nonresponsiveness.

Diagnosis

Because it's hard to obtain direct pathological evidence of Alzheimer's disease, diagnosis in a living person is made by ruling out other possible causes of dementia and is based on the criteria in the *DSM-IV-TR*. (See *Diagnostic criteria: Dementia of the Alzheimer's type*.)

Diagnostic criteria: Dementia of the Alzheimer's type

Dementia of the Alzheimer's' type is diagnosed when the person meets these criteria from the *Diagnostic and Statistical Manual of Mental Disorders*, Fourth Edition, Text Revision.

Multiple cognitive deficits

The person has multiple cognitive defects, manifested by *both* memory impairment (impaired ability to learn new information or to recall previously learned information) and at least one of the following conditions:

- aphasia (language disturbance)
- apraxia (impaired ability to perform motor activities despite intact motor function)
- agnosia (failure to recognise or identify objects despite intact sensory function)
- disturbance in executive functioning (planning, organising, sequencing and abstracting).

Each of these cognitive deficits cause significant impairment in social or occupational functioning and represent a marked decline from the person's previous level of functioning.

Other features

The disease course is characterised by a gradual onset and continuing cognitive decline. Also, the cognitive deficits don't stem from:

- other central nervous system conditions that cause progressive deficits in memory and cognition (such as cerebrovascular disease, Parkinson's disease, brain tumour, Huntington's disease or subdural haematoma)
- systemic conditions known to cause dementia (for instance, hypothyroidism, vitamin B_{12} or folic acid deficiency, niacin deficiency, hypercalcaemia, neurosyphilis or human immunodeficiency virus infection)
- substance-induced conditions.

In addition, the cognitive deficits don't occur exclusively during the course of delirium and aren't better accounted for by another Axis I disorder (such as major depressive disorder or schizophrenia).

Dementia of the Alzheimer's type may occur with or without a clinically significant behavioural disturbance, such as wandering or agitation.

Early vs. late onset

In early-onset Alzheimer's-type disease, symptoms are apparent by age 65 or younger. With late onset, symptoms become apparent only after age 65.

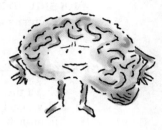

The full assessment

Diagnostic tests that aid diagnosis include:
• cognitive assessment evaluation, which typically shows cognitive impairment in Alzheimer's disease
• functional dementia scale, which may indicate the degree of dementia
• magnetic resonance imaging (MRI) of the brain, which typically shows structural and neurological changes
• mini–mental status examination, which reveals disorientation and cognitive impairment.

Treatment

Although no cure exists for Alzheimer's disease, certain drugs may be prescribed in an attempt to improve or stabilise the symptoms. Likewise, several care strategies and activities may minimise or prevent behavioural problems. Researchers continue to look for new treatments to alter the course of the disease and improve the quality of life.

Native habitat preferred

In most cases, institutional placement should be delayed until absolutely necessary. Some clinical trials for Alzheimer's disease have begun to use delay of institutionalisation as a primary outcome or as a longer-term outcome in follow-up studies.

> It's usually best for the person to live at home as long as possible.

Drug therapy

Drugs used to treat Alzheimer's disease include:
• anticholinesterase agents, such as donepezil, galantamine and rivastigmine, to improve cognitive functioning
• antipsychotic agents, such as haloperidol, to calm agitated behaviour
• benzodiazepines, such as lorazepam, to ease anxiety.
Agents under investigation for Alzheimer's disease include oestrogen, nonsteroidal anti-inflammatory agents, vitamin E, selegiline and ginkgo biloba. A vaccine is being studied in mice.

Experimental treatments

Hyperbaric oxygen treatment and tissue transplantation are being explored as treatments for people with Alzheimer's disease.

Psychotherapy

Brief psychotherapy techniques, such as reality orientation and memory retraining, may aid people during certain stages of Alzheimer's disease.

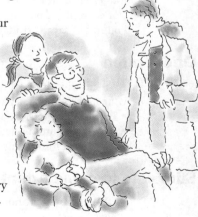

Preventive strategies

Alzheimer's disease prevention might target individuals at increased genetic risk. Specific measures may involve prophylactic nutritional agents (such as vitamin E) or cholinergic- or amyloid-targeting interventions.

Nursing interventions

These nursing interventions may be appropriate for a person with Alzheimer's disease:

Strive for safety

- Protect the person from injury. Remove hazardous items or potential obstacles to help maintain a safe environment.
- Monitor the person's food and fluid intake because he's at risk for poor nutrition.

Recommend routines

- To the extent possible, have the person follow a regular exercise routine, maintain normal social contacts with family and friends and continue intellectual activities.
- Encourage the person to see a doctor every 3–6 months.

Soften your speech

- Speak to the person calmly, using a soft, low-pitched voice.
- State your expectations simply and completely.
- Minimise confusion by maintaining consistent, structured verbal and nonverbal communication.

Affirm emotions

- If the person discusses an event that isn't happening or people who are no longer alive, affirm his emotions without adding to or refuting the fantasy. For example, if he talks about his dead mother coming to his birthday party, you might say, 'Birthdays are fun.'

Orient often

- Add orienting material to every conversation. Frequently tell the person your name and what you're going to do.
- Place a large clock and calendar in every room.
- Provide outdoor activities or a bed by the window.
- Redirect him to appropriate activities when behaviour problems occur.

Stimulate to some extent

- Decrease environmental stimuli, such as noise, excessive artificial light and television use.
- Provide frequent meaningful sensory input.
- Increase the person's social interaction to provide stimuli. But avoid placing him in large rooms with many people, such as dining rooms or group activity rooms.

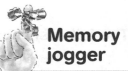

Memory jogger

How can you help keep a person with Alzheimer's disease safe? Just think of the word SAFE.

S Secure the area if the person wanders

A Arrange the room and furniture to accommodate the person's needs and disabilities

F Frequently orient the person to time, place and situation

E Easy access to self-care items is crucial

Monitor medications

- Check the person for drug side effects and drug interactions.
- Advise the person and his family that scientific evidence generally doesn't support claims that certain nonprescription products can improve mental functioning.
- Instruct the family to always check with the doctor before the person begins nonprescription agents, especially if he has heart or liver problems or is taking a drug for heart problems, hypertension, diabetes or mental illness.

Offer information

- Give the person and his family information about community resources, support groups and placement in a long-term care facility (if necessary).
- Refer the person to health care professionals skilled in caring for people with Alzheimer's disease.

Subdue stress

- Teach the person and his caregivers stress-management techniques.
- Provide support and education to home caregivers. Refer them to respite services as needed.
- If appropriate, suggest that his family consult mental health professionals for help in coping with caregiver stress, financial pressures and related issues.

Vascular dementia

Also called multi-infarct dementia, vascular dementia impairs cognitive functioning, memory and personality but doesn't affect the level of consciousness. The condition is caused by an irreversible alteration in brain function that results from damage or destruction of brain tissue – as when blood clots block small blood vessels in the brain.

Vascular dementia typically starts between ages 60 and 75. It accounts for an estimated 10–20% of dementias and affects more men than women. Approximately 20% of patients have both vascular dementia and Alzheimer's disease.

Think local, not global

Cerebral problems affect localised parts of the brain, sparing some brain function. Brain damage may be so slight that symptoms are barely noticeable. Over time, though, as more small vessels are blocked, the mental decline becomes obvious.

Causes

Vascular dementia occurs when small focal deficits, typically caused by a series of small strokes, accumulate. The condition tends to progress in stages and

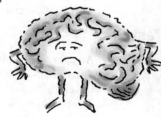

In vascular dementia, blockage of small blood vessels leads to brain damage and, ultimately, a gradual mental decline.

causes patchy distribution of cognitive problems. Lesions are usually in the frontal and subcortical parts of the brain.

Besides advanced age, contributing factors include:
- cerebral emboli or thrombosis
- diabetes
- heart disease
- high blood cholesterol level
- hypertension (leading to stroke)
- transient ischaemic attacks.

Signs and symptoms

Signs and symptoms of vascular dementia often develop progressively. They include:
- confusion
- problems with recent memory
- wandering or getting lost in familiar places
- loss of bladder or bowel control
- inappropriate emotional reactions, such as laughing or crying inappropriately
- difficulty following instructions
- problems handling money
- depression
- dizziness
- neurological symptoms lasting only a few days
- slurred speech
- leg or arm weakness.

Diagnosis

Diagnostic test results may include:
- cognitive assessment scale showing deterioration in cognitive ability
- global deterioration scale indicating degenerative dementia
- mini–mental status examination revealing disorientation and difficulty with recall
- MRI or computed tomography scan showing structural, vascular and neurological changes in the brain.

Test time

An abbreviated mental examination can detect memory problems and aid differential diagnosis, treatment and rehabilitation. To be most useful, the examination should be repeated periodically. (Be aware, though, that depressed people may do poorly on these tests even if they don't have a memory problem.)

In a typical mental exam, the person is asked to provide the following information:
- name
- date of birth

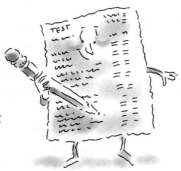

Diagnostic criteria: Vascular dementia

Vascular dementia is diagnosed when the person meets these criteria from the *Diagnostic and Statistical Manual of Mental Disorders*, Fourth Edition, Text Revision.

Multiple cognitive deficits

The person has multiple cognitive deficits manifested by both memory impairment (impaired ability to learn new information or to recall previously learned information) and one or more of the following cognitive disturbances:

- aphasia (language disturbance)
- apraxia (impaired ability to perform motor activities despite intact motor function)
- agnosia (failure to recognise or identify objects despite intact sensory function)
- disturbance in executive functioning (planning, organising, sequencing and abstracting).

Memory impairment and the other deficits present must significantly impair social or occupational functioning and represent a significant decline from the person's previous level of functioning.

Focal neurological indications

In addition, the person must have focal neurological signs and symptoms (such as exaggerated deep tendon reflexes, extensor plantar response, pseudobulbar palsy, gait abnormalities or arm or leg weakness) or laboratory evidence of cerebrovascular disease (such as multiple infarctions involving the cortex and underlying white matter) that are aetiologically related to the disturbance.

Other features

The cognitive deficits don't occur exclusively during the course of an episode of delirium.

- age
- date and time of day
- address
- name of the president
- years that World War I or II took place
- current location
- an address he was told 5 minutes earlier.
  He's also asked to count backward from 20 to 1.
  The official diagnosis of vascular dementia is based on the criteria in the *DSM-IV-TR*. (See *Diagnostic criteria: Vascular dementia*.)

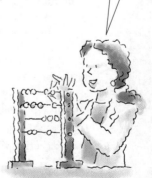

Assessing the person's ability to count backward helps diagnose vascular dementia.

Treatment

Treatment for vascular dementia may include:
- therapy for any underlying condition (such as hypertension, high cholesterol or diabetes), including dietary interventions, medications and smoking cessation
- drug therapy – for example, aspirin to decrease platelet aggregation and prevent clots.

Nursing interventions

The same interventions you would use for a person with ARCD or Alzheimer's disease apply to a person with vascular dementia. The main goal of interventions is to keep the person safe and oriented.

Sweeten the surroundings

- Monitor the environment to prevent overstimulation.
- Reduce unnecessary stimulation and make the environment as stable as possible. Avoid changing rooms and moving furniture or possessions around.
- Minimise factors that may contribute to confusion, such as dehydration, malnutrition and difficulty sleeping.

Orient at all times

- Orient the person to his surroundings to ease his anxiety.
- Provide frequent meaningful sensory input.
- Place a large clock and calendar in every room.
- Include orienting material in every conversation.
- Frequently tell the person your name and what you're going to do.

Avert injury

- Check the person often because he may be prone to falls, wandering and self-poisoning.
- Take extra safety measures regarding food and bath water temperature to avoid accidental burns.
- Teach the person and family members about proper diet, weight control and exercise to reduce cardiovascular risk factors.
- Frequently assess the person's need for medications, appropriateness of the dosage and side effects. Also, monitor him for drug interactions.

Quick quiz

1. A person with gradually occurring global impairments of cognitive functioning, memory and personality is most likely to have:

    A. age-related cognitive decline.
    B. Alzheimer's-type dementia.
    C. vascular dementia.
    D. dyskinesia.

Answer: B. A person with Alzheimer's-type dementia suffers global impairment of cognitive functioning, memory and personality. The dementia occurs gradually but with a continuous decline.

2. Age-related declines in intelligence, learning ability, short-term memory and reaction time may grow more significant by about age:

    A. 60.
    B. 65.
    C. 70.
    D. 75.

Answer: D. By about age 75, declines in intelligence, learning ability, short-term memory and reaction time may become significant.

3. An appropriate way to teach an older adult person is to use:
   A. audiotapes.
   B. pictures and simple wording.
   C. television programmes.
   D. musical recordings.

Answer: B. Because picture recognition doesn't seem to be affected by ageing, using pictures can help older adults with memory.

4. A drug used to treat Alzheimer's disease is:
   A. aspirin.
   B. chlorpromazine.
   C. donepezil.
   D. sertraline.

Answer: C. Donepezil and other anticholinesterase agents are currently used to treat Alzheimer's disease.

Scoring

✰✰✰ If you answered all four items correctly, marvy! Your mastery of older adults' mental disorders is magnificent!

✰✰ If you answered two or three items correctly, mazel tov! Your knowledge of mental disorders is maturing quite nicely.

✰ If you answered fewer than three items correctly, don't be melancholic! Just read the chapter again – your working memory is bound to improve.

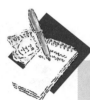

4 Schizophrenic disorders

Just the facts

In this chapter, you'll learn:

♦ phases and subtypes of schizophrenic disorders

♦ theories on the cause of schizophrenia

♦ assessment, diagnosis and treatment of people with schizophrenia

♦ nursing interventions for people with schizophrenia.

A look at schizophrenic disorders

Schizophrenia refers to a group of severe, disabling psychiatric disorders marked by withdrawal from reality, illogical thinking, possible delusions and hallucinations, and other emotional, behavioural or intellectual disturbances. These disturbances may affect everything from speech, effect and perception to psychomotor behaviour, interpersonal relationships and sense of self.

Schizophrenics may have trouble distinguishing reality from fantasy. Their speech and behaviour may frighten or mystify those around them.

Schizophrenia subtypes

Schizophrenia occurs in four subtypes – simple, hebephrenic, catatonic and paranoid.

Statistically speaking . . .

Approximately 1% of the population – 1 in every 100 people – develops schizophrenia during their lifetime. The disease affects equal numbers of men and women.

Schizophrenia is more prevalent than Alzheimer's disease, diabetes and multiple sclerosis.

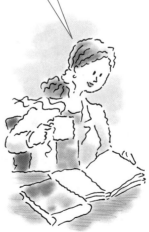

It says here that individuals with schizophrenia have trouble distinguishing reality from fantasy.

Functional fade-out

The person's overall disability depends mainly on the severity of cognitive impairment. Symptoms may impair the ability to hold a job, stay in school, maintain relationships and even perform self-care. All too often, the schizophrenic ends up unemployable, socially isolated and estranged from family and friends.

Life interrupted

Many schizophrenics neglect their personal hygiene and ignore their health needs. As a result, their life expectancy is about 10 years shorter than that of the general population. Approximately 10% of schizophrenics commit suicide.

Symptom start-up

Usually, schizophrenia symptoms arise gradually. But occasionally, they emerge over just a few days or a week.

The most common age at disease onset is late adolescence – although earlier and later onsets aren't unusual. In males, the disease typically starts in the late teens or early twenties; in females, in the twenties or early thirties.

Episodes and exacerbations

Between periods of exacerbation, some people have no disability, while others need continuous institutional care. With each acute episode, the prognosis worsens.

A few schizophrenics experience just a single psychotic episode, but only about one in five recovers from the disease completely. Most schizophrenics continue to suffer at least some symptoms lifelong.

Progress and promise

However, the outcome for people with this disorder has improved. Research has brought safer and better treatments. New discoveries into possible causes and cutting-edge brain-imaging techniques hold the promise of further insights and therapeutic advances. (See *Prognosis and probability*, page 124.)

Psychosocial and economic issues

Schizophrenia is a devastating illness – and the afflicted person isn't the only one who suffers. Family, friends and the entire community feel the effects. (See *The truth about schizophrenia and violence*, page 124.)

Denial

Few schizophrenics seek initial treatment on their own. Because of impaired thought processes and perceptual problems, many deny that they need help and resist seeking health care.

Prognosis and probability

Overall, about one-third of people with schizophrenia achieve significant and lasting improvement. Another third improve somewhat but have intermittent relapses and residual disability. The remaining third are severely and permanently incapacitated.

However, during any given 1-year period, the prognosis depends largely on the person's compliance with the prescribed drug regimen.

Good omens

Besides treatment compliance, other factors that portend a good prognosis include:

- late or sudden disease onset
- female sex
- relatively good preillness functioning
- minimal cognitive impairment
- paranoid schizophrenia subtype or many positive symptoms
- family history of mood disorders rather than schizophrenia.

Unfavourable outlook

Factors linked to a poor prognosis include:

- early age at onset
- poor preillness functioning
- family history of schizophrenia
- disorganised schizophrenia subtype with many negative symptoms.

Myth busters

The truth about schizophrenia and violence

Are schizophrenics harmless victims of mental illness or unpredictable perpetrators of violence?

Myth: Schizophrenics are more violent than other people.

Reality: Schizophrenics pose a relatively modest risk for violent behaviour. Although some threaten violence and have minor aggressive outbursts, few commit violent acts. In fact, schizophrenics are far less likely to behave violently than substance abusers.

Nonetheless, a schizophrenic who obeys hallucinatory voices telling him to attack someone poses a real danger. In rare cases, a depressed, isolated, paranoid schizophrenic attacks or kills someone he views as the cause of his problems.

Economic and social consequences

Schizophrenia is more prevalent among lower socioeconomic groups in urban areas – perhaps because its disabling effects often lead to unemployment and poverty.

It's also more common among single people. This may reflect the effects of the illness or its precursors on the person's social functioning.

Impact on the family

Schizophrenia profoundly affects the person's family. Although the person needs the understanding and support of family members, his behaviour may frighten those closest to him.

Family ferment

Few families are adequately prepared to deal with the stressors caused by chronic schizophrenia – among them, personality disintegration, hospital admissions and medication noncompliance. Also, family members may be uninformed about the disease.

Substance abuse

An estimated 50% of schizophrenics are substance abusers. Substance abuse may lead to noncompliance with prescribed medication, repeated illness relapses, frequent hospitalisations, declining function and loss of social support.

> About 50% of schizophrenics are substance abusers – which certainly doesn't aid recovery.

Possible causes of schizophrenia

Schizophrenia is a complex illness whose precise cause isn't known. Like many diseases, it probably results from the interplay of genetic, biochemical, anatomic and other factors.

Genetic factors

Experts have long known that schizophrenia runs in families. People who have a first-degree relative with the disease stand a 15% chance of developing it themselves – compared to a 1% chance among the general population.

Double jeopardy

Those at highest risk are the identical twins of schizophrenics and the children of two schizophrenic parents – roughly 50% will develop schizophrenia.

However, nearly two-thirds of diagnosed schizophrenics have no family history of the disease.

Predictable – not!

Most likely, multiple genes are involved in creating a predisposition to schizophrenia. Other factors (such as prenatal infections, perinatal complications and certain stressors) seem to influence disease development.

But researchers don't understand how the genetic predisposition is transmitted and can't predict whether a given person will develop the disease. (See *Vulnerability-stress theory*, page 126.)

> If one of us develops schizophrenia, the other one stands a 50% chance of getting it.

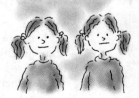

Vulnerability-stress theory

Some experts believe schizophrenia occurs when a biologically susceptible person experiences an environmental stressor. According to the vulnerability-stress theory, a stressful event (such as the death of a loved one, job loss or divorce) can trigger symptom onset in a vulnerable person.

Foetal forebodings

What causes this vulnerability in the first place? Some researchers blame such factors as:

- genetic predisposition
- viral infections of the central nervous system
- illness or complications during pregnancy, delivery or the neonatal period.

It's known, for instance, that the offspring of women who get influenza during the second trimester of pregnancy or experience maternal–foetal Rh incompatibility during a second or subsequent pregnancy are at increased risk for developing schizophrenia.

Genome jumble

Scientists are investigating several regions of the human genome to identify the genes involved in schizophrenia. So far, the strongest evidence points to chromosomes 13 and 6, although these findings haven't been confirmed.

Identifying the specific genes will yield significant clues into the brain abnormalities that produce and sustain the illness. This knowledge will guide the development of better treatments.

Biochemical theories

Scientists strongly suspect that schizophrenics have abnormalities in the chemical brain messengers called neurotransmitters – particularly dopamine and glutamate.

Dopamine theory

Most of the studies exploring the role of neurotransmitters in schizophrenia have focused on dopamine. According to the dopamine theory of schizophrenia, the disease results (at least in part) from an overactive dopamine system in the brain.

The dopamine theory might explain such symptoms as hallucinations, agitation, delusional thinking and grandiosity – forms of hyperactivity that have been linked to excessive dopamine activity.

Redundant receptors?

A recent study found that schizophrenics have an excess of dopamine-1 (D1) receptors in the frontal part of the cerebral cortex. Positron emission tomography scans showed that the more D1 receptors a schizophrenic had, the worse his symptoms were.

Another study found that schizophrenics had a higher percentage of active dopamine receptors than healthy people did. Also, post-mortem studies of schizophrenics have found increased numbers of dopamine receptors in the basal ganglia (masses of the grey matter in the cerebral hemispheres and upper brainstem).

Data dearth

Despite strong evidence supporting the dopamine theory, not all the data support it. About 20–30% of schizophrenics don't show high levels of dopamine activity. This suggests that other factors are involved in their disease process.

Other brain chemicals

Besides dopamine, schizophrenia may involve abnormalities of endorphins (peptide hormones that bind to opiate receptors in the brain) or other neurotransmitters, such as norepinephrine, serotonin, acetylcholine and gamma-aminobutyric acid. High norepinephrine levels have been linked to positive symptoms of schizophrenia, whereas increased dopamine activity seems to correlate to paranoid symptoms.

Glutamate guesswork

Some cognitive symptoms of schizophrenia may be associated with abnormalities of glutamate – a neurotransmitter involved in dopamine breakdown as well as learning and memory. Glutamate aids neuron migration during brain development and may play a role in the structural brain abnormalities found in some schizophrenics.

Structural brain abnormalities

Post-mortem examinations of schizophrenics' brains have found small changes in the distribution or number of brain cells. In living schizophrenics, scientists using neuroimaging techniques have discovered:
* enlarged ventricles
* reductions in the sizes of certain brain regions
* abnormalities in specific brain functions, including decreased metabolic activity in some brain regions.

However, these abnormalities weren't found in all schizophrenics – and *were* found in some people without the disease.

Developmental factors

Developmental neurobiologists suspect that schizophrenia results from faulty connections formed by neurons during foetal development. These errors may lie dormant until puberty, when the brain changes that occur normally at this time may interact adversely with the faulty connections. Researchers are trying to identify the prenatal factors that may influence the apparent abnormality.

Psychophysiological markers of schizophrenia

Adding to an already convincing body of evidence showing a genetic influence on schizophrenia, researchers have found abnormal eye-tracking movements in about 40–80% of people with schizophrenia and in 25–40% of their first-degree relatives.

Not so smooth pursuit

When tracking a moving object, such as a baseball in flight, the human eye uses a movement called smooth pursuit. The neuromuscular system produces pursuit movement by adjusting the moving eyeball's velocity to that of the object being viewed. This allows a stable image to be reflected onto the retina.

In schizophrenics, smooth-pursuit eye movements are interrupted inappropriately by rapid eye movements, such as those used to read or look around. Although this genetically driven abnormality doesn't directly relate to the cause or effects of schizophrenia, it may serve as a genetic marker and a predictor of possible disease development.

Other abnormalities

Studies also show that schizophrenics are more likely to have abnormal results on cognition and attention tests as well as deficient sensory gating (blocking of an incoming sensory message when other stimuli are occupying the person's attention). These markers, also found in first-degree relatives of schizophrenics, may signal vulnerability before the overt onset of illness.

Vulnerability markers

Proposed vulnerability markers for schizophrenia include psychophysiological deficits in eye tracking, information processing, attention and sensory inhibition. (See *Psychophysiological markers of schizophrenia*.)

Other possible causes

Many physical conditions have been linked to schizophrenia, including:
- maternal influenza during the second trimester of pregnancy
- birth trauma
- head injury
- epilepsy (especially of the temporal lobe)
- Huntington's chorea
- cerebral tumour
- stroke
- systemic lupus erythematosus
- myxoedema
- Parkinsonism
- Wilson's disease (a rare inherited disorder of poor copper metabolism)
- substance misuse

Viral aftermath

Some post-mortem studies of people with schizophrenia have found degenerative changes involving the neurons and neuroglia (supportive cells of the nervous system). This finding suggests that a healed viral or inflammatory infection may be involved in the disease development.

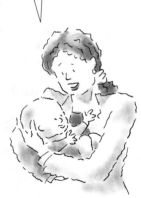

An infant whose mother had the flu during the second trimester of pregnancy has an increased risk for developing schizophrenia.

Assessment

Although behaviours and functional deficiencies may vary widely among people – and even in the same person at different times – some characteristic signs and symptoms usually are detectable during the assessment.

To assess a person for schizophrenia, gather a comprehensive history and conduct a physical examination. If necessary, obtain information from family, friends, teachers and others who know the person well.

Keep in mind that assessment findings will depend partly on the disease subtype, prevailing symptom type and illness phase. (See *Recognising schizophrenia*.)

Advice from the experts

Recognising schizophrenia

During the assessment interview, you may note characteristic signs and symptoms in a person with schizophrenia. Remember that specific findings vary with the schizophrenia subtype – simple, hebephrenic, catatonic, paranoid – and other factors.

Speech abnormalities

The person's speech may include:

- clang associations – words that rhyme or sound alike, used in an illogical, nonsensical manner (for example, 'It's the rain, train, pain')
- echolalia – meaningless repetition of words or phrases
- loose association and flight of ideas – rapid succession of incomplete ideas that aren't connected by logic or rationality
- word salad – illogical word groupings (for example, 'She had a star, barn, plant')
- neologisms – bizarre words that have meaning only for the person.

Thought distortions

Stay alert for evidence of:

- overly concrete thinking – inability to form or understand abstract thoughts
- delusions – false ideas or beliefs accepted as real by the person

- hallucinations – false sensory perceptions with no basis in reality
- thought blocking – sudden interruption in the train of thought
- magical thinking – a belief that thoughts or wishes can control other people or events.

Social interactions

Note whether the person exhibits:

- poor interpersonal relationships
- withdrawal and apathy – disinterest in objects, people or surroundings.

Other findings

In some schizophrenics, you also may assess:

- regression – return to an earlier developmental stage
- ambivalence – coexisting strong positive and negative feelings, leading to emotional conflict
- echopraxia – involuntary repetition of movements observed in others.

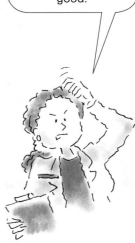

> How odd . . . they're called positive symptoms, but they sure aren't good.

Myth busters

Tall tales about schizophrenia

The behaviour of schizophrenics frightens and puzzles many people and has led to many misconceptions about the disease. Two of these misconceptions are addressed below.

Myth: The agitated psychomotor behaviour of some people with schizophrenia reflects excessive energy, which causes them to engage in violent acts.

Reality: Schizophrenics frequently show a lack of energy and have difficulty performing activities of daily living and interacting with other people.

Myth: A schizophrenic may experience either hallucinations or delusions, but not both.

Reality: People who experience positive symptoms of schizophrenia may have both hallucinations and delusions – especially delusions of paranoia or persecution.

Symptom categories

Many clinicians refer to positive and negative symptoms of schizophrenia. In most people with schizophrenia, one of these symptom clusters predominates. (See *Tall tales about schizophrenia*.)

Positive symptoms

Positive symptoms are deviant symptoms – symptoms that are present but should be absent. They include primarily delusions and hallucinations.

Keep in mind that in this context, 'positive' doesn't mean 'good'. Quite the contrary, positive symptoms are psychotic and show that the person has lost touch with reality.

Hallucinations

The most common feature of schizophrenia is hallucinations, which involve hearing, seeing, smelling, tasting or touching things that aren't actually there. For instance, the person may hear voices commenting on his behaviour, conversing with one another or making critical and abusive comments.

Delusions

Delusions are erroneous beliefs that usually grow out of misinterpretations of experience. They may cause the person to think that someone is reading his thoughts, plotting against him or monitoring him – or that he can control the minds of other people.

Delusional distinctions

Delusions fall into several categories. A person with a *persecutory* delusion, for instance, thinks he's being tormented, followed, tricked or spied on.

A person with a *reference* delusion may think that passages in books, newspapers, television shows, song lyrics or other environmental cues are directed at him.

In delusions of *thought withdrawal* or *thought insertion*, the person believes others can read his mind, his thoughts are being transmitted to others or outside forces are imposing their thoughts or impulses on him.

• *Thought disorder* refers to confused thinking and speech, ranging from mildly disorganised speech to incoherent ramblings. The person makes loose associations, jumping from one idea to another and wandering further and further from the original topic. He may have trouble carrying on conversations with others.

• Bizarre behaviour may include childlike silliness, agitation and inappropriate appearance, hygiene or conduct. The person may move slowly, repeat rhythmic gestures or walk in circles. He may be unable to make sense of everyday sights, sounds and feelings.

Negative symptoms

Negative (deficit) symptoms reflect the absence of normal characteristics. They include apathy, lack of motivation, blunted affect, poverty of speech, anhedonia and asociality.

• *Apathy* refers to a lack of interest in people, things and activities.

• *Lack of motivation* renders the person unable to start and follow through with activities.

• *Blunted affect* refers to flattening of the emotions. The person's face may appear immobile and inexpressive. As schizophrenia progresses, blunted affect may grow more pronounced. (But keep in mind that inability to show emotions doesn't mean inability to *feel* emotions.)

• *Poverty of speech* refers to speech that is brief and lacks content. The person gives terse replies to questions, creating the impression of inner emptiness.

• *Anhedonia* is diminished capacity to experience pleasure.

• *Asociality* refers to avoidance of relationships. A schizophrenic may withdraw socially because he's depressed, feels relatively safe when alone or is completely caught up in his own feelings and fears he can't manage the company of others. (See *Linking symptoms to brain abnormalities*.)

Disease phases

Schizophrenia usually progresses in three distinct phases – prodromal, active and residual.

Prodromal phase

During the *prodromal phase*, which may arise a year or so before the first hospital admission, the person shows a clear decline from his previous level of functioning.

Linking symptoms to brain abnormalities

Brain scans suggest that the positive and negative symptoms of schizophrenia may be linked to structural brain abnormalities in different parts of the brain.

Generally, positive symptoms are associated with temporal lobe abnormalities, while negative symptoms are linked to abnormalities in the frontal cortex and the ventricles. Also, studies of regional brain glucose and oxygen use found diminished activation in the prefrontal cortex and mesolimbic regions in people with negative symptoms and cognitive dysfunction.

A low profile

He may withdraw from friends, hobbies and other interests. He may exhibit peculiar behaviour, neglect personal hygiene and grooming and lack energy and initiative. His work or school performance may deteriorate.

Active phase

During the *active phase* (commonly triggered by a stressful event), the person has acute psychotic symptoms, such as hallucinations, delusions, incoherence or catatonic behaviour. Functional deficits worsen.

Symptomatic periods may occur episodically (with identifiable exacerbations and remissions) or continuously (with no identifiable remissions).

Number of acute episodes

Up to one-third of schizophrenics have just one acute episode and no more. Others have repeated, acute exacerbations of the active phase. With each acute episode, the prognosis worsens.

Residual phase

During the *residual phase*, which follows the active phase, symptoms resemble those of the prodromal phase. However, blunted affect and impaired role functioning may be more pronounced. Some psychotic symptoms, such as hallucinations, may persist but without strong affect.

During the residual phase, the illness pattern may become established, disability levels may stabilise or late improvements may appear.

Remissions

Although few schizophrenics return to their full preillness functioning level, full remissions have occurred.

Disease course

The course of schizophrenia varies among people and depends largely on compliance with prescribed antipsychotic drug regimen.

Mild course

The person with a mild disease course is usually stable. He always complies with drug treatment, has just one or two major relapses by age 45 and experiences only a few mild symptoms.

Moderate course

Typically, the person with a moderate disease course takes drugs as prescribed most of the time but isn't fully compliant. He has several major relapses by age 45 and increased symptoms during stressful periods. Between relapses, his symptoms persist.

Severe, unstable course

The person with a severe disease course doesn't comply with his drug regimen – or discontinues it entirely. He has frequent relapses and is stable only for brief periods between relapses. He experiences bothersome symptoms and needs help with activities of daily living. He's also likely to have other problems (such as substance abuse) that make recovery more difficult.

Symptoms over time

During the first 5 years of the illness, the person's level of functioning may deteriorate. Social and work skills may decline, cognitive deficits grow more pronounced and self-care neglect may worsen progressively. Also, negative symptoms may grow more severe.

In the most common disease course, acute episodes are followed by residual impairment. During the first few years of schizophrenia, impairment between episodes commonly increases.

Respite and relief

After the first 5 years, the disability level tends to plateau. Some evidence suggests that illness severity may lessen later in life, particularly among women.

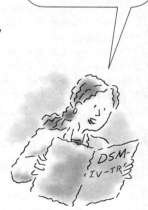

> The patient has stopped taking his meds? Oh, my – he may be destined for a severe disease course.

Diagnosis

A mental status examination, psychiatric history and careful clinical observation form the basis for diagnosing schizophrenia.

For a thorough evaluation, the person should undergo physical and psychiatric examinations to rule out other possible causes of symptoms – including physical disorders, substance-induced psychosis and primary mood disorders with psychotic features.

The stamp of authority

Official diagnosis is based on the criteria in the *Diagnostic and Statistical Manual of Mental Disorders*, Fourth Edition, Text Revision (*DSM-IV-TR*). (See *Diagnostic criteria: Schizophrenia*, page 134.)

> This book certainly makes it easier to diagnose schizophrenia.

Diagnostic test results

No diagnostic test definitively confirms schizophrenia. To support a diagnosis, the doctor may order a dexamethasone suppression test, which fails to show suppression in some schizophrenics. (However, some clinicians question the test's accuracy.) Other tests may be done to rule out disorders that can cause psychosis, including vitamin deficiencies, uraemia, thyrotoxicosis and electrolyte imbalances.

The following tests may show structural brain abnormalities that suggest schizophrenia:
• computed tomography (CT) scans and magnetic resonance imaging (MRI), which may show enlarged ventricles and other findings characteristic of schizophrenia
• ventricular-brain ratio (VBR) analysis, which may find an elevated VBR in people with schizophrenia.

Diagnostic criteria: Schizophrenia

The general diagnosis of schizophrenia applies if the person meets the criteria in the *Diagnostic and Statistical Manual of Mental Disorders,* Fourth Edition, Text Revision.

Characteristic symptoms

Two or more of the following signs and symptoms are present for a significant part of a 1-month period (or less, if successfully treated):

- delusions
- prominent hallucinations (throughout the day for several days or several times a week for several weeks, with each hallucinatory experience lasting more than a few moments)
- disorganised speech – for example, frequent derailment or incoherence
- grossly disorganised or catatonic behaviour
- negative symptoms – for example, flat affect, inability to make decisions or inability to speak.

The diagnosis requires just *one* of the above symptoms if:

- delusions are bizarre (involving a phenomenon that the person's culture would consider implausible)
- hallucinations consist of a voice issuing a running commentary on the person's behaviour or thoughts
- hallucinations consist of two or more voices talking to each other.

Social and occupational dysfunction

For a significant period during the course of the disturbance, one or more major areas of functioning (such as work, interpersonal relationships or self-care) are markedly below the level achieved before the onset of the disturbance.

When the disturbance begins in childhood or adolescence, the dysfunction takes the form of failure to achieve the expected level of interpersonal, academic or occupational development.

Duration

Continuous signs and symptoms of the disturbance last at least 6 months. During at least one of these 6 months, the person has characteristic, active-phase signs and symptoms (or less, if treated successfully).

During the prodromal or residual periods, signs of the disturbance may appear only as negative symptoms or as two or more characteristic symptoms in a less severe form (for example, odd beliefs or unusual perceptual experiences).

Exclusion of schizoaffective and mood disorders

Schizoaffective disorder and mood disorder with psychotic features have been ruled out for either of these reasons:

- No major depressive, manic or mixed episodes have occurred concurrently with active-phase symptoms.
- If mood disorder episodes have occurred during active-phase symptoms, their total duration has been relatively brief compared with the duration of the active and residual periods.

Exclusion of substance effects and general medical conditions

The disturbance doesn't stem from direct physiological effects of a substance or a general medical condition.

Relationship to a pervasive developmental disorder

If the person has a history of autistic disorder or another pervasive developmental disorder, the additional diagnosis of schizophrenia is appropriate only if prominent delusions or hallucinations also are present for at least 1 month (or less, if successfully treated).

Views of the ventricles

In up to 40% of schizophrenics, CT scans show structural brain abnormalities, such as:
- lateral ventricular enlargement (common in males but not females)
- enlargement of the sulci, or fissures on the cerebral surface
- atrophy of the cerebellum.

More recently, MRIs have found certain abnormalities in the brain's amygdala, limbic system, frontal cortex, temporal lobes, hippocampus, basal ganglia and thalamus. A reported deviation in schizophrenics is decreased blood flow to the thalamus, which may cause a flood of sensory information.

Mysterious asymmetry

In normal healthy people, brain scans reveal functional cerebral asymmetries. But for reasons not understood, this asymmetry is reversed in many schizophrenics' brains.

General treatment

Regardless of which schizophrenia subtype the person has, antipsychotic drugs (sometimes called neuroleptics) are the mainstay of treatment. Continuous prophylactic antipsychotic drug therapy can reduce the 1-year relapse rate to about 30%. Without prophylactic drugs, 70–80% of people who have had one schizophrenia episode experience a subsequent one within the next 12 months.

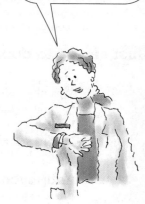

The sooner a schizophrenic begins treatment, the faster and more fully he's likely to respond.

Value of early treatment

Schizophrenics tend to develop psychotic symptoms an average of 12–24 months before they present for medical care. The interval between symptom onset and the first treatment correlates with the speed and quality of the initial treatment response and severity of negative symptoms. People treated soon after diagnosis tend to respond more quickly and fully than those who don't begin drug therapy until later in the disease course.

Mixed modalities

Despite their importance, though, drugs alone are rarely sufficient. For most people, drug therapy must be combined with:
- psychosocial treatment and rehabilitation
- compliance promotion programmes
- vocational counselling
- psychotherapy
- appropriate use of community resources.
    Some schizophrenics also may be candidates for electroconvulsive therapy (ECT).

Treatment goals

Treatment goals for the person with schizophrenia include:
- reducing the severity of psychotic symptoms
- preventing recurrences of acute episodes and the associated functional decline
- meeting the person's physical and psychosocial needs
- helping him function at the highest level possible. (See *Myths about dependence*, page 136.)

Myth busters

Myths about dependence

Many people have the notion that schizophrenics are too inept to manage everyday life.

Myth: People with schizophrenia are incapable of making life decisions and need the help of a legal guardian.

Reality: Although some schizophrenics need guidance through certain periods, only a small minority must depend on others to make decisions and care for them. Most handle their own affairs successfully.

Drug therapy

Antipsychotic drugs control symptoms adequately in most schizophrenics. The wide choice of drug treatment options available today has improved peoples' chances for remission and recovery.

Just say no to dopamine

Antipsychotic drugs appear to work at least in part by blocking postsynaptic dopamine receptors. These drugs have multiple benefits, including:
- reducing positive symptoms, such as hallucinations and delusions
- easing thought disorders
- relieving anxiety and agitation
- maximising the person's level of functioning.

Antipsychotic drug categories

Three categories of antipsychotics are available – conventional antipsychotics, clozapine and newer atypical antipsychotics.

Conventional antipsychotics

Conventional antipsychotics have been in use the longest. Chlorpromazine was the first antipsychotic used. Although effective in managing positive symptoms of schizophrenia, it doesn't relieve negative symptoms.

Other conventional antipsychotics include:
- fluphenazine
- haloperidol
- perphenazine
- thiothixene
- trifluoperazine.

Largely because of their side effects, these drugs are becoming obsolete. (See *Side effects of antipsychotic drugs*, page 137.) However, people who do well on them and avoid troublesome side effects are usually advised to continue them.

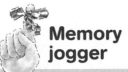

Memory jogger

The word PRESSURE can help you remember the treatment goals for a schizophrenic person.

P Psychiatric medications administered properly and monitored

R Realistic perceptions and self-expectations developed

E Environmental situations managed effectively

S Safety needs addressed

S Self-care performed adequately

U Use of community resources on an ongoing basis

R Relationships developed and sustained

E Establishment and maintenance of family involvement in care

Side effects of antipsychotic drugs

People with schizophrenia must take antipsychotic drugs for a long time – usually for life. Unfortunately, some of these drugs may cause unpleasant side effects.

Sedative, anticholinergic and extrapyramidal effects

High-potency conventional antipsychotics (such as haloperidol) cause minimal sedation and anticholinergic effects, such as rapid pulse, dry mouth, inability to urinate and constipation.

But these drugs carry a high incidence of extrapyramidal (motor) effects. The most common motor effects are dystonia, Parkinsonism and akathisia.

- *Dystonia* refers to prolonged, repetitive muscle contractions that may cause twisting or jerking movements – especially of the neck, mouth and tongue. It's most common in young males, usually appearing within the first few days of drug treatment.
- Drug-induced *Parkinsonism* results in bradykinesia (abnormally slow movements), muscle rigidity, shuffling gait, stooped posture, flat facial affect, tremors and drooling. It may emerge 1 week to several months after drug treatment begins.
- *Akathisia* causes restlessness, pacing and an inability to rest or sit still.

Intermediate-potency conventional antipsychotics (such as molindone) have a moderate incidence of extrapyramidal effects. Low-potency agents (such as chlorpromazine) are highly sedative and anticholinergic but cause few extrapyramidal effects.

Orthostatic hypotension

Low-potency antipsychotics may cause orthostatic hypotension (low blood pressure when standing).

Tardive dyskinesia

With prolonged use, antipsychotics may cause tardive dyskinesia – a disorder characterised by repetitive, involuntary, purposeless movements. Signs and symptoms include grimacing, rapid eye blinking, tongue protrusion and smacking, lip puckering or pursing and rapid movements of the hands, arms, legs and trunk.

Symptoms may persist long after the person stops taking the antipsychotic drug. With careful management, though, some symptoms eventually lessen or even disappear.

Neuroleptic malignant syndrome

In up to 1% of people, antipsychotic drugs cause neuroleptic malignant syndrome. This life-threatening condition leads to fever, extremely rigid muscles and altered consciousness. It may occur hours to months after drug therapy starts or the dosage is increased.

Drug depots

Some noncompliant patients may receive depot formulations of fluphenazine or haloperidol. These long-acting I.M. doses release the drug gradually for a maximum of 4 weeks.

Clozapine

Introduced in 1990, clozapine was the first atypical antipsychotic. It has proven to be effective in an estimated 25–50% of people who don't respond to conventional antipsychotics. The drug controls a wider range of signs and symptoms (including negative symptoms) than conventional agents and causes few or no adverse motor effects.

Agranulocytosis and other adversities

However, clozapine may cause agranulocytosis – a potentially fatal blood disorder marked by a low white blood cell count and pronounced neutrophil depletion. People receiving it should undergo routine blood monitoring to detect the disorder. When caught early, it's reversible.

Other side effects of clozapine include drowsiness, sedation, hypotension, weight gain, excessive salivation, hyperglycaemia, tachycardia, dizziness and seizures.

Newer atypical antipsychotics

The introduction of newer atypical antipsychotics has given new hope to many schizophrenics. Called atypical because they work differently than conventional antipsychotics, they're much less likely to cause the distressing motor effect called tardive dyskinesia.

Currently available atypical antipsychotics include:
- olanzapine
- quetiapine
- risperidone
- ziprasidone
- palperidone
- amisulpride
- zotepine.

People should take these drugs for a trial of 4–8 weeks to assess their efficacy. For acute treatment, rapid symptom resolution is the goal. For maintenance, people should receive the lowest dose that prevents symptoms.

Atypicals' advantages

Newer atypical antipsychotics offer many benefits:
- They have a selective affinity for brain regions involved in schizophrenia symptoms.
- They relieve positive symptoms.
- They improve negative symptoms more effectively than conventional antipsychotics.
- They enhance the brain's serotonin levels while stabilising dopamine levels.
- They may improve neurocognitive deficits.
- They're more effective in treating refractory schizophrenia.
- They're less likely to cause motor adverse effects.
- They produce little or no prolactin elevation (a possible side effect of conventional antipsychotics.)

Other drugs

Antidepressants and anxiolytics may be used to control associated signs and symptoms in some people. Mood-stabilising agents, such as lithium, carbamazepine and valproic acid, may be given to manage negative symptoms. Benzodiazepine may be prescribed for people who are substance abusers.

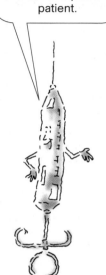

A depot formulation of fluphenazine or haloperidol may be given I.M. to a noncompliant patient.

Better symptom coverage, fewer side effects, higher serotonin levels – atypical antipsychotics sound pretty impressive.

Home is where the help is

A stable place to live plays an important role in treating schizophrenia. Depending on the individual's geographic location, a wide range of residential options may be available.

Crisis resolution and home treatment

Crisis resolution and home treatment teams offer intensive therapeutic interventions with clinical staff who can provide 24-hour supervision and treatment. These teams may be a good choice for individuals experiencing acute episodes or during the stabilisation phase that follows an acute episode. For relapsing individuals, these teams may help them avoid the need for hospitalisation.

Group homes

Group homes are supportive group living situations run by qualified and unqualified staff. Usually, the staff provides supervision during the day, with one staff member sleeping over at night. These homes may be recommended for individuals in long-term recovery and maintenance.

Supported or supervised apartments

Supported or supervised apartments usually have a specially trained on-site residential manager who provides support, assistance and supervision. Alternatively, a mental health professional or family member may provide these services.

These apartments are useful for individuals in long-term recovery and maintenance. They help the individual remain autonomous while providing sufficient care to minimise the chance of relapse and reduce the need for hospitalisation.

Family living

For some individuals, living with family members may be the best long-term arrangement. For others, it may be needed only during acute episodes. Support and advocacy groups can provide families with information and support.

Independent living

During long-term recovery and maintenance, independent living is recommended for most individuals. Of course, this may be impossible during acute episodes and for individuals with a more severe disease course.

Psychosocial treatment and rehabilitation

Besides antipsychotic drugs, most people need support to overcome the illness and deal with the isolation, stigma and fear it often brings. Experts recommend psychosocial treatment, rehabilitation services and special living arrangements to aid in the various stages of recovery. (See *Home is where the help is*.)

Psychosocial treatment

Key components of psychosocial treatment for people with schizophrenia include:
- teaching the person and their family about the disease and its treatment
- collaborative decision-making
- monitoring of drug therapy and symptoms
- assistance with obtaining prescribed drugs, services and resources (such as disability income)
- supervision of financial resources, as needed
- training and assistance with activities of daily living
- peer support and self-help groups
- psychotherapy.

Psychotherapy

By itself, individual or group psychotherapy has little value in treating schizophrenia. But for many people, adjunctive psychotherapy provides emotional support, reinforces health-promoting behaviours, aids adjustment to the illness and helps them make the most of their abilities. Typically, psychotherapy is used during the maintenance phase or during the stabilisation phase that follows an acute episode.

Go it alone or hang with a gang?

Generally, the focus of individual therapy is reality based and supportive. Group therapy, on the other hand, is aimed at encouraging socialisation and social and coping skills and resolving interpersonal conflicts. It also promotes reality testing.

Family psychotherapy and teaching

Because schizophrenia is so disruptive to the family, all family members may benefit from psychotherapy. Such therapy can reduce guilt and disappointment, improve acceptance of the person and his behaviour and teach the family stress-management skills. For people who live with their families, psychoeducational family interventions can reduce the relapse rate.

Rehabilitation

Rehabilitation may be particularly important for people who need to sharpen their job skills, want to work and have only a few remaining symptoms.

A range of rehab

During the long-term recovery and maintenance phases of the illness, three types of rehabilitation programmes may be used.

 Psychosocial rehabilitation programmes help people improve their work skills so they can get and keep jobs.

 Psychiatric rehabilitation teaches people the skills they need to define and achieve their personal goals regarding education, work, socialisation and living arrangements.

 Vocational rehabilitation involves work assessment and training to help people prepare for full-time employment.

Electroconvulsive therapy

ECT sometimes is used to treat people with acute schizophrenia and those who can't tolerate or don't respond to medication. It has been effective in reducing depressive and catatonic symptoms of schizophrenia.

Preserving the schizophrenics' rights

Remember that people with schizophrenia have much the same rights as other people in hospital.

Memory jogger

If you have trouble recalling the rights of people with schizophrenia just think of the word RIGHTS.

R Refusal of nonemergency treatment

I Individualised care

G Grievances addressed as they occur

H Health alternatives given

T Treatment obtained in the least restrictive setting

S Security of the person's civil rights

Simple schizophrenia

This is a form of schizophrenia having an insidious onset during late adolescence.

Signs and symptoms

The person gradually becomes socially withdrawn, apathetic and detached; he may develop an abnormal anxiety about his health. Family members may become worried about the changes they see and this leads to conflict between the person and his family.

The basic nursing interventions for people with schizophrenia are appropriate for people with simple schizophrenia.

Hebephrenic schizophrenia

This is similar to simple schizophrenia with respect to emotional and motivational deficits. The presentation is of a very emotionally and behaviourally disturbed person. This type of schizophrenia usually develops between the ages of 15 and 30.

Signs and symptoms

There is a greater degree of thought disorder with bizarre delusions and hallucinations and behavioural disturbances. It may be accompanied by mood swings and incongruity of affect (inappropriate emotions and desires).

As the disease progresses, there is a marked disintegration of personality, he becomes more withdrawn and may develop strange mannerisms and fragmentation of thought and speech.

The basic nursing interventions for people with schizophrenia are appropriate for people with hebephrenic schizophrenia.

Catatonic schizophrenia

A rare disease form, catatonic schizophrenia is marked by a tendency to remain in a fixed stupor for long periods. Periodically, this state may yield to brief spurts of extreme excitement. Many catatonic schizophrenics have an increased potential for destructive, violent behaviour.

Signs and symptoms

A catatonic schizophrenic may remain mute and refuse to move about or tend to his personal needs. He may show bizarre mannerisms, such as facial grimacing and sucking mouth movements.

Diagnostic criteria: Catatonic schizophrenia

Catatonic schizophrenia is diagnosed when the person meets these criteria from the *Diagnostic and Statistical Manual of Mental Disorders,* Fourth Edition, Text Revision.
At least two of the following conditions are dominant:

- lack of motor movements, as shown by stupor, catalepsy (lack of response to external stimuli and muscular rigidity) or waxy flexibility (in which the person's arms and legs can be moved into various positions and maintained there for unusually long periods)
- excessive motor activity (seemingly purposeless movements not influenced by external stimuli)
- extreme negativism (such as resisting instructions or staying in a rigid posture against efforts to be moved)

- or mutism (failing to speak when speech is expected or demanded)
- peculiar voluntary movements, such as posturing (voluntarily assuming bizarre or inappropriate postures), stereotyped movements or prominent mannerisms or grimacing
- echolalia (repeating words or phrases spoken by others) or echopraxia (imitating others' movements).

Contortions and repetitions

Other signs and symptoms of catatonic schizophrenia include:
- rapid swings between stupor and excitement (extreme psychomotor agitation with excessive, senseless or incoherent shouting or talking)
- bizarre postures, such as holding the body (especially the arms and legs) rigidly in one position for a long time
- diminished sensitivity to painful stimuli
- negative symptoms
- echolalia – repeating words or phrases spoken by others
- echopraxia – imitating others' movements.

Diagnosis

A person is diagnosed with catatonic schizophrenia if other possible causes of his symptoms are ruled out and if he meets the criteria listed in the *DSM-IV-TR*. (See *Diagnostic criteria: Catatonic schizophrenia.*)

Treatment

Many experts recommend ECT and benzodiazepines (such as diazepam or lorazepam) for catatonic schizophrenics. Conventional antipsychotic drugs should be avoided as they may worsen catatonic symptoms. The role of atypical antipsychotics in treating catatonic schizophrenia requires further evaluation.

Nursing interventions

Certain nursing interventions are appropriate for all people with schizophrenia, regardless of which disease subtype they have. (See *General nursing interventions for people with schizophrenia*, pages 143 and 144.)

For catatonic schizophrenics, you may find the additional guidelines below helpful.

Advice from the experts

General nursing interventions for people with schizophrenia

You can use the nursing interventions given below when caring for any person with schizophrenia – regardless of which schizophrenia subtype he has.

Establishing trust and rapport

- Expect the person to put you through a rigorous testing period before he shows evidence of trust. Don't tease or joke with him.
- Don't touch him without first telling him exactly what you're going to do. For example, clearly explain, 'I'm going to put this cuff on your arm so I can take your blood pressure.'
- If necessary, postpone procedures that require physical contact with hospital staff until the person is less suspicious or agitated.
- Use an accepting, consistent approach. Don't avoid or overwhelm the person. Keep in mind that short, repeated contacts are best until trust has been established.
- Use clear, unambiguous language. Otherwise, the person may interpret your words the wrong way. (For example, if you tell him, 'This procedure will be done on the floor', he may become frightened, thinking he's being told to lie down on the floor.)
- Maintain a sense of hope for possible improvement, and convey this to the person.

Maximising the level of functioning

- Assess the person's ability to carry out activities of daily living.
- Avoid promoting dependence. Meet the person's needs, but do for him only what he can't do for himself.
- Reward positive behaviour and work with him to increase his sense of his own responsibility in improving his level of functioning.

Promoting social skills

- Encourage the person to engage in meaningful interpersonal relationships.
- Provide support in assisting him to learn social skills.

Ensuring safety

- Maintain a safe environment with minimal stimulation.
- As needed, use physical restraints according to national and local policy to ensure the person's and others' safety.
- Monitor the person's nutritional status. Weigh him regularly if he isn't eating. If he thinks his food is poisoned, let him prepare his own food when possible, or offer him foods in closed containers that he can open. If you give liquid medication in a unit-dose container, allow him to open the container.
- If the person expresses suicidal thoughts, institute suicide precautions. Document his behaviour and your precautions.
- If he expresses homicidal thoughts (for example, 'I have to kill my mother'), initiate homicidal precautions. Notify the doctor and the potential victim. Document the person's comments and who was notified.

Keeping it real

- Engage the person in reality-oriented activities that involve human contact, such as inpatient social skills training groups, outpatient day care and sheltered workshops.
- Provide reality-based explanations for distorted body images or hypochondriacal complaints.
- Clarify private language, autistic inventions or neologisms. Tell the person that other people don't understand what he says.

(continued)

General nursing interventions for people with schizophrenia *(continued)*

Dealing with hallucinations

- If the person is hallucinating, explore the content of the hallucinations. If he has auditory hallucinations, determine if they're command hallucinations that place him or others at risk. Tell him you don't hear the voices but you know they're real to him.
- Avoid arguing about the hallucinations. If possible, change the subject.

Promoting compliance and monitoring drug therapy

- Administer prescribed drugs to manage schizophrenia symptoms or ease anxiety.
- Encourage the person to comply with the medication regimen to prevent relapse.
- If he's taking a drug that requires monitoring of blood levels, stress the importance of returning to the hospital or outpatient clinic for regular monitoring.
- Regularly assess the person for side effects of medication. Document and report these promptly.
- Instruct a person taking a slow-release drug formulation when to return for the next dose. Urge him to keep the appointment.

Encouraging family involvement

- Involve the person's family in his treatment, particularly as his altered thought processes may make teaching difficult.
- Teach family members how to recognise an impending relapse (nervousness, insomnia, decreased ability to concentrate and loss of interest). Suggest ways in which they can manage the person's symptoms.

Establish a presence

- Spend time with the person even if he's mute and unresponsive. Remember – despite appearances, he's acutely aware of his environment. Your presence can be reassuring and supportive.
- Assume he can hear. Speak to him directly and don't talk about him in his presence.

Reach toward reality

- Emphasise reality during all person contacts to reduce distorted perceptions.
- Offer reality orientation. You might say, for instance, 'The leaves on the trees are turning brown and the air is cooler. It's autumn!'
- Verbalise for the person the message that his behaviour seems to convey. Encourage him to do the same.
- Tell the person directly, specifically and concisely what needs to be done. Don't give him a choice. Instead, say, 'It's time to go for a walk. Let's go.'

Hold off harm

- Assess for signs and symptoms of physical illness. Keep in mind that if he's mute, he won't complain of pain or physical symptoms.
- Remember that if he's in a bizarre posture, he may be at risk for pressure ulcers or decreased circulation. Provide range-of-motion exercises or walk him every 2 hours.

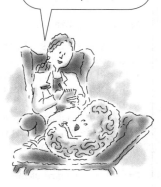

This may shock you, but electroconvulsive therapy is sometimes used to treat catatonic schizophrenia.

- During periods of hyperactivity, try to prevent him from experiencing physical exhaustion and injury.
- As appropriate, meet his needs for adequate food, fluid, exercise and elimination. Follow orders with respect to nutrition, urinary catheterisation and enema use.
- Stay alert for violent outbursts. If these occur, get help promptly to intervene safely for yourself, the person and others.

Paranoid schizophrenia

Persecutory or grandiose delusional thought content and, possibly, delusional jealousy characterise paranoid schizophrenia. Some people also have gender identity problems, such as fears of being thought of as homosexual or of being approached by homosexuals. Stress may worsen the person's symptoms.

The good news is that paranoid schizophrenia may cause only minimal impairment in the person's level of functioning – as long as he doesn't act on delusional thoughts.

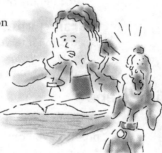

I've been studying this chapter so long, I think I may be hallucinating. Is it my imagination, or is a dog barking at me?

Hearing things, but not incoherent

Although paranoid schizophrenics may experience frequent auditory hallucinations related to a single theme, they typically lack some of the symptoms of other schizophrenia subtypes – notably, incoherence, loose associations, flat or grossly inappropriate affect and catatonic or grossly disorganised behaviour.

On the one hand . . .

Paranoid schizophrenics tend to be less severely disabled and more responsive to treatments than other schizophrenics are.

On the other hand . . .

Those with late disease onset and good preillness functioning (the very people who have the best prognosis) are at the greatest risk for suicide. Because they're capable of feeling grief and anguish, they may be more prone to act in despair, based on their realistic recognition of the disease's effects and implications.

Signs and symptoms

Signs and symptoms of paranoid schizophrenia include:
- persecutory or grandiose delusional thoughts
- auditory hallucinations
- unfocused anxiety
- anger

- tendency to argue
- stilted formality or intensity when interacting with others
- possible violence.

Diagnosis

Paranoid schizophrenia is diagnosed if other causes of the person's symptoms are ruled out and if he meets the *DSM-IV-TR* criteria for the disorder. (See *Diagnostic criteria: Paranoid schizophrenia*.)

Treatment

As with most other schizophrenia subtypes, treatment of paranoid schizophrenia typically involves:
- antipsychotic drugs
- psychosocial therapies and rehabilitation, including group and individual psychotherapy.
  For details on these therapies, see 'General treatment', page 135.

Nursing interventions

Besides the interventions described in *General nursing interventions for people with schizophrenia*, pages 143 and 144, the following guidelines may be useful when caring for a paranoid schizophrenic.

First steps

- Build trust, and be honest and dependable. Don't threaten or make promises you can't fulfil.
- Be aware that brief person contacts may be most useful initially.
- When the person is newly admitted, minimise his contact with the staff.

Don't come on strong

- Don't touch the person without telling him first exactly what you're going to do.
- Approach him in a calm, unhurried manner.
- Avoid crowding him physically or psychologically. He may strike out to protect himself.
- Respond neutrally to his condescending remarks. Don't let him put you on the defensive, and don't take his remarks personally.
- If he tells you to leave him alone, do leave – but make sure you return soon.
- Set limits firmly but without anger. Avoid a punitive attitude.
- Be flexible and give the person some control.

Cut back on contacts

- Anticipate the need for reduced social contact to increase the person's comfort level.
- Consider postponing procedures that require physical contact with hospital staff if the person becomes suspicious or agitated.

Diagnostic criteria: Paranoid schizophrenia

Paranoid schizophrenia is diagnosed when the person meets these criteria from the *Diagnostic and Statistical Manual of Mental Disorders,* Fourth Edition, Text Revision.

- The person is preoccupied with one or more delusions or frequent auditory hallucinations.
- Disorganised speech, disorganised or catatonic behaviour, or flat or inappropriate affect aren't prominent.

Focus on facts

• If the person is hallucinating, explore the content of the hallucinations. If he hears voices, find out whether he thinks he must do what they command. Tell him you don't hear the voices, but you know they're real to him.

• Don't try to combat the person's delusions with logic. Instead, respond to feelings, themes or underlying needs – for example, 'It seems you feel you've been treated unfairly' (persecution).

• Offer simple, matter-of-fact explanations about environmental safeguards, medications and facility policies.

Create a safe haven

• If the person expresses suicidal thoughts or says he hears voices telling him to harm himself, institute suicide precautions. Document his behaviour and your precautions.

• If he expresses homicidal thoughts, institute homicide precautions. Notify the doctor and the potential victim. Document the person's comments and the names of those notified.

• Make sure the person's nutritional needs are met. If he thinks his food is poisoned, let him make his own food when possible, or offer foods in closed containers that he can open himself.

• Monitor the person for adverse drug reactions. Document and report these promptly.

Contain conversations

• Don't tease, joke, argue with or confront the person. Remember – his distorted perceptions will cause him to misinterpret such actions in a way that's derogatory to himself.

• Let him talk about anything he wishes initially, but keep the conversation light and social, and avoid engaging in power struggles.

Quick quiz

1. Flattening of emotions refers to:
   A. anhedonia.
   B. asociality.
   C. blunted affect.
   D. regression.

Answer: C. Blunted affect is the flattening of emotions. The person's face may be immobile and inexpressive, with poor eye contact.

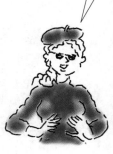

Chill out . . . Approach the person with schizophrenia calmly, and give him space.

Be a good listener. Let the person talk about anything he wants – at least initially.

2. False ideas or beliefs that the person accepts as real are called:
    A.   delusions.
    B.   hallucinations.
    C.   illusions.
    D.   magical thinking.

Answer: A. Delusions are false ideas or beliefs accepted as real by the person. Among schizophrenics, delusions of grandeur, persecution and reference are common.

3. A newly admitted person can't take care of his personal needs, shows insensitivity to painful stimuli and exhibits negativism, rigidity and posturing. The most appropriate diagnosis is:
    A.   paranoid schizophrenia.
    B.   simple schizophrenia.
    C.   hebephrenic schizophrenia.
    D.   catatonic schizophrenia.

Answer: D. Catatonic schizophrenia is characterised by the inability to take care of personal needs, diminished sensitivity to painful stimuli, negativism, rigidity and posturing.

4. A schizophrenic person who began taking haloperidol 1 week ago now exhibits jerking movements of the neck and mouth. These are signs of:
    A.   dystonia.
    B.   psychosis.
    C.   akathisia.
    D.   Parkinsonism.

Answer: A. Haloperidol and other high-potency conventional antipsychotics cause a high incidence of dystonia and other extrapyramidal adverse effects. Dystonia is marked by prolonged, repetitive muscle contractions that cause twisting or jerking movements – especially of the neck, mouth and tongue.

5. A positive symptom of schizophrenia is:
    A.   hallucination.
    B.   blunted affect.
    C.   anhedonia.
    D.   asociality.

Answer: A. Characterised by an excess or distortion of normal functions, positive symptoms of schizophrenia include hallucinations and delusions.

Scoring

✰✰✰ If you answered all five items correctly, spectacular! We hereby declare you the Grand Sage of Schizophrenia!

✰✰ If you answered three or four items correctly, good show! You're exhibiting superior schizophrenia savvy.

✰ If you answered fewer than three items correctly, don't get paranoid! We'll just chalk it up to a few faulty dopamine receptors.

5 Mood disorders

Just the facts

In this chapter, you'll learn:

♦ effects of mood disorders on functioning

♦ proposed causes of mood disorders

♦ how to assess a person's suicide risk

♦ types of bipolar and depressive disorders

♦ assessment and interventions for people with mood disorders.

A look at mood disorders

Mood disorders are disturbances in the regulation of mood, behaviour and affect that go beyond the normal fluctuations that most people experience. In the United Kingdom 1 person in 100 will suffer from mood disorders. Throughout the world, mood disorders are a leading cause of disability.

This chapter discusses bipolar disorders and depressive disorders. These potentially disabling mood disorders can affect every aspect of a person's life – thought processes, emotions, behaviour and even physical health.

Many people with mood disorders have coexisting mental and physical disorders. For instance, about half of those with major depressive disorder also suffer from an anxiety disorder.

Mood and affect

Mood refers to a pervading feeling. With a mood disorder, a person's mood becomes so intense and persistent that it interferes with social and psychological functioning.

Special affects

Affect refers to the outward expression of emotion attached to ideas – including but not limited to facial expression and vocal modulation. Variations in affect are termed the *range of emotional expression*.

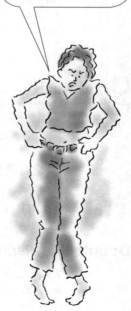

149

People with mood disorders may exhibit various abnormalities in affect, such as:

- blunted affect – severe reduction in the intensity of outward emotional expression
- flat affect – complete or almost complete absence of outward expressional expression
- restricted affect – reduction in the intensity of outward emotional expression
- inappropriate affect – affect that doesn't match the situation or the content of the verbalised message (for instance, laughter when describing a loved one's death)
- labile affect – rapid and easily changing affective expression, unrelated to external events or stimuli.

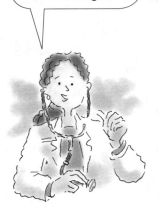

Flat affect – that's one thing I've never been accused of having.

Challenges in caring for people with mood disorders

Caring for people with mood disorders poses numerous challenges.
- Mood disorders may cause primarily somatic (physical) symptoms, so they may be mistaken for physical illnesses.
- The person may neglect self-care because of lowered motivation and energy levels.
- Mood disorders may alter family and social relationships and lead to frustration, anger and guilt. As a result, the person may be the victim or perpetrator of abuse.
- If the person is unable to work because of the mood disorder, financial hardship may occur.
- A seriously depressed person may be at risk for suicide.

Causes

Theories regarding the causes of mood disorders centre on genetic, biological and psychological factors.

Genetic factors

Genetics appear to play a major role in mood disorders. Major depressive disorder and bipolar disorders occur much more often in first-degree relatives than in the general population.

Double the displeasure

Also, studies of identical twins show that when one twin is diagnosed with major depression, the other twin has more than a 70% chance of developing it. Research is underway to pinpoint the specific genetic underpinnings of the various mood disorders.

Biological factors

Biological research into the roots of mood disorder focuses on deficiencies or abnormalities in the brain's chemical messengers – neurotransmitters such as norepinephrine, serotonin, dopamine and acetylcholine. The success of drugs that affect neurotransmitter levels in treating mood disorders supports the theory that these illnesses have biological roots.

Psychological theories

Cognitive, behavioural and psychoanalytic theories also offer explanations for mood disorders.

Cognitive theory

Cognitive theory suggests that people who suffer from depression process information in a characteristically negative way. They view themselves and the world in a negative light and believe these negative perceptions will continue in the future.

Behavioural theory

According to the learned helplessness theory, people may become depressed after a negative event, such as a loved one's death or loss of a job, if the event makes them feel helpless. The perceived lack of control over life events dampens motivation, self-esteem and initiative. Lack of social support and ineffective stress-management and problem-solving skills increase the risk of depression after stressful events.

Psychoanalytical theory

According to psychoanalytical theory, depression results from a harsh superego (the 'conscience' of the unconscious mind) and feelings of loss and aggression. Loss – especially at an early age – makes a child more susceptible to depression later in life.

Anger turned inwards

The child interprets the loss as rejection and a sign that he's unworthy of love. He may feel aggressive towards those who have rejected him, but realises that these aggressive feelings could lead to further rejection. So, he pushes those feelings out of awareness and turns them against himself – and becomes depressed.

A child who feels rejected may ultimately turn his anger inwards.

Bipolar disorders

Bipolar disorders (also called manic-depressive disorders) are mood disorders marked by severe, pathological mood swings. Typically, the person experiences extreme highs (mania or hypomania) alternating with extreme

Myth busters

Bipolar disorder and psychotic symptoms

Many people are confused about the potential for psychotic symptoms in people with bipolar disorder.

Myth: People with bipolar disorder never experience psychotic symptoms.

Reality: Some people with bipolar disorder have rapidly alternating moods, severe impairment in functioning and psychotic features that necessitate hospitalisation.

lows (depression). Interspersed between the highs and the lows are periods of normal mood.

Variations in the pattern of highs and lows can occur. For instance, some people experience only acute episodes of mania.

Millions of moody people

Men and women are affected equally with bipolar disorder. Women, however, are likely to have more depressive episodes, while men experience more manic episodes. (See *Bipolar disorder and psychotic symptoms*.)

Onset usually occurs between ages 20 and 30, although symptoms sometimes arise in late childhood or early adolescence. Roughly 50% of people with bipolar disorder have difficulties in work performance and psychosocial functioning.

Episodes and residuals

Most people with bipolar disorder have recurring episodes of mania and depression across the life span, with symptom-free periods between episodes. Up to one-third experience residual symptoms and a small percentage have chronic, unremitting symptoms despite treatment.

Mania and hypomania

The highs of bipolar disorder may involve either mania or hypomania. *Mania* is characterised by:

- elation
- euphoria
- agitation or irritability
- hyperexcitability
- hyperactivity

- rapid thought and speech
- exaggerated sexuality
- decreased sleep.

Not quite so manic

Hypomania refers to an expansive, elevated or agitated mood that resembles mania but is less intense and lacks psychotic symptoms. For some people, hypomania doesn't cause problems in social activities or work. In fact, it may feel good, bringing high energy, confidence and enhanced social functioning and productivity.

You call that progress?

For others, however, hypomanic episodes can be troublesome. Without proper treatment, these episodes may progress to severe mania or switch to depression.

Psychotic symptoms

Some people with bipolar disorder have severe episodes of mania or depression that involve psychotic symptoms, such as hallucinations (hearing, seeing, touching, smelling or tasting things that aren't actually there) or delusions (false beliefs not influenced by logical reasoning or explained by a person's usual cultural concepts). These people may be misdiagnosed with schizophrenia. (For information on schizophrenia, see Chapter 4).

Implications

The impulsive behaviour of a manic episode may have far-reaching emotional and social consequences – divorce, child abuse, joblessness, bankruptcy and promiscuity, to name a few.

STDs and suicide

People with bipolar disorders have an increased incidence of sexually transmitted diseases (STDs) and unwanted pregnancies. Hyperactivity and sleep disturbances may lead to exhaustion and poor nutrition.

Bipolar disorder also increases the suicide risk. A suicide attempt may occur impulsively during a manic episode or after a depressive episode resolves.

Classification

Bipolar disorder occurs in three major types.
- *Bipolar I disorder* is the classic and most severe disease form. The person has manic episodes or mixed episodes (with symptoms of both mania and depression) that alternate with major depressive episodes. The depressive phase may immediately precede or follow a manic phase, or it may be separated from the manic phase by months or years.
- In *bipolar II disorder*, the person doesn't experience severe mania but instead has milder episodes of hypomania that alternate with depressive episodes.

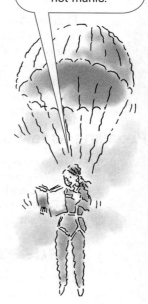

I may be high right now, but I'm not manic.

- In *cyclothymic disorder*, the person has a history of numerous hypomanic episodes intermingled with numerous depressive episodes that don't meet the criteria for major depressive episodes.

Rapid cycling

Ten to 20% of people with bipolar disorder have rapid cycling. In this variant, four or more distinct periods of depression, mania, hypomania or mixed states occur within a 12-month period. Periods of normal mood may be brief or even absent.

The vast majority of rapid cyclers are women. Rapid cycling tends to develop later in the course of illness.

Pedalling as fast as they can

The more rapid the cycling, the more numerous the mood swings. Some sufferers experience multiple illness episodes within a single week. Some ultra-rapid cyclers have several mood swings in a single day.

Experts believe any person with bipolar disorder can 'switch' to a rapid cycling pattern – but most return to their normal bipolar pattern in time.

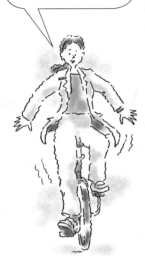

For someone with rapid-cycling bipolar disorder, mood swings come fast and furious.

Causes

The precise cause of bipolar disorder isn't known. However, genetic, biochemical and psychological factors probably play a role.

Genetic factors

Twin, family and adoption studies strongly suggest that bipolar disorder has a genetic component. First-degree relatives of a person with bipolar disorder are about seven times more likely than the general population to develop the disorder. In affected families, researchers have found autosomal dominant inheritance.

Biochemical factors

Experts think bipolar disorder stems at least in part from neurotransmitter abnormalities or imbalances. Some studies suggest the illness involves sensitivity of receptors on nerve cells.

Precipitating events

Stressful life events, such as a serious loss, chronic illness or financial problems, may trigger a bipolar episode in people who are predisposed to the disorder. Other possible triggers include:

- treatment of depression with an antidepressant drug, which may cause a switch to mania
- sleep deprivation
- hypothyroidism.
  However, bipolar episodes can occur with no obvious trigger.

Signs and symptoms

Bipolar disorder can be difficult to diagnose. Assessment findings vary with the illness phase.

During the manic phase

Signs and symptoms that may appear during the manic phase include:
- expansive, grandiose or hyperirritable mood
- increased psychomotor activity, such as agitation, pacing or hand wringing
- excessive social extroversion
- short attention span
- rapid speech with frequent topic changes (flight of ideas)
- decreased need for sleep and food
- impulsivity
- impaired judgement
- easy distractibility
- rapid response to external stimuli, such as background noise or a ringing telephone.

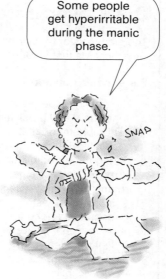

Some people get hyperirritable during the manic phase.

SNAP

Maximal mania

With severe mania, the person may have delusions, paranoid thinking and an inflated sense of self-esteem ranging from uncritical self-confidence to marked grandiosity.

During the depressive phase

During a depressive episode, the person may report or exhibit:
- low self-esteem
- overwhelming inertia
- social withdrawal
- feelings of hopelessness, apathy or self-reproach
- difficulty concentrating or thinking clearly (without obvious disorientation or intellectual impairment)
- psychomotor retardation (sluggish physical movements and activity)
- slowing of speech and responses
- sexual dysfunction
- sleep disturbances (such as difficulty falling or staying asleep or early-morning awakening)
- decreased muscle tone
- weight loss
- slow gait
- constipation.

Diagnosis

The diagnosis of bipolar disorder is confirmed if the person meets the criteria in the *Diagnostic and Statistical Manual of Mental Disorders*, Fourth Edition, Text Revision (*DSM-IV-TR*). (See *Diagnostic criteria: Bipolar disorder*, pages 156 and 157.)

Diagnostic criteria: Bipolar disorder

The diagnosis of bipolar disorder is confirmed when the person meets these criteria from the *Diagnostic and Statistical Manual of Mental Disorders*, Fourth Edition, Text Revision.

For a manic episode

- The person experiences a distinct period of abnormally and persistently elevated, expansive or irritable mood that lasts at least 1 week (or, if hospitalisation is needed, for any duration).
- During the mood disturbance period, at least three of these symptoms persist (four, if the mood is only irritable) and are present to a significant degree:
  - inflated self-esteem or grandiosity
  - decreased need for sleep
  - increased talkativeness
  - flight of ideas or a subjective experience that thoughts are racing
  - distractibility
  - increased goal-directed activity or psychomotor agitation
  - excessive involvement in pleasurable activities with a high potential for painful consequences.
- Symptoms don't meet the criteria for a mixed episode.
- The mood disturbance is severe enough to cause any of these results:
  - marked impairment in occupational functioning or in usual social activities or relationships
  - hospitalisation to prevent harm to self or others
  - evidence of psychotic features.
- Symptoms don't result from the direct physiological effects of a substance or a general medical condition.

For a hypomanic episode

- The person experiences a distinct period of abnormally and persistently elevated, expansive or irritable mood lasting at least 4 days. The mood is clearly different from the usual nondepressed mood.
- During the mood disturbance period, at least three of these symptoms persist (four, if the mood is only irritable) and are present to a significant degree:
  - inflated self-esteem or grandiosity

- decreased need for sleep
- increased talkativeness
- flight of ideas or a subjective experience that thoughts are racing
- distractibility
- increased goal-directed activity or psychomotor agitation
- excessive involvement in pleasurable activities that have a high potential for painful consequences.
- The episode is associated with an unequivocal change in functioning not seen during asymptomatic periods.
- Others can recognise the mood disturbance and the change in functioning.
- The episode isn't severe enough to markedly impair social or occupational functioning or to necessitate hospitalisation to prevent harm to self or others. Also, no psychotic features appear.
- Symptoms don't result from the direct physiological effects of a substance or a general medical condition.

For bipolar I disorder, single manic episode

- The person experiences only one manic episode and has had no past major depressive episodes.
- The manic episode isn't better explained by schizoaffective disorder and isn't superimposed on schizophrenia, schizophreniform disorder, delusional disorder or psychotic disorder not otherwise specified.

For bipolar I disorder, most recent episode hypomanic

- The person is currently experiencing or most recently experienced a hypomanic episode.
- He previously had at least one manic episode or mixed episode.
- Mood symptoms cause clinically significant distress or impairment in social, occupational or other important areas of functioning.

Diagnostic criteria: Bipolar disorder (*continued*)

- The first two exacerbations of the mood episode described previously aren't better explained by schizoaffective disorder and aren't superimposed on schizophrenia, schizophreniform disorder, delusional disorder or psychotic disorder not otherwise specified.

For bipolar I disorder, most recent episode manic

- The person is currently experiencing or most recently experienced a manic episode.
- He previously had at least one major depressive episode, manic episode or mixed episode.
- The first two exacerbations of the mood episode described previously aren't better explained by schizoaffective disorder and aren't superimposed on schizophrenia, schizophreniform disorder, delusional disorder or psychotic disorder not otherwise specified.

For bipolar I disorder, most recent episode mixed

- The person is currently experiencing or most recently experienced a mixed episode.
- He previously had at least one major depressive episode, manic episode or mixed episode.
- The first two exacerbations of the mood episode described previously aren't better explained by schizoaffective disorder and aren't superimposed on schizophrenia, schizophreniform disorder, delusional disorder or psychotic disorder not otherwise specified.

For bipolar I disorder, most recent episode depressed

- The person is currently experiencing or most recently experienced a major depressive episode.
- He previously had at least one manic episode or mixed episode.
- The first two exacerbations of the mood episode described previously aren't better explained by schizoaffective disorder and aren't superimposed

on schizophrenia, schizophreniform disorder, delusional disorder or psychotic disorder not otherwise specified.

For bipolar I disorder, most recent episode unspecified

- Except for duration, the person meets or most recently met the criteria for a manic, hypomanic, mixed or major depressive episode.
- He previously had at least one manic episode or mixed episode.
- Mood symptoms cause clinically significant distress or impairment in social, occupational or other important areas of functioning.
- The first two exacerbations of the mood episode described previously aren't better explained by schizoaffective disorder and aren't superimposed on schizophrenia, schizophreniform disorder, delusional disorder or psychotic disorder not otherwise specified.
- The first two exacerbations of the mood episode didn't result from the direct physiological effects of a substance or a general medical condition.

For bipolar II disorder

- The person currently has, or his history includes, one or more major depressive episodes.
- He currently has, or his history includes, at least one hypomanic episode.
- He has never had a manic or a mixed episode.
- The first two exacerbations of the mood episode described previously aren't better explained by schizoaffective disorder and aren't superimposed on schizophrenia, schizophreniform disorder, delusional disorder or psychotic disorder not otherwise specified.
- Symptoms cause clinically significant distress or impairment in social, occupational or other important areas of functioning.

Treatment

Treatment of bipolar disorder requires drug therapy. Lithium is highly effective in both preventing and relieving manic episodes. It curbs accelerated thought processes and hyperactive behaviour without the sedating effect of antipsychotic drugs. Lithium also may prevent the recurrence of depressive episodes (although it's ineffective in treating acute depression).

> Lithium can be tricky because of its narrow margin of safety.

Not much wiggle room

Lithium has a narrow margin of safety and can easily cause toxicity. Treatment must begin cautiously with a low dose, which is adjusted slowly as needed. The person must maintain therapeutic blood levels for 7–10 days before the desired effects appear, so the doctor may prescribe antipsychotic drugs in the interim for sedation and symptomatic relief. (See *Lithium alert.*)

Other drugs

The doctor may prescribe valproic acid for rapid cyclers or for people who can't tolerate lithium. Carbamazepine may be useful in the prophylaxis of bipolar disorder in service users who are unresponsive to lithium; it seems particularly effective in people with rapid-cycling bipolar disorder (four or more affective episodes a year).

Advice from the experts

Lithium alert

For a person who's receiving lithium, blood level monitoring is crucial because of the drug's narrow therapeutic margin. In fact, lithium shouldn't be used if the person can't have regular blood tests. In addition, because lithium is excreted by the kidneys, it shouldn't be given to service users with renal impairment.

Blood levels should be checked 8–12 hours after the first dose, two or three times weekly for the first month and then weekly to monthly during maintenance therapy.

Person teaching

- Instruct the person to maintain a fluid intake of 2,500–3,000 ml/day to promote adequate lithium excretion.
- Teach him that the lithium may cause sodium depletion, especially during initial therapy until he achieves consistent blood levels. Instruct him not to make dietary changes that might alter his sodium intake because this might reduce lithium elimination and increase the toxicity risk.
- Inform the person that raising his salt intake may increase his lithium excretion – which could lead to the return of mood symptoms. So stress the need to maintain adequate salt and water intake and to eat a normal, well-balanced diet. Remind him that sodium loss (which can result from diarrhoea, illness, extreme sweating or other conditions) may alter lithium levels.
- Teach the person and family to watch for evidence of toxicity – diarrhoea, vomiting, tremors, drowsiness, muscle weakness and ataxia. Instruct him to withhold one dose and call the doctor if toxic symptoms occur – but not to stop taking the drug abruptly.

Flip-flop effect

Antidepressants occasionally are prescribed to treat depressive symptoms. They must be used cautiously, however, because they may trigger a manic episode in people with bipolar disorders.

Nursing interventions

Appropriate nursing interventions vary with the phase of bipolar disorder.

During a manic episode

• Provide for the person's physical needs. Involve him in activities that require gross motor movements.
• Encourage him to eat. He may jump up and walk around the room after every mouthful but will sit down again if you remind him. If he can't sit still long enough to finish a meal, offer high-calorie finger foods, sandwiches, and cheese and crackers to supplement his diet.
• Suggest short daytime naps, and help with personal hygiene. As symptoms subside, encourage him to assume responsibility for personal care.
• Provide diversionary activities suited to a short attention span. Firmly discourage the person if he tries to overextend himself.

Mission: Harmony

• Maintain a calm environment and protect the person from overstimulation, such as from large groups, loud noises and bright colours.
• Provide emotional support and set realistic goals for behaviour.
• Tactfully divert the conversation if it becomes intimately involved with other service users or staff.
• Avoid reinforcing socially inappropriate or suggestive comments.

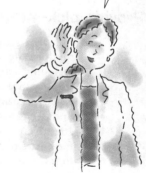

Listen to the person's requests with a neutral attitude.

Limit setting and listening

• In a calm, clear, self-confident manner, set limits for the person's demanding, hyperactive, manipulative and acting-out behaviours. Don't leave an opening for him to test or argue with you.
• Listen to requests attentively and with a neutral attitude, but avoid power struggles if the service user pressures you for an immediate answer. Explain that you'll seriously consider the request and respond later.
• Collaborate with other staff members to provide consistent responses to the service user's manipulations or acting out.
• Anticipate the need for excessive verbalisation.

No Oscars for acting out

• Watch for early signs of frustration – when the person's anger escalates from verbal threats to hitting an object.
• Tell the person firmly that threats and hitting are unacceptable and indicate that he needs help to control his behaviour. Inform him that the

staff will help him move to a quiet area and help him control his behaviour so that he won't hurt himself or others. Staff members who have practised as a team can work effectively to prevent acting-out behaviour or to remove and confine the person.

• Alert the care team promptly when acting-out behaviour escalates. It's safer to have help available before you need it than to try controlling an anxious or frightened person by yourself.

• When the acting-out incident ends and the person is calm and in control, discuss his feelings with him and offer suggestions to prevent recurrence.

Minding medications

• Advise the person to take lithium with food or after meals to avoid stomach upset.

• Because lithium may impair mental and physical function, caution the person against driving or operating dangerous equipment.

• Teach the person to discontinue lithium and notify the doctor if he experiences toxicity symptoms, such as diarrhoea, abdominal cramps, vomiting, unsteadiness, drowsiness, muscle weakness, frequent urination or tremors.

During a depressive episode

• Provide for the person's physical needs. If he's too depressed to care for himself, help with personal hygiene.

• Encourage him to eat, or feed him if necessary. If he's constipated, add high-fibre foods to his diet; offer small, frequent meals; and encourage physical activity.

• To help the person sleep, give him back rubs or warm milk at bedtime.

Provide pick-me-ups

• Keep in mind that a depressed person needs continual positive reinforcement to improve his self-esteem. Provide a structured routine, including activities to boost confidence and promote interaction with others (for instance, group therapy). Keep reassuring him that his depression will lift.

• Assume an active role in communicating. Encourage the person to talk or to write down his feelings if he's having trouble expressing them. Listen attentively and respectfully. If he seems sluggish, give him time to formulate his thoughts. Record your observations and conversations to assist in evaluating his condition.

• Avoid overwhelming the person with expectations.

Injury aversion

• To prevent self-injury or suicide, remove harmful objects (such as glass, belts, rope and bobby pins) from the person's environment.

• Institute suicide precautions as dictated by facility policy.

• Observe the person closely, and strictly supervise his medications.

Medication teaching

- If the person is taking lithium, instruct him to maintain a normal diet with normal salt and water intake. Inform him that restricting sodium intake increases lithium toxicity.
- Teach the person the importance of continuing his medication regimen even if he doesn't feel a need for it.
- If the person is taking an antidepressant, watch for signs and symptoms of mania.

Cyclothymic disorder

In cyclothymic disorder, short periods of mild depression alternate with short periods of hypomania. Between the depressive and manic episodes, brief periods of normal mood occur. The person never goes more than 2 months without symptoms of depression or hypomania.

In many people with cyclothymic disorder, manic episodes emerge over a few days to weeks – although onset within hours is possible.

Cyclothymic disorder affects up to 1% of the population, striking men and women equally. Typically, onset occurs in the teens or early twenties.

Mood indigo

Both the depressive and hypomanic periods of cyclothymic disorder are shorter and less severe than in bipolar I or II disorder. Also, delusions don't occur, and few people required hospitalisation.

Nonetheless, mood swings may impair social and occupational functioning. Also, many people progress to a more severe form of bipolar illness. Approximately 30% experience a full-blown manic episode or major depression, with a consequent change in diagnosis to bipolar I or II disorder.

Damage and instability

Hypomanic periods of cyclothymic disorder may enhance a person's achievement in business and artistic endeavours – but also may damage interpersonal and social relationships. The person's instability may lead to an uneven work and academic history, impulsive and frequent changes of residence, repeated romantic or marital breakups and an episodic pattern of alcohol and drug abuse. Many people with cyclothymic disorder self-medicate with alcohol or illegal drugs.

Signs and symptoms

General features of cyclothymia include:
- an odd, eccentric or suspicious personality
- dramatic, erratic or antisocial personality features
- inability to maintain enthusiasm for new projects

- a pattern of pulling close and then pushing away in interpersonal relationships
- abrupt changes in personality from cheerful, confident and energetic to sad, blue or mean.
  Other signs and symptoms vary with the illness phase.

During the hypomanic phase
The person experiencing the hypomanic phase may report or exhibit:
- insomnia
- hyperactivity
- inflated self-esteem
- increased productivity and creativity
- over-involvement in pleasurable activities, including sex
- physical restlessness
- rapid speech.

During the depressive phase
Signs and symptoms during the depressive phase may include:
- insomnia or hypersomnia
- feelings of inadequacy
- decreased productivity
- social withdrawal
- loss of libido
- loss of interest in pleasurable activities
- lethargy
- depressed speech
- crying.

> Physical restlessness is a possible sign of hypomania.

Causes

Most likely, genetic factors influence the development of cyclothymic disorder. Many people have a family history of bipolar disorder, major depression, substance abuse or suicide.

Diagnosis

The doctor must rule out various disorders to accurately diagnose cyclothymia. Medical disorders that can mimic cyclothymia include:
- acquired immunodeficiency syndrome
- Cushing's disease
- epilepsy
- Huntington's disease
- hyperthyroidism
- premenstrual syndrome
- migraines
- multiple sclerosis
- neoplasm
- postpartum depression

- stroke
- systemic lupus erythematosus
- trauma
- uraemia
- vitamin deficiency
- Wilson's disease.

Copycat conditions

Psychiatric disorders that can mimic cyclothymic disorder include:
- mood disorder caused by substance abuse or a general medical condition
- bipolar I or II disorder with rapid cycling
- borderline personality disorder.

The diagnosis is confirmed if the person meets the criteria in the *DSM-IV-TR*. (See *Diagnostic criteria: Cyclothymic disorder*.)

Treatment

Pharmacological options for cyclothymic disorder include:
- lithium
- carbamazepine
- valproic acid
- verapamil.

Other therapies may include individual psychotherapy and couple or family therapy, which can help people deal with relationship problems associated with the disorder.

Diagnostic criteria: Cyclothymic disorder

The person is diagnosed with cyclothymic disorder if he meets these criteria from the *Diagnostic and Statistical Manual of Mental Disorders,* Fourth Edition, Text Revision.

Characteristic features

- For at least 2 years, the person experiences numerous periods with hypomanic symptoms as well as numerous periods with depressive symptoms that don't meet the criteria for a major depressive episode.
- During this 2-year period, the person hasn't been without the previously described symptoms for more than 2 months at a time.
- No major depressive, manic or mixed episode occurred during the first 2 years of the disturbance. (After the first 2 years of cyclothymic disorder, superimposed manic or mixed episodes may occur; in this case, both bipolar I disorder and cyclothymic disorder may be diagnosed. If superimposed major depressive episodes also occur, both bipolar II disorder and cyclothymic disorder may be diagnosed.)

Other features

- Symptoms aren't better explained by schizoaffective disorder and aren't superimposed on schizophrenia, schizophreniform disorder, delusional disorder or psychotic disorder.
- Symptoms don't result from the direct physiological effects of a substance or a general medical condition.
- Symptoms cause clinically significant distress or impairment in social, occupational or other important areas of functioning.

Nursing interventions

These nursing interventions may be appropriate for people with cyclothymic disorder.

- Explore ways to help the person cope with frequent mood changes.
- Encourage vocational opportunities that allow flexible work hours.
- Urge a person with artistic ability to pursue a career in the arts, where mood changes may be better tolerated.

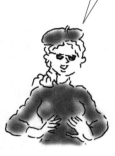

Some roses are red, dude. And violets are blue. If you're cyclothymic, the art world's calling you.

Major depressive disorder

Major depressive disorder (also called unipolar major depression) is a syndrome of a persistent sad mood lasting 2 weeks or longer. The feeling of sadness is accompanied by:

- feelings of guilt, helplessness or hopelessness
- poor concentration
- sleep disturbances
- lethargy
- appetite loss
- anhedonia (inability to feel pleasure)
- loss of mood reactivity (failure to feel a mood uplift in response to something positive)
- thoughts of death.

Major depression often goes undiagnosed, and those who have it commonly receive inadequate treatment.

Beyond sad to bad

In major depressive disorder, sad feelings go beyond – and last longer than – 'normal' sadness or grief. Also, some symptoms of severe depression (such as disinterest in pleasurable activities, hopelessness and loss of mood reactivity) rarely accompany 'normal' sadness.

In harm's way

Major depression can profoundly alter a person's social, family and occupational functioning. Suicide – the most serious complication – can occur if feelings of worthlessness, guilt and hopelessness are so overwhelming that the person no longer considers life worth living.

Nearly 15% of people with untreated depression commit suicide. Most of them sought help from a doctor within 1 month of death.

What a bummer

At some time in their lives, about 8% of the population experience major depressive disorder. The incidence of major depression rises with age. Onset usually occurs in early adulthood, with recurrences throughout the person's lifetime.

It's baaaaack!

Recurrences may follow a prolonged symptom-free period or may occur sporadically. For some people, they come in clusters. For others, recurrences grow more frequent with age.

About 50% of those affected have their first episode of depression at about age 40 – but this may be shifting downwards to the 30s. More than 50% of people who have one episode go on to have at least two more. An untreated episode can last from 1 month to a year – or even longer.

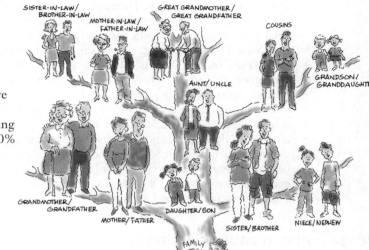

Causes

Genetic, biochemical, physical, psychological and social factors have been implicated in major depression. The relationship between psychological stress, stressful life events and depression onset is unclear. However, the person's history often reveals a specific personal loss or severe stress. According to one theory, the stressor interacts with the person's predisposition to provoke major depression.

Genetic basis

Depression is two to three times more common in people with first-degree relatives with the disorder, indicating a genetic vulnerability. Although some researchers believe a single depression gene exists, mounting evidence suggests several genes may be involved in depression.

Biochemical defects

The neural networks of the brain's prefrontal cortex and basal ganglia may be the primary defect sites in major depressive disorder.

The serotonin, neuroendocrine and hypothalamic–pituitary–adrenal regulation systems may also be involved in development of depression. Differences in biological rhythms may also play a role, as seen by changes in circadian rhythms and various neurochemical and neurohormonal factors.

Finally, some researchers are homing in on abnormal cortisol levels as a factor in depression. In the dexamethasone suppression test, about 50% of people with depression fail to suppress cortisol levels.

Organic causes

Health care professionals must distinguish major depression from depression caused by a specific event or a recognisable organic condition. Secondary depression can result from a wide range of physical disorders, including:

- metabolic disturbances, such as hypoxia and hypercalcaemia
- endocrine disorders, such as diabetes and Cushing's disease
- neurological diseases, such as Parkinson's disease and Alzheimer's disease
- cancer (especially of the pancreas)
- viral and bacterial infections, such as influenza and pneumonia
- cardiovascular disorders, such as heart failure
- pulmonary disorders, such as chronic obstructive lung disease
- musculoskeletal disorders, such as degenerative arthritis
- GI disorders, such as irritable bowel syndrome
- genitourinary problems, such as incontinence
- collagen vascular diseases, such as lupus
- anaemias.

Drugs that can cause depression

Drugs prescribed for certain medical and psychiatric conditions can cause depression; examples include:

- antihypertensives
- psychotropics
- anti-Parkinsonian drugs
- narcotic and nonnarcotic analgesics
- numerous cardiovascular medications
- oral antidiabetics
- antimicrobials
- steroids
- chemotherapeutic agents
- cimetidine.
  Alcohol use may also contribute to depression.

Signs and symptoms

During the assessment interview, a person with major depression may seem unhappy or apathetic. He may report such changes as:

- feeling 'down in the dumps'
- increased or decreased appetite
- sleep disturbances (for example, insomnia or early awakening)
- disinterest in sex
- difficulty concentrating or thinking clearly
- easy distractibility
- indecisiveness
- low self-esteem
- poor coping
- constipation or diarrhoea.

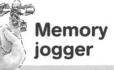

Memory jogger

Can't remember the things that may predispose a service user to suicide? The term RISK FACTORS can guide you.

R Relationship difficulties

I Intense feelings of hopelessness or helplessness

S Sex differences (females make more suicide attempts; males succeed more often)

K Kinship supports are weak or nonexistent

F Family abuse or other types of abuse

A Age extremes (those under age 19 and over age 65 are at highest risk)

C Chronic or debilitating health problems

T Thinking is distorted

O Overreacts to stress

R Revenge or rage present

S Substance abuse

The person may report that symptoms are worse in the morning.

During the physical examination, you may note agitation (such as hand wringing or restlessness) or psychomotor retardation (slow movements). With severe depression, the person may have delusions of persecution or guilt, which can have an immobilising effect.

Psychosocial clues

The psychosocial history may reveal life problems or losses that may explain or contribute to depression. Or, the medical history may implicate a physical disorder or use of a prescription drug or other substances that can cause depression.

A danger to oneself

Stay alert for clues to suicidal thoughts, a preoccupation with death or previous suicide attempts. Many people are reluctant to verbalise suicidal thoughts unless prompted, so you may need to assess the person's suicide risk by asking direct questions.

A person who has specific suicide plans or significant risk factors (such as a history of a suicide attempt, profound hopelessness, concurrent medical illness, substance abuse or social isolation) should be referred to a mental health specialist for immediate care. (See *Obstacles to detecting depression*, page 168.)

Diagnosis

The doctor may administer psychological tests, such as the Beck Depression Inventory, to determine symptom onset, severity, duration and progression.

Memory jogger

For a depressed person, positive OUTCOMES include:

O Overwhelming feelings of grief and loss are processed

U Uses problem-solving and reasoning skills to handle stressors

T Talks with others willingly and appropriately

C Cognitive distortions are decreased or eliminated

O Overcomes thoughts of physically harming self

M Maintains a positive sense of self

E Eats nutritionally balanced meals and snacks

S Sleeps 6–8 hours each night

Bridging the gap

Obstacles to detecting depression

Always consider the person's cultural background and values when assessing for signs and symptoms of depression. In most parts of the world, depression and other mood disorders are viewed as social or moral problems – not as mental health problems appropriate to discuss with health care providers.

Even in the United Kingdom, many people from both mainstream and immigrant cultures feel that depression implies a moral weakness. As a result, they're likely to deny or minimise their emotional distress and express it instead as more socially acceptable somatic (physical) symptoms.

Diagnostic criteria: Major depressive disorder

The service user is diagnosed with major depressive disorder if he meets these criteria for a single major depressive episode from the *Diagnostic and Statistical Manual of Mental Disorders,* Fourth Edition, Text Revision.

Characteristic symptoms

At least five of these symptoms are present nearly every day during the same 2-week period, and represent a change from the service user's previous functioning (one symptom must be either depressed mood or loss of interest in previously pleasurable activities):

- depressed mood most of the day, as indicated by either subjective account or others' observation
- markedly diminished interest or pleasure in all, or almost all, activities, most of the day
- significant weight loss or gain when not dieting, or a decrease or increase in appetite (in children, consider failure to make expected weight gains)
- insomnia or hypersomnia
- psychomotor agitation or retardation
- fatigue or loss of energy
- feelings of worthlessness or excessive or inappropriate guilt

- diminished ability to think or concentrate, or indecisiveness
- recurrent thoughts of death, recurrent suicidal ideation with no specific plan, a suicide attempt or a specific plan for committing suicide.

Other features

- Symptoms don't meet the criteria for a mixed episode.
- Symptoms cause clinically significant distress or impairment in social, occupational or other important areas of functioning.
- Symptoms don't result from the direct physiological effects of a substance or a general medical condition.
- Symptoms aren't better explained by bereavement; they last longer than 2 months, or they're characterised by marked functional impairment, morbid preoccupation with worthlessness, suicidal ideation, psychotic symptoms or psychomotor retardation.

The dexamethasone suppression test may show failure to suppress cortisol secretion in people with depression (although this test has a high false-negative rate). Toxicology screening may suggest drug-induced depression. The diagnosis is confirmed if the person meets the criteria in the *DSM-IV-TR*. (See *Diagnostic criteria: Major depressive disorder*.)

Treatment

The primary treatments for major depressive disorder are pharmacological therapy, electroconvulsive therapy (ECT) and psychotherapy.

Pharmacological therapy

Medication is the most effective means of achieving remission and preventing relapse. Combining medication with psychotherapy can improve the treatment outcome by helping the person cope with low self-esteem and demoralisation.

Types of antidepressants

Generally, antidepressant drugs work by modifying the activity of relevant neurotransmitter pathways. These agents fall into several categories:

* selective serotonin reuptake inhibitors (SSRIs)
* serotonin/norepinephrine reuptake inhibitors (SNRIs)
* atypical antidepressants
* tricyclic antidepressants (TCAs)
* monoamine oxidase inhibitors (MAOIs)
* other antidepressants.

No ideal antidepressant exists for all service users. The doctor must consider the service user's metabolism, possible side effects, agents that have been effective with family members and potential for toxicity (if suicidal overdose is a concern).

Whichever drug is prescribed, the service user's response should be reevaluated after the first 2 months of therapy, with dosage changes made as needed. After remission, drug therapy should continue for at least 6–9 months. (See *Matching the treatment to the culture*.)

Selective serotonin reuptake inhibitors

SSRIs include citalopram, fluoxetine, fluvoxamine, paroxetine and sertraline. These agents inhibit serotonin reuptake and may inhibit the reuptake of other neurotransmitters as well.

SSRIs have become the first-choice treatment for most people. They lack most of the disturbing side effects associated with TCAs and MAOIs.

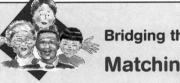

Bridging the gap

Matching the treatment to the culture

No matter what the diagnosis, always consider the person's cultural and religious background. Some people, for instance, may have cultural or religious reasons for not complying with the prescribed medication regimen. They may oppose taking medication for fear they'll become addicted. They may refuse medications in the belief that Western medicine is too strong for their bodies.

When this occurs, consider possible alternative treatments.

Serotonin/norepinephrine reuptake inhibitors

SNRIs, such as venlafaxine, inhibit norepinephrine uptake. They're generally used as second-line agents for service users with major depressive disorder.

Atypical antidepressants

Atypical antidepressants include trazodone and mirtazapine. These drugs' mechanisms of action aren't well understood. Trazadone inhibits serotonin and norepinephrine reuptake. Mirtazapine is thought to inhibit serotonin and norepinephrine reuptake while blocking two specific serotonin receptors.

Although effective in certain service users, atypical antidepressants generally are used as second-line agents.

Tricyclic antidepressants

An older class of antidepressants, TCAs inhibit the reuptake of norepinephrine, serotonin and dopamine and cause a gradual decline in beta-adrenergic receptors.

Specific TCAs include:
- amitriptyline
- amoxapine
- clomipramine
- doxepin
- imipramine
- nortriptyline
- trimipramine.

Although TCAs can be effective, they may cause intolerable side effects. Consequently, they generally aren't used as first-line agents.

Monoamine oxidase inhibitors

MAOIs, such as phenelzine and tranylcypromine, increase norepinephrine, serotonin and dopamine levels by inhibiting MAO, an enzyme that inactivates them. They may have additional actions that contribute to their antidepressant effect.

MAOIs may be prescribed for people with atypical depression (for example, depression marked by an increased appetite and increased sleep, rather than anorexia and insomnia) or for people who don't respond to TCAs.

Although often effective, MAOIs carry a high risk of side effects and dangerous interactions with various foods and medications. Consequently, they're rarely used today – although conservative doses may be combined with a TCA for people refractory to either type of drug alone.

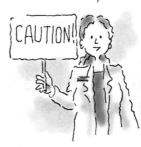

MAOIs can cause serious side effects and dangerous interactions with foods and other drugs.

Other antidepressants

Other antidepressants, such as mirtazapine, have varying mechanisms of action. They're generally used as second-line agents. (See *Pharmacological therapy for mood disorders*, pages 171, 172 and 173.)

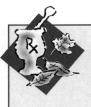

Meds matters

Pharmacological therapy for mood disorders

This chart highlights several of the drugs used to treat mood disorders.

Drug	Side effects	Contraindications	Nursing considerations
Monoamine oxidase inhibitor (MAOI)			
Isocarboxazid	• Blurred vision • Constipation • Dry mouth • Drowsiness or insomnia • Fatigue • Hepatic dysfunction (jaundice, malaise, right upper abdominal quadrant pain, change in stool colour or consistency) • Hypertensive crisis • Hypomania • Muscle twitching • Orthostatic hypotension • Skin rash • Vertigo • Weakness • Weight gain	• Cardiovascular or cerebrovascular disease • Confusion, uncooperativeness • Elderly or debilitated people • Glaucoma • Heart failure • History of severe headaches • Impaired renal function • Liver disease • Paranoid schizophrenia • Pregnancy	• Monitor service user's blood pressure every 2–4 hours during initial therapy. Instruct service user to change positions slowly. • Assess for signs and symptoms of hypertensive crisis. • Monitor fluid intake and output. • Monitor service user for suicidal risk. • Caution service user not to ingest foods and beverages containing tyramine, caffeine, or tryptophan. Warn him that ingesting tyramine can cause a hypertensive crisis. Give him a list of foods and beverages that contain substances that include aged cheeses, sour cream, beer, Chianti, aged sherry, pickled herring, liver, canned figs, raisins, bananas, avocados, chocolate, soy, smoked fish, sausage, bologna, fava beans, yeast extracts, meat tenderisers, coffee and colas. • Instruct service user to avoid, epinephrine, local anaesthetics, decongestants, cough medicines, diet pills and most over-the-counter agents. • Teach service user to wear medical identification jewellery. • Advise service user to go to the Accident & Emergency department immediately if hypertensive crisis develops.
Tricyclic antidepressant			
Amitriptyline Imipramine	• Agranulocytosis • Arrhythmias • Blurred vision • Bone marrow depression • Constipation • Dry mouth • Oesophageal reflux • Galactorrhoea • Hallucinations • Heart failure	• Concomitant use of MAOIs • Recent myocardial infarction (MI) • Renal or hepatic disease	• Supervise service user's drug ingestion. • Monitor blood pressure and pulse for signs of orthostatic hypotension. • Monitor liver function and complete blood counts. • Institute suicide precautions as needed. • Know that special monitoring is required if service user poses a suicide risk or has a history of angle-closure glaucoma or seizure disorder. • Instruct service user to change positions slowly. • Tell service user to avoid driving or hazardous machinery if drowsiness occurs.

(continued)

Pharmacological therapy for mood disorders (*continued*)

Drug	Side effects	Contraindications	Nursing considerations
Tricyclic antidepressant (continued)			
	• Increased or decreased libido • Jaundice and fatigue • Mania • MI • Orthostatic hypotension or hypertension • Palpitations • Shock • Slowed intracardiac conduction • Urinary hesitancy • Weight gain		• Instruct service user to avoid alcohol and over-the-counter agents unless the doctor approves. • Inform service user that the drug may take up to 4 weeks to become effective.
Selective serotonin reuptake inhibitor			
Fluoxetine	• Dry mouth • Insomnia • Nausea • Nervousness • Rash • Vertigo • Weight loss	• Within 14 days of taking an MAOI	• Know that this drug is usually given in the morning with or without food. • Monitor service user for weight loss if nausea occurs. • Know that service user should wait 5 weeks after stopping fluoxetine before starting an MAOI. • Tell service user to avoid alcoholic beverages. • Instruct service user to report side effects to the doctor, especially rash or itching.
Anticonvulsant (for treatment of bipolar disorder)			
Divalproex sodium	• Abdominal cramps • Diarrhoea or constipation • Double vision or seeing 'spots' • Increased urination • Indigestion • Nausea • Prolonged bleeding time • Sedation • Skin rashes • Vomiting	• Liver disease	• Monitor liver function tests and platelet counts. • Instruct service user to take the drug with meals if stomach upset occurs. • Urge service user to report excessive bruising or unexplained bleeding. • Caution service user not to discontinue the drug abruptly. • Instruct service user not to crush tablets. • Caution service user to avoid alcohol while taking this drug.

Pharmacological therapy for mood disorders (*continued*)

Drug	Side effects	Contraindications	Nursing considerations
Antimanic drug			
Lithium carbonate	• Below 1.5 mmol/l: fine hand tremors, dry mouth, increased thirst, increased urination, nausea • 1.5–2.0 mmol/l: vomiting, diarrhoea, muscle weakness, ataxia, dizziness, confusion, slurred speech • 2.0–2.5 mmol/l: persistent nausea and vomiting, blurred vision, muscle twitching, hyperactive deep tendon reflexes • 2.5–3.0 mmol/l: myoclonic twitches or movements of an entire limb, choreathetoid movements, urinary and faecal incontinence • Above 3.0 mmol/l: seizures, cardiac arrhythmias, hypotension, peripheral vascular collapse, death	• Early pregnancy	• Monitor serum drug levels. • Instruct service user not to chew extended-release preparations but to swallow them whole. • Supervise service user during administration to ensure that the medication is swallowed. • To relieve dry mouth or increased thirst, instruct service user to increase fluids or eat sugarless gum or boiled sweets. • If service user has increased urination, suggest limiting fluids after 8 p.m. Evaluate for diabetes insipidus, dilute urine or low specific gravity. • For nausea, suggest service user take the drug with food. • Instruct service user to maintain adequate sodium intake. • Inform service user that metallic taste may occur while taking this drug. • Teach service user to take the drug even when feeling better and not to stop it abruptly. • Instruct service user to monitor weight weekly. • Caution service user not to take the drug with alcohol. • Instruct service user to notify the doctor if severe vomiting or diarrhoea occur. • Instruct female service user to use a reliable form of contraception while on this drug. • Tell service user to get the doctor's approval before taking any new medications. • Instruct service user not to stop taking the drug without discussing it with the doctor.

Electroconvulsive therapy

In ECT, a tiny electrical current is applied to the person's brain through electrodes. The current produces a seizure lasting from 30 seconds to 1 minute.

A quicker picker-upper

Although controversial, ECT sometimes is used to treat severe depression when psychotherapy and medication aren't effective, when ECT poses a lower risk than other treatments or when the service user is at immediate risk of suicide. ECT produces faster results than antidepressant drugs.

Get ready, get set . . .

The service user fasts for 6–8 hours before ECT. Just before the session, dentures, glasses, hearing aids, contact lenses and hairpins are removed and the service user is asked to go to the toilet. He receives various drugs, including:
- atropine or glycopyrronium bromide to reduce secretions, prevent aspiration and reduce the risk of bradycardia
- a short-acting general anaesthetic
- a muscle relaxant
- oxygen.

A bite block is inserted to prevent tongue biting during the seizure, and the service user is connected to devices that monitor his brain waves, heart rhythm and arterial oxygen saturation.

. . . Get zapped

Then a 1-second electrical current is applied to the brain through electrodes placed above the temples. The current produces a brief seizure.

In a typical course of treatment for major depression, the service user receives 2 or 3 ECT treatments a week, for a total of 6–12 treatments. Contraindications include recent myocardial infarction, a history of stroke and intracranial lesions.

Psychotherapy

Short-term psychotherapy can aid in relieving major depression. Many psychiatrists believe the best results occur from combining individual, family or group psychotherapy with medication.

After the acute episode of depression resolves, a person with a history of recurrent depression may be maintained on a low dose of an antidepressant drug as a preventive measure.

Nursing interventions

These nursing interventions may be appropriate for a person with major depression.
- Provide for the person's physical needs. If he's too depressed to perform self-care, help him with personal hygiene. Encourage him to eat, or feed him if necessary. If he's constipated, add high-fibre foods to his diet; offer small, frequent meals; and encourage physical activity and fluid intake. Give him warm milk or back rubs at bedtime to improve sleep.
- Record all observations and conversations with the person. They're valuable in evaluating his response to treatment.
- Plan activities for times when the person's energy level peaks.

Connection and communication

- Assume an active role in initiating communication.
- Share your observations of the person's behaviour. You might say, 'You're sitting all by yourself, looking sad. Is that how you feel?'

- The person may think and react sluggishly, so speak slowly and allow ample time for him to respond.
- Avoid feigned cheerfulness, but don't hesitate to laugh with him and point out the value of humour.
- Encourage the person to talk about and write down his feelings. Show him he's important by listening attentively and respectfully, avoiding interruptions and remaining nonjudgemental.

> With this beastly mood you're in, you need a lot of TLC.

Structure and socialisation

- Provide a structured routine, including noncompetitive activities, to build the person's self-confidence and promote interaction with others. Urge him to socialise and join group activities.
- Try to spend some time with the person each day so that he doesn't become isolated. Avoid long periods of silence, which tend to increase anxiety.

Self-help suggestions

- Reassure the person he can help ease depression by expressing his feelings, engaging in pleasurable activities and improving his grooming and hygiene.
- Teach the person about depression. Emphasise that effective methods are available to relieve symptoms.
- Help him recognise distorted perceptions, and link them to his depression. When he learns to recognise depressive thought patterns, he can consciously begin to substitute self-affirming thoughts.

Inklings of suicide

- Ask the person if he thinks of death or suicide. Such thoughts signal an immediate need for consultation and assessment. Failure to detect suicidal thoughts early may encourage a suicide attempt.
- Be aware that the suicide risk rises as depression lifts. (See *Recognising suicide potential*, page 176.)

> Alcohol is a big no-no for a service user during TCA or SSRI therapy.

Medication edification

- If the person is taking an antidepressant, stress the need for compliance, and review side effects. For drugs that produce strong anticholinergic effects (such as amitriptyline and amoxapine), suggest using sugarless gum or hard boiled sweets to relieve dry mouth. For sedating antidepressants (such as amitriptyline and trazodone), warn the person to avoid activities that require alertness, including driving and operating mechanical equipment.
- Some antidepressants lower the seizure threshold, so monitor the person for seizures.
- Inform the person that antidepressants may take several weeks to produce the desired effect.
- Caution the service user taking a TCA or an SSRI to avoid drinking alcoholic beverages or taking other central nervous system depressants during therapy.

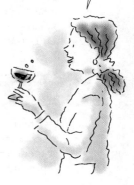

Advice from the experts

Recognising suicide potential

A person with a mood disorder may be at risk for attempting suicide. Stay alert for:

- overwhelming anxiety (the most frequent trigger for a suicide attempt)
- withdrawal and social isolation
- saying farewell to friends and family
- putting affairs in order
- giving away prized possessions
- sending covert suicide messages and death wishes
- expressing obvious suicidal thoughts ('I'd be better off dead')
- describing a suicide plan
- hoarding medications
- talking about death and a feeling of futility
- behaviour changes, especially as depression begins to subside.

Taking action

If you think the person is at risk for suicide, take these steps:

- Keep communication lines open. Maintaining personal contact may help the suicidal person feel he isn't alone or without resources or hope. Continuity of care and consistency of primary nurses also can help him maintain emotional ties to others – the ultimate technique for preventing suicide.
- To ensure a safe environment, check for dangerous conditions, such as exposed pipes, windows without safety glass and access to the roof or open balconies.
- Remove belts, sharp objects such as razors, knives, nail files and clippers, suspenders, light cords and glass from the service user's room.
- Make sure an acutely suicidal person is observed around the clock. Stay alert when he uses a sharp object (as when shaving), takes medications or uses the bathroom (to prevent hanging or other injury). Assign him a room near the nurses' station and with another service user.

FYI on MAOIs

- If the service user is taking a MAOI, emphasise that he must avoid foods that contain tyramine, caffeine or tryptophan. Warn him that ingesting tyramine can cause a hypertensive crisis. Give him a list of foods and beverages that contain these substances, which include aged cheeses, sour cream, beer, Chianti, sherry, pickled herring, liver, canned figs, raisins, bananas, avocados, chocolate, soy sauce, fava beans, yeast extracts, meat tenderisers, coffee and colas.

Dysthymic disorder

Dysthymic disorder, or dysthymia, refers to mild depression that lasts at least 2 years in adults or 1 year in children. The depression is relatively mild or moderate, and most service users aren't certain when they first became depressed.

Despite its relative mildness, dysthymic disorder may impair functioning at home, in school or at work. However, hospitalisation rarely is needed unless suicidal intent is present.

Dysthymic disorder may affect up to 3% of the population. It's twice as common in women as in men and more prevalent among the poor and the unmarried.

Depressed? Who – me?

This disorder often goes unrecognised by those experiencing it, as well as by their family and friends. People with dysthymic disorder may not consider themselves depressed. Because of the mild symptoms – which may be physical rather than emotional – people typically see a mental health professional only if dysthymia progresses to major depression.

Even when recognised, dysthymia is hard to treat. Recovery is slower if the condition becomes chronic and goes untreated.

Additional agonies

An estimated 75% of service users with dysthymic disorder have a coexisting psychiatric or medical disorder, such as heart disease, cancer, diabetes or another psychiatric disorder (for instance, substance abuse or an anxiety disorder).

Causes

Biological, psychological and medical factors may play a role in dysthymic disorder. Many people with dysthymic disorder have below-normal serotonin levels, so it's likely that serotonin is involved in development of this disorder.

As with many other psychiatric disorders, personality problems and multiple stressors, combined with inadequate coping skills, may increase a person's vulnerability to this disorder.

Signs and symptoms

Signs and symptoms of dysthymic disorder include:
• persistent sad, anxious or empty mood
• loss of interest in activities previously enjoyed
• excessive crying
• increased feelings of guilt, helplessness or hopelessness
• weight or appetite changes
• sleep difficulties
• poor school or work performance
• social withdrawal
• conflicts with family and friends
• increased restlessness and irritability
• poor concentration
• inability to take decisions

- reduced energy level
- thoughts of death or suicide, or suicide attempts
- physical symptoms, such as headache or backache.

Diagnosis

The person may be diagnosed with dysthymic disorder after a careful psychiatric examination and medical history are performed by a psychiatrist or other mental health professional. The diagnosis is confirmed if the person meets the criteria in the *DSM-IV-TR*. (See *Diagnostic criteria: Dysthymic disorder*.)

Treatment

Short-term psychotherapy teaches the person more constructive ways of communicating with family, friends and co-workers. It also allows ongoing assessment of suicidal ideation and suicide risk.

Behavioural therapy may be used to reeducate the person in social skills and help him make attitude changes. Group therapy can help him change maladaptive social functioning.

A person who's under a lot of stress and lacks the skills to cope may be destined for dysthymia.

Diagnostic criteria: Dysthymic disorder

Dysthymic disorder is diagnosed if the person meets these criteria from the *Diagnostic and Statistical Manual of Mental Disorders,* Fourth Edition, Text Revision.

Depression symptoms

For at least 2 years, the person experiences a depressed mood most of the day for more days than not, as indicated either by his own account or by others' observation.

During the period of depression, at least two of these symptoms are present:

- poor appetite or overeating
- difficulty sleeping or increased need for sleep
- low energy or fatigue
- low self-esteem
- poor concentration or difficulty taking decisions
- feelings of hopelessness.

Other features

- During the 2-year period, the person has never been without depression or the previously described symptoms for more than 2 months at a time.

- The person didn't experience major depressive disorder during the first 2 years of the disturbance. Or, if major depressive disorder did occur, he had a full remission (with no significant signs or symptoms for 2 months) before dysthymic disorder developed.
- The person has never had a manic, hypomanic or mixed episode and has never met the criteria for cyclothymic disorder.
- The disorder doesn't occur within the course of a chronic psychotic disorder, such as schizophrenia.
- Symptoms don't stem directly from substance abuse, other medication use or a general medical condition (such as hypothyroidism).
- Symptoms cause multiple functional impairments, such as impaired social and occupational functioning.

Pharmacological treatment of dysthymic disorder may involve antidepressants, such as SSRIs or TCAs. People who exhibit pessimism, disinterest and low self-esteem typically respond to antidepressant drugs.

Nursing interventions

These nursing interventions may be appropriate for a service user with dysthymic disorder.

* Provide supportive measures, such as reassurance, warmth, availability and acceptance – even if the service user becomes hostile.
* Teach the service user about the illness and prescribed antidepressant medication.
* Urge him to engage in activities that enhance his sense of accomplishment.
* Encourage positive health habits, such as eating well-balanced meals, avoiding drugs and alcohol (which can worsen depression) and getting physical exercise (which can lift his mood).

Post-natal depression

Post-natal depression (PND) is one of the most common and most severe complications after childbirth. About half of new mothers feel weepy, flat and unsure of themselves on the third or fourth day after having a baby. This is known as the 'baby blues' and passes after a few days. Most cases of PND start within a month of giving birth, but it can start up to 6 months afterwards. One in 10 mothers develops PND.

Causes

There is no single cause, although a number of different stresses may add up to cause it. These include:

* a history of depressive illness (including previous PND)
* not having a supportive partner
* having a premature or sick baby
* loss of own mother at a young age
* several recent life stresses such as bereavement, unemployment, housing or financial problems.

PND can start for no obvious reason without any of these stresses. Having any of these problems does not mean the mother will definitely develop PND.

Signs and symptoms

* Depressed mood. Feeling low, unhappy, irritable and tearful; having difficulty concentrating; and feeling worse at particular times of the day such as mornings or evenings.
* Sleep disturbance. Feeling constantly tired but unable to sleep, waking early.
* Negative self-perception. Feeling unable to cope, and having feelings of inadequacy, guilt and self-blame.

- Thoughts of harming self or baby. The incidence of nonaccidental injury to the baby is not significantly raised at this time. It is recognised in law that if infanticide occurs during PND or in the first year following childbirth, the mother is deemed to have acted whilst the balance of her mind was disturbed. Infanticide is rare.
- Rejection of the baby, both physically and emotionally.
- Anxiety. Excessive worrying about how much weight the baby is putting on, worrying about 'snuffles', worrying about the baby crying or being too quiet or worrying about if he has stopped breathing. Anxiety about the baby being left alone, in case he comes to harm. Feeling detached from the baby. Unable to work out baby's needs. Worries about own health needs.
- Impaired or loss of libido.

Treatment

A questionnaire such as the Edinburgh Postnatal Depression Scale can be used to help health visitors and GPs identify PND. Most women will get better without treatment after a number of weeks or months; however, this can mean a lot of suffering. It is important to get help as soon as possible to relieve the depression, to support the relationship between mother and child and to help the child's development in the long term.

Talking treatments can help; many GP practices have counsellors or trained health visitors to talk to. More specialist psychological treatments such as cognitive behavioural therapy may be appropriate.

Antidepressant medication may be useful, but care must be taken in breastfeeding mothers.

Quick quiz

1. Severe pathological mood swings, from hyperactivity and euphoria to sadness and depression, occur in:
    A. dysthymic disorder.
    B. cyclothymic disorder.
    C. bipolar disorder.
    D. depressive disorder.

Answer: C. Severe pathological mood swings occur in bipolar disorder. The mood swings of cyclothymic disorder are much milder.

2. In a person who's predisposed to bipolar disorder, a bipolar episode may be triggered by:
    A. hypothyroidism.
    B. hyperthyroidism.
    C. antimanic drugs.
    D. antiseizure drugs.

Answer: A. In a person who's predisposed to bipolar disorder, hypothyroidism may trigger a disease episode.

3. Rapid cycling refers to bipolar disorder with:
  A. one or more episodes of depression or mania in 1 year.
  B. two or more episodes of depression or mania in 1 year.
  C. four or more episodes of depression or mania in 1 year.
  D. no episodes of depression.

Answer: C. Rapid cycling is a bipolar disorder in which four or more episodes of depression and mania occur within a 12-month period.

4. ECT may be used to treat:
  A. dysthymic disorder.
  B. major depressive disorder.
  C. cyclothymic disorder.
  D. bipolar I disorder.

Answer: B. ECT sometimes is used to treat major depression as well as certain psychotic disorders.

5. A service user who has been prescribed lithium should be taught to:
  A. limit fluids to 1,500 ml daily.
  B. maintain a high fluid intake.
  C. restrict sodium intake.
  D. exercise outside in hot weather.

Answer: B. A service user taking lithium must maintain a high fluid intake.

Scoring

☆☆☆ If you answered all five items correctly, you should be feeling elated! Your performance was grandiose!

☆☆ If you answered three or four items correctly, feel free to indulge in an episode of hypomania. Your insight into mood disorders is expansive.

☆ If you answered fewer than three items correctly, don't get depressed. By the end of the next chapter, your mood should stabilise.

6 Anxiety disorders

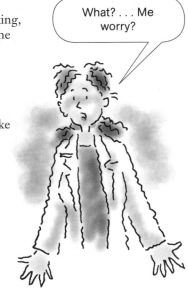

Just the facts

In this chapter, you'll learn:

- ◆ positive and negative effects of anxiety
- ◆ how anxiety disorders impair functioning
- ◆ proposed causes of anxiety disorders
- ◆ how to distinguish acute stress disorder from post-traumatic stress disorder
- ◆ assessment and intervention for people with anxiety disorder.

A look at anxiety disorders

Anxiety disorders are a group of conditions marked by extreme or pathological anxiety or dread. Sufferers experience disturbances of thinking, mood, behaviour and physiological activity. Many feel anxious most of the time, with no apparent reason.

The anxiety may be so uncomfortable that they stop doing certain everyday activities to avoid the feeling of dread. Some have terrifying bouts of intense anxiety that immobilise them. To relieve overwhelming feelings of anxiety, impending catastrophe, guilt, shame, helplessness or worthlessness, sufferers cling to maladaptive behaviours, which only make their symptoms worse.

This chapter discusses eight anxiety disorders:

- panic disorder
- agoraphobia
- generalised anxiety disorder (GAD)
- post-traumatic stress disorder (PTSD)
- acute stress disorder
- social phobia
- specific phobia
- obsessive–compulsive disorder (OCD).

The anatomy of anxiety

From time to time, everyone experiences worry, uncertainty or apprehension – particularly when confronting a stressful event such as a job interview or a first date. Mild or moderate anxiety rarely threatens one's coping ability. In fact, it can motivate us to try new things and take risks. In that sense, it's useful and productive.

The degree of anxiety experienced and the ability to perceive it accurately and channel it appropriately determine if the anxiety will help or hinder the person's level of functioning. Someone who perceives anxiety as severe will feel threatened – and either avoid it or become overwhelmed by it.

Sure – this is risky and makes me a little anxious. But I thrive on that feeling.

Treatable, but usually not treated

Anxiety disorders are highly treatable – but only about one-third of sufferers receive treatment. Left untreated, these disorders become chronic and can grow progressively worse, increasing the risk for suicide and other serious complications.

Oodles of anxiety

The most common type of mental health disorder, anxiety disorders, occur in all human cultures. People with anxiety disorders are three to five times more likely than the general population to visit a doctor and six times more likely to be hospitalised for a mental health disorder.

Anxiety disorders can occur at any age. They affect twice as many women as men.

Over and above anxiety

Anxiety disorders are often accompanied by other mental health illnesses, especially mood disorders and substance abuse – as well as medical disorders. Health care providers must stay alert for this possibility. (See *Plain talk about anxiety disorders*, page 184.)

Causes

Anxiety disorders are thought to result from a combination of genetic, biochemical, neuroanatomic and psychological factors – plus life experiences.

Genetic factors

Research shows that some anxiety disorders are inherited. Many of them – including panic disorder, OCD, GAD and major phobias – run in families.

Researchers are looking for specific genetic factors that might explain or contribute to an inherited risk. Some studies are focusing on possibly defective genes that regulate specific chemical messengers in the brain (neurotransmitters), such as serotonin and dopamine.

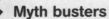

Myth busters

Plain talk about anxiety disorders

Here's a reality check to help you stay on course when caring for people with anxiety disorders.

Myth: All anxiety disorders cause psychological symptoms, but only panic attacks cause physiological symptoms.

Reality: Both physiological and psychological symptoms accompany all levels of anxiety, from mild to severe.

Myth: With post-traumatic stress disorder, people who frequently talk about their trauma tend to relive the traumatic experience.

Reality: Talking about the trauma with a mental health professional can help the person acknowledge the traumatic event, learn coping strategies and obtain support during the recovery process.

Biochemical factors

Some experts believe that people with anxiety disorders have a biological vulnerability to stress, which makes them more susceptible to environmental stimuli. Neurotransmitter imbalances and breathing abnormalities may also contribute to anxiety disorders.

CO_2 sensitivity

Some studies suggest that people with anxiety disorders are hypersensitive to the effects of carbon dioxide, which is released from the lungs during exhalation. The hypersensitivity may be aggravated in crowded spaces, such as aeroplanes or lifts.

In hypersensitive people, exposure to carbon dioxide aggravates anxiety symptoms. Over time, they may develop a pattern of impaired breathing and a sense of panic that evolves into a full-fledged anxiety disorder.

Neuroanatomic factors

Scientists are using magnetic resonance imaging (MRI) and other neuroimaging techniques to locate the brain areas or abnormalities associated with anxiety responses. So far, they've identified brain atrophy, underdeveloped frontal and temporal lobes and abnormalities involving the amygdala (which regulates fear, memory and emotion) and the hippocampus (which plays a role in emotion and memory storage).

Psychological factors

Some theories suggest that certain anxiety disorders arise when unconscious defence mechanisms become overwhelmed and dysfunctional.

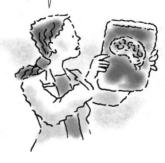

MRI scans have found brain abnormalities in some people with anxiety disorders.

Fear in the family

The family's role in phobias is also under investigation. Several studies show a strong correlation between a parent's fears and those of their children. In other words, a child 'learns' fears by observing the parent's fearful reaction to an object or situation.

Traumatic life events

Traumatic events can trigger anxiety disorders; the most obvious example is PTSD. Also, panic disorders have been associated with anxiety following separation and loss.

Some experts, however, believe that only someone who's vulnerable because of psychological, genetic or biochemical factors will develop an anxiety disorder in response to trauma. Some people may even have a biological propensity for specific phobias (such as a fear of snakes) that's triggered by a single exposure.

Medical conditions

Some anxiety disorders are associated with particular medical conditions, although no causal relationship has been established.

Risk factors

In addition to female gender, risk factors for anxiety disorders include:
- younger than age 45
- marital separation or divorce
- history of childhood physical or sexual abuse
- low socioeconomic status.

Panic disorder

Panic disorder represents anxiety in its most severe form. In this disorder, the person has recurrent, unexpected panic attacks that cause intense apprehension and feelings of impending doom. Between attacks, she persistently worries about having additional panic attacks and the consequences of the attacks, and may change her behaviour because of them. The frequency of panic attacks and the high level of anxiety may cause functional impairments. (See *Differentiating fear, anxiety and panic*.)

Thirty minutes of terror

Panic attacks occur suddenly, with no warning. They usually build to peak intensity within 10–15 minutes and rarely last longer than 30 minutes. However, repeated attacks may continue to recur for hours.

During the attack, the person may fear she's dying, going crazy or losing control of her emotions or behaviour. She has a strong urge to escape or flee the place where the attack began. If she experiences chest pain or shortness of breath, she may go to the Accident & Emergency department or seek some other type of urgent assistance.

Advice from the experts

Differentiating fear, anxiety and panic

When assessing a person for anxiety disorders, keep in mind the key differences among fear, anxiety and panic:

- Fear is a response to external stimuli.
- Anxiety is a response to internal conflict.
- Panic is an extreme level of anxiety.

The frequency and severity of panic attacks vary from one person to the next. Attacks may arise once a week or in clusters separated by months. Because they occur spontaneously – without exposure to a known anxiety-producing situation – the person worries about when the next one will occur and may restrict her lifestyle to avoid them.

Agoraphobia to boot

At some point, about 50% of those with panic disorder develop severe avoidance, warranting a separate diagnosis of panic disorder with agoraphobia. (See 'Agoraphobia', page 191.) However, panic disorder can occur without a history of agoraphobia.

A person who has panic disorder with agoraphobia may be unable to carry out normal daily activities and may grow so fearful that she's unable to leave home.

Panic tally

Roughly 2–4% of the general population experiences panic disorder at some time in their lives. The disorder affects about twice as many women as men.

The most common age of onset is from late adolescence to mid-adulthood. The earlier the onset, the greater the risk of coexisting illnesses, chronic, and impairment. Panic disorder rarely begins after age 50.

Affliction overlap

For many sufferers, panic disorder is complicated by major depressive disorder (50–65% lifetime comorbidity). The tendency to self-medicate with alcohol or anxiolytic drugs may result in alcoholism and substance abuse disorders (20–30% comorbidity).

Many people with panic disorder have additional anxiety disorders – including social phobia (up to 30% comorbidity), GAD (up to 25%), specific phobia (up to 20%) and OCD (up to 10%).

Causes

Although intense stress or a sudden loss may trigger panic disorder, the underlying cause of the disorder probably involves a combination of genetic, biochemical and other factors.

Genetic factors

Panic disorder tends to run in families. Up to 17% of people have first-degree relatives with the disorder. It also occurs to a much higher degree in identical twins, supporting the theory of a genetic basis.

Biochemical abnormalities

Higher norepinephrine levels have been found in people with panic attacks, suggesting a defect in the body's catecholamine system.

Autonomic factors

Some researchers believe that people with panic disorder may have a heightened sensitivity to somatic (physical) symptoms. This sensitivity, in turn, may trigger the autonomic system, which then sets off a series of events leading to a panic attack.

Cognitive and behavioural factors

Learning theory, which proposes that a person misinterprets symptoms, may explain some cases of panic disorder. The person fears that mild anxiety symptoms are the start of a major physical illness. The exaggerated fear triggers a panic attack.

Psychological factors

Some psychoanalysts think panic disorder results from failure to resolve the early childhood conflict of dependence versus independence.

Medical conditions

Panic disorder has been linked to migraine, obstructive sleep apnoea, mitral valve prolapse, irritable bowel syndrome, chronic fatigue syndrome and premenstrual syndrome.

Life events

Intensely stressful life events or multiple stressors can contribute to panic disorder.

Risk factors

Such physical illnesses as asthma, cardiovascular disease and GI disorders may predispose a person to panic disorder by causing fear. The first experience of one of these conditions may be so frightening that it causes a panic attack.

Signs and symptoms

Panic attacks can produce various physical and cognitive signs and symptoms. These include:
- palpitations and rapid heart beat
- sweating
- generalised weakness or trembling
- shortness of breath or rapid, shallow breathing
- sensations of choking, smothering or a lump in the throat
- chest pain or pressure
- abdominal pain, nausea, heartburn, diarrhoea or other GI distress
- dizziness, tingling sensations or light-headedness
- chills, pallor or flushing
- diminished ability to focus or think clearly, even with direction

- fidgeting or pacing
- rapid speech
- exaggerated startle reaction.

Diagnosis

Because some physical conditions and drug effects can mimic panic disorder, the doctor may order tests to rule out an organic or pharmacological basis for symptoms. For example, serum glucose measurements can rule out hypoglycaemia, urine catecholamine and vanillylmandelic acid tests can exclude pheochromocytoma, and thyroid function tests can eliminate hyperthyroidism. Urine and serum toxicology tests can rule out the presence of psychoactive substances capable of triggering panic attacks, such as barbiturates, caffeine and amphetamines.

An official diagnosis is warranted if the person meets the criteria in the *Diagnostic and Statistical Manual of Mental Disorders*, Fourth Edition, Text Revision (*DSM-IV-TR*). (See *Diagnostic criteria: Panic disorder*.)

Diagnostic criteria: Panic disorder

Panic disorder is diagnosed when the person meets these criteria from the *Diagnostic and Statistical Manual of Mental Disorders*, Fourth Edition, Text Revision.

Panic attacks

- One or more panic attacks occurred unexpectedly and weren't triggered by situations in which the person was the focus of other people's attention.
- The panic attacks were followed by a period of at least a month of persistent fear of having another attack.
- During a panic attack, at least four of these signs and symptoms developed abruptly and reached a peak within 10 minutes:
  - shortness of breath or smothering sensations
  - dizziness or faintness
  - palpitations or tachycardia
  - trembling or shaking
  - sweating
  - feelings of choking
  - nausea or abdominal distress
  - depersonalisation (a sense of being detached from the self)
  - or derealisation (feelings of unreality)
  - numbness or tingling sensations
  - hot flashes or chills
  - chest pain or discomfort
  - fear of dying or going crazy.

Other features

- The panic attacks don't result from direct physiological effects of a substance or a general medical condition (such as hyperthyroidism).
- The attacks aren't better explained by another mental disorder.

With or without agoraphobia

Panic disorder may occur with or without agoraphobia. When it occurs with agoraphobia, the person has the symptoms described previously, plus fear or avoidance of any place outside of the home or a 'safe' zone.

Treatment

Panic disorder is highly treatable with a combination of teaching, cognitive or behavioural therapies and relaxation techniques. Some people also require medication.

Teaching
Teaching the person about the disorder and its physiological effects can help her overcome it. Many people experience some relief simply by understanding exactly what panic disorder is and how many others suffer from it.

Cognitive therapy
Cognitive restructuring can be helpful for people who worry that their panic attacks mean they're going crazy or are about to have a heart attack. This method teaches them to replace those negative thoughts with more realistic, positive ways of viewing the attacks. It also helps them identify and evaluate the thoughts that precede anxiety and then restructure them to gain a more realistic perception.

Trigger talk
Through cognitive therapy, the person can identify possible triggers for the panic attacks, such as a particular thought or situation or even a slight change in the heartbeat. Once she understands that the panic attack is separate and independent of the trigger, that trigger starts to lose some of its power to induce an attack.

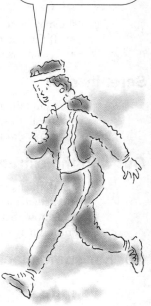

I'm not just jogging. I'm trying to induce tachycardia as part of my interoceptive exposure.

Panic interrupted
In a technique called *interoceptive exposure*, a therapist guides the person through repeated exposure to the sensations she experiences during a panic attack (such as palpitations or dizziness). The feared sensations may be produced using such methods as controlled hyperventilation or physical exertion (such as running up a flight of stairs to cause tachycardia). Through this approach, she learns that these sensations needn't progress to a full-blown attack.

Behavioural therapy
Behavioural therapy typically involves desensitisation, which resembles interoceptive exposure but lacks the cognitive component.

Baby steps
Behavioural therapy also can help the person deal with the situational avoidance associated with panic attacks. In one behavioural technique, a trained therapist helps the person break down a fearful situation into small, manageable steps. The person then performs the steps one at a time until she can master the most difficult step.

Relaxation techniques

Relaxation techniques help the person cope with a panic attack by easing physical symptoms and directing her attention elsewhere. These techniques include:

- deep-breathing exercises, which also reduce the risk of hyperventilation (a contributing factor for anxiety)
- progressive relaxation, which involves conscious tightening and relaxation of the skeletal muscles in a sequential fashion
- positive visualisation or guided imagery, in which the person elicits peaceful mental images or some other purposeful thought or action, promoting feelings of relaxation, renewed hope and a sense of being in control of a stressful situation
- listening to calming music.

Pharmacological therapy

For some people, the doctor may prescribe anxiolytic drugs (especially benzodiazepines) or antidepressants. Combining an anxiolytic drug with an antidepressant promotes rapid stabilisation of panic symptoms. Some people also benefit from beta blockers, which control irregular heartbeats.

Nursing interventions

These nursing interventions may be appropriate for people with panic disorder.

During a panic attack

- Stay with the person until the attack subsides. If left alone, she may grow even more anxious.
- Avoid touching her until you've established rapport. Unless she trusts you, she may be too stimulated or frightened to find touch reassuring.
- If the person loses control, guide her to a smaller, quieter area.
- Avoid insincere expressions of reassurance.

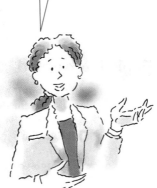

Keep a panicky person away from crowds, bright lights and noise.

Serenity now

- Maintain a calm, serene approach.
- Speak in short, simple sentences, and slowly give the person one direction at a time. Avoid giving lengthy explanations and asking too many questions.

Out with the extraneous

- Reduce external stimuli, such as groups of people.
- Provide a safe environment, and prevent harm to the person or others.
- Know that the person's perceptual field may be narrowed, and excessive stimuli may overwhelm her. Dim bright lights as necessary.

Cut her some slack

- Encourage the person to express her feelings and to cry, if necessary.
- Allow her to pace around the room to help her expend energy.

Between panic attacks

- Encourage the person to discuss her fears. Help her identify situations or events that trigger the attacks.
- Discuss alternative coping mechanisms.
- Monitor therapeutic and side effects of prescribed medications. Teach the person how to recognise side effects.
- Instruct the person to notify the doctor before discontinuing medication because abrupt withdrawal could cause severe symptoms.

Agoraphobia

Agoraphobia is the intense fear or avoidance of situations or places that may be difficult or embarrassing to leave, or in which help might not be available. Sufferers worry they won't be able to get somewhere safe and may fear they'll have a panic attack or panic symptoms (such as dizziness, vomiting, loss of control or difficulty breathing). Eventually, they begin to avoid situations where they feel uncomfortable.

Holed up at home

Without treatment, agoraphobia may get worse. In extreme cases, the person becomes a prisoner in her home, too fearful to leave her 'safe' zone. In less severe cases, she's able to engage in activities or travel if a trusted companion goes along.

Many experts view agoraphobia as an adverse behavioural outcome of repeated panic attacks and the subsequent worry, preoccupation and avoidance. However, agoraphobia sometimes occurs without a history of panic disorder. (See 'Panic disorder', page 185.)

As safe zones go, a bubble bath isn't bad.

Scary territory

Among people with agoraphobia, common fears include large public spaces (such as parks, shopping centres, theatres and supermarkets), crowds and places where the person feels trapped (such as aeroplanes or driving in rush-hour traffic or on a bridge). Most people can verbalise what they fear and where they fear it, although some know only that they have a sense of dread.

Factoring in fear

Nearly 6% of adults develop agoraphobia at some point in their lives. The disorder is twice as common in women as men. Age of onset is usually in the twenties or thirties.

People with agoraphobia have higher depression and suicide rates than the general population and may be prone to alcohol and sedative abuse.

Causes

The exact cause of agoraphobia isn't known. Theories include biochemical imbalances (especially related to neurotransmitters) and environmental factors. The disorder may run in families, suggesting a genetic basis.

Signs and symptoms

The person's avoidance of the feared situation significantly impairs daily functioning. She may report or exhibit:
- fear and avoidance of open spaces or public places
- concern that help might not be available in public places.

If the person also has panic disorder, she may express concern that a panic attack in public will lead to embarrassment or the inability to escape. (For symptoms of a panic attack, see 'Panic disorder', page 185.)

Diagnosis

Agoraphobia without panic disorder is diagnosed when the person meets the criteria in the *DSM-IV-TR*. (See *Diagnostic criteria: Agoraphobia without panic disorder*.)

Treatment

The doctor may prescribe a selective serotonin reuptake inhibitor (SSRI), such as paroxetine (SSRIs are first-line antidepressants). If SSRI proves ineffective, then the doctor may prescribe a tricyclic antidepressant (TCA), such as imipramine. In severe cases it may be necessary to use a short course of benzodiazepines (diazepam) or beta blocker (propranolol).

Diagnostic criteria: Agoraphobia without panic disorder

Agoraphobia without panic disorder is diagnosed when the person meets these criteria from the *Diagnostic and Statistical Manual of Mental Disorders*, Fourth Edition, Text Revision.

- The person experiences agoraphobia (intense fear or avoidance of situations that may be hard to leave or in which help might not be available) related to the fear of developing paniclike symptoms (for instance, dizziness or diarrhoea).
- The person has never met the criteria for panic disorder.
- The disturbance doesn't result from the direct physiological effects of a substance or a general medical condition. If an associated general medical condition is present, then the fear of developing paniclike symptoms exceeds that usually associated with the medical condition.

The overexposure cure

The mainstay of treatment for agoraphobia is desensitisation, which gradually exposes the person to the situation that triggers fear and avoidance. Such exposure helps her learn to cope with the situation and break the mental connection between the situation and anxiety. The person may receive anxiolytic medications to reduce anxiety during desensitisation sessions.

Some people may also benefit from relaxation techniques as well as psychotherapy, in which they discuss underlying emotional conflicts with a therapist or support group.

Nursing interventions

For a person with agoraphobia, these nursing interventions may be appropriate.
- Encourage the person to discuss the feared object or situation.
- Collaborate with the person and multidisciplinary team to develop and implement a systematic desensitisation programme that exposes the person gradually to the feared situation in a controlled environment.
- Provide training in assertiveness skills to reduce submissive and fearful responses. Such strategies allow the person to experiment with new coping skills and encourage her to discard ineffective ones.
- Administer anxiolytic or antidepressant medications, as prescribed.

Generalised anxiety disorder

Occasional anxiety is a normal part of life. However, in GAD, the anxiety is persistent, overwhelming, uncontrollable and out of proportion to the stimulus.

Effects of GAD range from mild to severe and incapacitating. To relieve anxiety, many sufferers self-medicate with alcohol and anxiolytic drugs.

Constant worrying can feel like the weight of the world on your shoulders.

Egad, that's a lot of GAD

GAD affects an estimated 3% of the general population, occurring more often in women than men. Age of onset is typically in the early 20s, but all age groups – including children and the elderly – are affected.

Usually, GAD emerges slowly, although occasionally it's triggered by a stressful event. GAD tends to be chronic, with periods of exacerbation and remission.

Medley of maladies

Up to 25% of people with GAD go on to develop panic disorder. Many also have other mental health disorders, such as social phobia, specific phobia, depression or dysthymic disorder.

Untreated, GAD can cause constant, unremitting tension that ultimately results in immunosuppression, leaving the person more susceptible to physical illnesses.

Causes

The exact cause of GAD is unknown. As with other anxiety disorders, genetic, biochemical, psychosocial and other factors are suspected.

Genetic factors

Genetic predisposition may contribute to GAD. According to one theory, people with GAD may have a genetic vulnerability to increased anxiety.

Biochemical abnormalities

Imbalances in serotonin and gamma-aminobutyric acid (GABA), an amino acid, may play a key role in susceptibility to GAD. Serotonin seems to be vital to feelings of well-being, while GABA helps prevent nerve cells from overfiring.

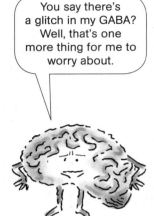

You say there's a glitch in my GABA? Well, that's one more thing for me to worry about.

Psychosocial and environmental factors

Children of anxious parents may learn to see the world as dangerous and uncontrollable, predisposing them to GAD.

Death of a loved one, illness, job loss or divorce can increase a person's stress level and may trigger anxiety attacks. However, experts believe stress is merely a trigger for GAD, not the cause.

Risk factors

Risk factors for GAD include unresolved conflicts, a tendency to misinterpret events and such behaviours as shyness and avoidance of new situations.

Signs and symptoms

Signs and symptoms of GAD fall into three general categories – excessive physiological arousal, distorted cognitive processes and poor coping.

Excessive physiological arousal

With excessive physiological arousal, the person may report or exhibit:
- shortness of breath
- tachycardia or palpitations
- dry mouth
- sweating
- nausea or diarrhoea
- inability to relax
- muscle tension, aches and spasms
- irritability
- fatigue
- restlessness

- trembling
- headache
- cold, clammy hands
- insomnia.

Distorted cognitive processes
Signs and symptoms of distorted cognitive processes include:
- poor concentration
- unrealistic assessment of problems
- excessive anxiety and worry over minor matters
- fears of grave misfortune or death.

Poor coping
A person with poor coping may exhibit:
- avoidance
- procrastination
- poor problem-solving skills.

Diagnosis

Because anxiety is the central feature of many mental disorders, the person should undergo a mental health evaluation to rule out phobias, OCD, depression and acute schizophrenia.

The diagnosis of GAD is confirmed if the person meets the criteria in the *DSM-IV-TR*. (See *Diagnostic criteria: Generalised anxiety disorder*.)

Diagnostic criteria: Generalised anxiety disorder

The diagnosis of generalised anxiety disorder is confirmed when the person meets these criteria from the *Diagnostic and Statistical Manual of Mental Disorders*, Fourth Edition, Text Revision.

Anxiety and associated symptoms

- Excessive anxiety and worry about a number of events or activities occur more days than not for at least 6 months.
- The person has difficulty controlling the worry.
- The anxiety and worry are associated with at least three of these symptoms:
  - restlessness or feeling keyed up or on edge
  - easy fatigue
  - difficulty concentrating or mind going blank
  - irritability
  - muscle tension
  - sleep disturbances (difficulty falling or staying asleep or restless, unsatisfying sleep).

Other features

- The focus of the anxiety and worry isn't confined to the features of an Axis I disorder (a major mental disorder, such as schizophrenia).
- The anxiety, worry or physical symptoms cause clinically significant distress or impairment in social, occupational or other important areas of functioning.
- The disturbance doesn't result from the direct physiological effects of a substance or a general medical condition.
- The disturbance doesn't occur exclusively during a mood disorder, psychotic disorder or pervasive developmental disorder.

Treatment

For people with mild anxiety, nonpharmacological methods should be tried first. Relaxation techniques and biofeedback can decrease arousal. Psychotherapy helps the person identify and deal with the cause of anxiety, anticipate her reactions and plan effective responses to deal with anxiety.

Other treatment options include cognitive therapy and medications.

Cognitive therapy

Cognitive therapy reduces cognitive distortions by teaching the person how to restructure her thoughts and view her worries more realistically.

Worry ledger

In one cognitive therapy approach, the person is taught to record her worries and list evidence that justifies or contradicts each one. She also learns that 'worrying about worry' maintains anxiety and that avoidance and procrastination are ineffective problem-solving techniques.

Biofeedback training

Biofeedback training eases physical symptoms of anxiety by teaching the person how to become aware of – and then consciously control – various body functions (including blood pressure, heart and respiratory rates, skin temperature and perspiration). Using a biofeedback device, the person learns when changes in these functions occur. With adequate training, she can repeat this response at will, even when not hooked up to the biofeedback device.

Pharmacological therapy

Drugs may be considered if anxiety significantly impairs the person's daily functioning. Benzodiazepines reduce anxiety by decreasing vigilance and easing somatic symptoms (for instance, muscle tension). Therefore, they only mask the symptoms not treat the anxiety, often resulting in profound psychological addiction.

Pass the Valium

Some people may require some short-term additional pharmacological support, which could include the use of either a beta blocker such as propanolol or benzodiazepine. To avoid addiction challenges benzodiazepines should not be prescribed longer than 2–4 weeks.

Other medications

Buspirone, TCAs (such as imipramine) and SSRIs may be used in some cases.

Buspirone may be prescribed for people with chronic anxiety and those who relapse after benzodiazepine therapy. It's also the initial drug of choice for anxious people with a history of substance abuse. Unlike benzodiazepines, which treat somatic symptoms, buspirone treats the worry associated with GAD.

Should I be worried about having such a long list of worries?

Hangin' in there

Buspirone appears to be as effective as benzodiazepines in treating GAD. It causes less sedation and rarely leads to physical dependence or tolerance. However, onset of action takes several weeks, so people should be told to expect a delay in symptom relief.

Nursing interventions

When caring for a person with GAD, these nursing interventions may be appropriate.
• Stay with the person when she's anxious. Remain calm and nonjudgemental. Suggest activities that distract her from her anxiety.
• Encourage her to discuss her feelings.
• Reduce environmental stimuli.

Stress-busting strategies

• Teach the person progressive muscle relaxation, guided imagery, deep-breathing or other relaxation techniques. Besides easing anxiety, these methods reduce the risk of hyperventilation, help her focus on something other than her anxiety, and interrupt the flow of negative or stressful thoughts.
• Provide nutrition counselling to reduce stress. Advise the person to avoid caffeine and alcohol, for instance.
• To help manage anxiety, instruct the person in time-management skills, such as making lists, setting realistic goals, and grouping tasks in batches.
• Make appropriate referrals to a mental health professional. Dissuade the person from visiting the Accident & Emergency department for symptom relief because of the frantic atmosphere.

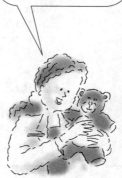

This is kind of embarrassing, but my teddy bear helps me to relax and get my mind off my anxiety.

Drug discussions

• Administer anxiolytic medications, as prescribed.
• Inform the person and her family that these drugs may cause adverse reactions, such as drowsiness, fatigue, ataxia, blurred vision, slurred speech, tremors and hypotension. Instruct her to report these to the doctor.
• Advise the person not to discontinue medications except with the doctor's approval, because abrupt withdrawal could cause severe symptoms.

Post-traumatic stress disorder

PTSD may occur after someone experiences or witnesses a serious traumatic event, such as wartime combat, a natural disaster, rape, murder or torture. The disorder is characterised by persistent and recurrent flashbacks, reliving the event, or nightmares of the event – along with avoidance of reminders of it.

Impairments caused by PTSD can be mild or severe, affecting nearly every aspect of the person's life. PTSD sufferers are irritable, anxious, fatigued, forgetful and socially withdrawn. Those who survived a catastrophe that took many lives may also have survivor guilt.

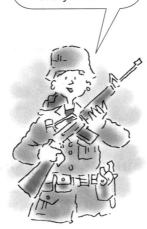

A person with PTSD may become hypervigilant and easily startled.

Inordinately alert

To avoid stimuli that trigger memories of the traumatic event, the person with PTSD may become hypervigilant, easily aroused and easily startled.

Sooner or later

PTSD can be acute or chronic. Acute PTSD is diagnosed if symptoms appear within 6 months of the trauma. If symptoms begin later, delayed or chronic PTSD is diagnosed. About half of PTSD cases remit within 6 months.

PTSD by the numbers

Women are more likely to be affected than men. (See *Post-traumatic stress disorder: Not just for war veterans*.)

People with PTSD are at increased risk for developing other anxiety-, mood- and substance-related disorders – especially alcohol abuse.

Causes

Obviously, a traumatic event is the trigger for PTSD. Some people, however, may be biochemically predisposed to the disorder. According to one theory,

---

Myth busters

Post-traumatic stress disorder: Not just for war veterans

When some people hear the term post-traumatic stress disorder (PTSD), the image of a male war veteran pops into mind. However, the typical victim is more likely to be female.

Myth: Most PTSD victims are war veterans.

Reality: Although about 15% of Vietnam veterans were still suffering from PTSD 19 years after combat exposure, the highest rates of PTSD occur in women. The estimated lifetime prevalence of PTSD is 7.8%. Women (10.4%) are twice as likely as men (5%) to have PTSD at some point in their lives.

In women, the traumatic events most often linked with PTSD are rape, sexual assault, physical attacks, being threatened with a weapon and childhood physical abuse. In men, the most common traumatising events are rape, combat exposure, childhood neglect and childhood physical abuse.

the alpha-2-adrenergic receptor response that inhibits stress-induced release of norepinephrine is impaired in people with PTSD. This results in progressive behavioural sensitisation and generalisation to stimulus cues from the original trauma, with responses of increased sympathetic activity.

Risk factors

Risk factors for PTSD include:
* limited social supports
* high anxiety levels
* low self-esteem
* neurotic and extroverted characteristics
* history of mental health disorders
* previous diagnosis of an acute stress disorder that failed to resolve within 1 month.

Although preexisting psychopathology may predispose a person to this disorder, PTSD can develop in anyone – especially if the stressor is extreme. Genetic factors may also play a role.

Signs and symptoms

Common signs and symptoms of PTSD may include:
* anger
* poor impulse control
* chronic anxiety and tension
* avoidance of people, places and things associated with the traumatic experience
* emotional detachment or numbness
* depersonalisation (a sense of loss of identity as a person)
* difficulty concentrating
* difficulty falling or staying asleep
* hyperalertness, hyperarousal and exaggerated startle reflex
* inability to recall details of the traumatic event
* labile affect (rapid, easily changing affective expression)
* social withdrawal
* decreased self-esteem
* loss of sustained beliefs about people or society
* hopelessness
* sense of being permanently damaged
* relationship problems
* survivor's guilt.

No thanks for the memories

Although the person may be unable to recall specific aspects of the traumatising event, she may experience it in flashbacks, dreams or thoughts when cues to the event occur.

The psychosocial history may reveal early life experiences, interpersonal factors, military experiences or other incidents that suggest the precipitating event.

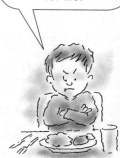

If they keep serving me this awful food, they'll traumatise me for life!

Diagnostic criteria: Post-traumatic stress disorder

The diagnosis of post-traumatic stress disorder is made when the person's signs and symptoms meet these criteria from the *Diagnostic and Statistical Manual of Mental Disorders*, Fourth Edition, Text Revision.

Exposure to trauma

The person was exposed to a traumatic event in which both of these situations occurred:

- The person experienced, witnessed or was confronted with an event that involved actual or threatened death or serious injury or a threat to the physical integrity of the self or others.
- The person's response involved intense fear, helplessness or horror.

Reexperiencing of the trauma

The person persistently reexperiences the traumatic event in at least one of these ways:

- recurrent and intrusive distressing recollections of the event, such as images, thoughts or perceptions
- recurrent distressing dreams of the event
- acting or feeling as if the traumatic event were recurring (such as a sense of reliving the experience, illusions, hallucinations and dissociative episodes that occur even on awakening or when intoxicated)
- intense psychological distress at exposure to internal or external cues that symbolise or resemble some aspect of the traumatic event.

Avoidance of reminders

The person persistently avoids stimuli associated with the trauma. She also experiences numbing of general responsiveness (not present before the traumatic event), as shown by at least three of these criteria:

- efforts to avoid thoughts or feelings associated with the trauma
- efforts to avoid activities, places or people that arouse recollections of the trauma
- inability to recall an important aspect of the traumatic event
- markedly diminished interest in significant activities
- feeling of detachment or estrangement from other people
- restricted range of affect – for instance, inability to love others
- sense of a foreshortened future.

Increased arousal

The person has persistent symptoms of increased arousal (not present before the trauma), as shown by at least two of these criteria:

- difficulty falling or staying asleep
- irritability or angry outbursts
- difficulty concentrating
- hypervigilance
- exaggerated startle response.

Other features

- The duration of the disturbance is at least 1 month.
- The disturbance causes clinically significant distress or impairment in social, occupational or other important areas of functioning.

Diagnosis

The person is diagnosed with PTSD if she meets the criteria for he disorder listed in the *DSM-IV-TR*. (See *Diagnostic criteria: Post-traumatic stress disorder*.)

Treatment

Nonpharmacological treatment options include interoceptive exposure, desensitisation, relaxation techniques and psychotherapy.

Individual psychotherapy gives the person a chance to talk through the traumatic experience with a nonthreatening person and thus gain some perspective. Promoting feelings of loss, grief and anxiety may aid in resolving the emotional numbness associated with PTSD.

Group therapy helps the person realise she isn't alone. A skilled group therapist can assist group members in confronting stressful feelings in a supportive environment.

Pharmacological treatment

To relieve PTSD symptoms, the doctor may prescribe an SSRI such as paroxetine or sertraline (for women). In severe cases the doctor may prescribe a TCA such as amitripyline or even a monoamine oxidase inhibitor (MAOI) such as phenelzine.

Other treatments

When indicated, the person should undergo alcohol or drug rehabilitation. Also, more positive coping strategies should be explored and practised.

Nursing interventions

These nursing interventions may be appropriate for people with PTSD.
- Establish trust by accepting the person's current level of functioning and assuming a positive, consistent, honest and nonjudgemental attitude.
- Encourage the person to express her grief, complete the mourning process and gain coping skills to relieve anxiety and desensitise her to memories of the traumatic event.
- Use crisis intervention techniques as needed.

Anger adjustment

- Deal constructively with the person's displays of anger. Encourage her to assess angry outbursts by identifying how the anger escalates.
- Help the person regain control over angry impulses by identifying situations in which she lost control and by talking about past and precipitating events.
- Provide a safe, staff-monitored room where the person can safely deal with urges to commit physical violence or self-abuse by displacement (such as pounding and throwing clay or destroying selected items).
- Encourage her to move from physical to verbal expressions of anger.

Perspective correctives

- Help the person relieve shame and guilt precipitated by real actions (such as killing or mutilation) that violated a consciously held moral code.
- Help her put her behaviour into perspective, recognise her isolation and self-destructive behaviour as forms of atonement and accept forgiveness from herself and others.
- Carefully review the healing process with the person. Remind her not to equate setbacks with treatment failure.

Prescription erudition

- Administer medications, as prescribed.
- Teach the person about prescribed medications and side effects. Advise her not to discontinue medication without first consulting the doctor.
- Evaluate her response to the prescribed drug regimen.
- Be aware that although benzodiazepines are fast acting, they may lose their effectiveness with prolonged use.

Reference rendering

- Refer the person to clergy and community resources as appropriate.
- Refer her to group therapy with other victims for peer support and forgiveness.

Acute stress disorder

Acute stress disorder is a syndrome of anxiety and behavioural disturbances that occurs within 4 weeks of an extreme trauma, such as combat, rape or a near-death experience in an accident. Generally, symptoms start during or shortly after the trauma and impair functioning in at least one key area.

Unlike PTSD, acute stress disorder resolves within 4 weeks. (If symptoms last longer than 4 weeks, the diagnosis may change to PTSD.) Acute stress disorder may begin as early as 2 days after the trauma.

Progression to depression

Prognosis depends on such factors as severity and duration of the trauma and the person's level of functioning. With immediate psychological care and much social support, recovery may be more rapid. If untreated, acute stress disorder may progress to PTSD, substance abuse or major depression.

Causes

Exposure to trauma is the major precipitant of acute anxiety disorder. The trauma may involve serious physical or emotional injury or threats to one's life.

Signs and symptoms

Clinical features of acute stress disorder include:
- generalised anxiety
- hyperarousal
- avoidance of reminders of the traumatic event
- persistent, intrusive recollections of the traumatic event in flashbacks, dreams or recurrent thoughts or visual images
- irritability
- physical restlessness

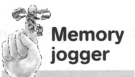

Memory jogger

The word *acute* is the key to remembering the difference between acute stress disorder and post-traumatic stress disorder (PTSD). Both cause similar symptoms but differ in their timing: Acute stress disorder happens shortly after the trauma (acute); PTSD takes a bit longer to emerge (delayed).

- sleep disturbances
- exaggerated startle reflex
- poor concentration.

Outside oneself

A hallmark of acute stress disorder is dissociation – a defence mechanism in which the person separates anxiety-provoking thoughts and emotions from the rest of the psyche. The world may seem dreamlike or unreal to her, or she may feel she's observing herself from a distance or that a body part has somehow changed.

Dissociation may be accompanied by poor memory of the traumatic event or even complete amnesia of it.

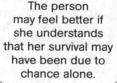

When I'm feeling outside myself like this, it usually means I'm experiencing acute stress.

Diagnosis

The person has a recent history of trauma. Physical examination helps rule out organic causes of signs and symptoms.

The person is diagnosed with acute stress disorder if she meets the criteria in the *DSM-IV-TR*. (See *Diagnostic criteria: Acute stress disorder*, page 204.)

Treatment

Treatment of acute stress disorder may include social supports, psychotherapy, cognitive or behavioural therapy and pharmacotherapy. A person experiencing hyperarousal may benefit from relaxation techniques and deep-breathing exercises.

Supportive counselling or short-term psychotherapy helps the person examine the trauma in a supportive environment, strengthen previously helpful coping mechanisms and learn new coping strategies.

Cognitive or behavioural therapy may involve trauma education, cognitive restructuring of the traumatic event to help the person see it from a different perspective and gradual reexposure with less avoidance.

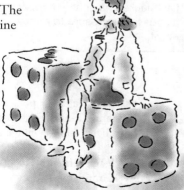

The person may feel better if she understands that her survival may have been due to chance alone.

When all else fails . . .

Drugs may be used if nonpharmacological methods aren't effective. The doctor may prescribe anxiolytic agents, beta blockers (such as clonidine or propranolol) or antipsychotic agents though the evidence of efficacy is weak.

Nursing interventions

These nursing interventions may be appropriate for people with acute stress disorder.
- Encourage the person to discuss the stressful event and identify it as traumatic. This validates that the situation was indeed beyond her personal control.
- Urge her to talk about her anxiety and her feelings about the trauma. This helps her cope with the reality of the event.

Diagnostic criteria: Acute stress disorder

The diagnosis of acute stress disorder is made when the person's signs and symptoms meet these criteria from the *Diagnostic and Statistical Manual of Mental Disorders*, Fourth Edition, Text Revision.

Exposure to trauma

A traumatic event occurred in which both of these situations took place:

- The person experienced, witnessed or was confronted with an event that involved actual or threatened death or serious injury, or a threat to the physical integrity of self or others.
- The person's response involved intense fear, helplessness or horror.

Dissociative symptoms

During or after the traumatic event, the person experienced three or more of these dissociative symptoms:

- subjective sense of numbing, detachment or absence of emotional responsiveness
- reduced awareness of surroundings (for instance, feeling as though in a daze)
- derealisation (a sense of unreality or loss of reality)
- depersonalisation (a sense of loss of identity as a person)
- dissociative amnesia (inability to recall an important aspect of the trauma).

Reexperiencing of the trauma

The person persistently reexperiences the traumatic event in at least one of these ways:

- recurrent images, thoughts, dreams, illusions, flashbacks or a sense of reliving the experience
- distress on exposure to reminders of the traumatic event.

Avoidance of reminders

The person avoids stimuli that trigger recollections of the trauma (such as thoughts, feelings, people, places, activities and conversations).

Anxiety or arousal symptoms

The person has pronounced symptoms of anxiety or increased arousal, such as difficulty sleeping, irritability, poor concentration, hypervigilance, exaggerated startle response or motor restlessness.

Other features

- The disturbance causes clinically significant distress or impairment in social, occupational or other important areas of functioning or impairs the person's ability to pursue a necessary task, such as obtaining required help.
- The disturbance lasts at least 2 days and no more than 4 weeks, and occurs within 4 weeks of the traumatic event.
- The disturbance doesn't result from the direct physiological effects of a substance or a general medical condition.
- The disturbance isn't better explained by brief psychotic disorder.
- The disturbance isn't merely an exacerbation of a preexisting Axis I disorder (a major mental disorder, such as schizophrenia) or a preexisting Axis II disorder (such as a personality disorder).

- Encourage the person to identify any feelings of survivor guilt, inadequacy or blame. Expressing these feelings helps her understand that her survival may have been due to chance and not related to any personal action or inaction by her.
- Teach relaxation techniques, such as progressive muscle relaxation.
- Administer anxiolytic medications, as prescribed.

Social phobia

Social phobia (sometimes called social anxiety disorder) refers to marked, persistent fear or anxiety in social or performance situations. The anxiety causes the sufferer to avoid these situations whenever possible out of fear that she'll be embarrassed or ridiculed. Common situations that provoke anxiety include speaking or eating in public and using a public toilet.

Spotlight shunners

Many people with social phobia are concerned that others will see their anxiety symptoms (such as sweating or blushing) or will judge them to be weak, stupid or crazy. Some fear they'll faint, lose bowel or bladder control or go mentally blank.

Even when around familiar people, they may feel overwhelmed, fearing that others are watching their every move and making negative judgements about them.

Expecting the worst

Social phobias generally are associated with anticipatory anxiety for days or weeks before the dreaded event. Such anxiety may further handicap the person's performance and heighten embarrassment.

Could you be specific?

Social phobia may be limited to one specific situation, such as speaking in public. In its most severe form, it's generalised to the point that the person has symptoms almost anytime she's near other people.

The disorder can be debilitating, preventing the person from going to work or school on some days. It can cause loss of a job or job promotion out of fear of speaking in public, or result in continual inconvenience – for instance, from fear of using a public lavatory.

People with social phobia have high rates of alcohol abuse and other mental health conditions (such as depression and eating disorders).

Numeric rundown

Social phobia is more common in women; the disorder typically starts in childhood or adolescence. It rarely develops after age 25. For many sufferers, it's linked with the traits of shyness and social inhibition.

Once the disorder is established, complete remission is unlikely without treatment. Severity of symptoms and impairments typically fluctuates with job or academic demands and the stability of the person's social relationships.

Causes

Preliminary studies suggest that social phobia runs in families. Biological and environmental factors may also play a role.

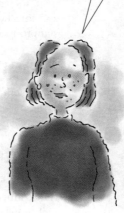

School wouldn't be so bad if the other kids weren't there.

Scientists exploring biological aspects of the disorder believe there may be a physiological or hormonal basis for increased sensitivity to disapproval. Others are investigating the role of the amygdala, a brain structure that controls fear responses.

Lessons in shyness

Some experts are keying in on environmental influences. Theories that focus on social modelling or observational learning, for example, propose that a person acquires fear from observing the behaviour and consequences of others.

Signs and symptoms

Signs and symptoms of social phobia may include:
• fear or avoidance of eating, writing or speaking in public; being stared at; or meeting strangers
• pronounced sensitivity to criticism
• low self-esteem
• scholastic underachievement because of test anxiety.
  Physical manifestations may include:
• blushing
• profuse sweating
• trembling
• nausea or stomach upset
• difficulty talking.

Worried about looking worried

Visible signs of social phobia, such as blushing or profuse sweating, heighten the person's fear of disapproval and may become an additional focus of fear. Thus, a vicious cycle may begin: The more the person worries about experiencing symptoms of social phobia, the greater her chance of developing symptoms.

Diagnosis

No specific test can diagnose social phobia. An official diagnosis is confirmed if the person meets the criteria in the *DSM-IV-TR*. (See *Diagnostic criteria: Social phobia*, page 207.)

Treatment

A mental health professional may use desensitisation therapy to gradually reintroduce the feared situation while coaching the person on relaxation techniques.

Relaxation techniques, such as progressive muscle relaxation, deep-breathing exercises or listening to calming music, may be helpful, too. By role-playing in guided imagery, the person rehearses ways to relax while confronting a feared object or situation.

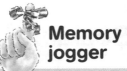

Memory jogger

FEAR can cue you in to signs and symptoms of phobias.

F Fear of an object or a situation

E Emotional conflict occurring unconsciously

A Avoidant behaviour demonstrated

R Reacts with severe anxiety

Diagnostic criteria: Social phobia

The diagnosis of social phobia is made when the person meets these criteria from the *Diagnostic and Statistical Manual of Mental Disorders*, Fourth Edition, Text Revision.

Fear of social situations

- The person has a marked and persistent fear of one or more social or performance situations that involve exposure to unfamiliar people or possible scrutiny by others. She fears she'll act in a way or show anxiety symptoms that will be humiliating or embarrassing.
- Exposure to the feared social situation almost always provokes anxiety, which may take the form of a panic attack.
- The person acknowledges that the fear is excessive or unreasonable.
- The person avoids the feared social or performance situation, or endures it with intense anxiety or distress.
- Avoidance, anxious anticipation or distress in the feared social or performance situation interferes significantly with the person's normal routine, occupational or academic functioning, social activities or relationships – or the person has marked distress about having the phobia.

Other features

- In people under age 18, the disorder lasts at least 6 months.
- Fear or avoidance doesn't result from the direct physiological effects of a substance or a general medical condition.
- Fear or avoidance isn't better explained by another mental disorder (such as panic disorder, separation anxiety disorder, body dysmorphic disorder or schizoid personality disorder).
- If a general medical condition or another mental disorder is present, the person's fear isn't related to it.
- Generalised social phobia is specified if the person's fears include most social situations.

A model for behaviour

Modelling behaviour and assertiveness training also can be valuable. In modelling behaviour, the person observes someone modelling, or demonstrating, appropriate behaviour when confronted with the feared situation.

Thought police

A behavioural technique called negative thought stopping can reduce the frequency and duration of disturbing thoughts by interrupting them and substituting competing thoughts. In thought stopping, the person is taught to recognise negative thoughts and then use an intense distracting stimulus (such as snapping a rubber band around the wrist) to stop the thought. With practice, the person can control thoughts without this distracting stimulus.

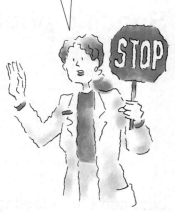

Stop right there, negative thought! I'm making a citizen's arrest!

Pharmacological therapy

The doctor may prescribe such drugs as benzodiazepines, SSRIs, MAOIs, TCAs or beta blockers. Beta blockers (such as propranolol) slow the heart rate, lower blood pressure and reduce nervous tension, sweating, panic and shakiness.

Be aware that relapse rates are high when medication is used as the sole treatment for social phobia.

Nursing interventions

These nursing interventions may be appropriate for people with social phobia.
- No matter how illogical the person's phobia seems, avoid the urge to trivialise her fears. Remember that her behaviour represents an essential coping mechanism. A facile pep talk or ridicule may alienate her or worsen her low self-esteem.
- Keep in mind that the person fears criticism. Encourage her to interact with others and provide continuous support and positive reinforcement.
- Teach the person progressive muscle relaxation, guided imagery or thought-stopping techniques as appropriate.

When the going gets tough . . .

- Ask the person how she normally copes with the fear. When she's able to face the fear, encourage her to verbalise and explore her personal strengths and resources with you.
- Suggest ways to channel energy and relieve stress, such as running and creative activities.

. . . The tough go shopping

- Don't let the person withdraw completely. If she's being treated as an outpatient, then suggest small steps to overcome her fears, such as planning a brief shopping trip with a supportive family member or friend.
- To increase self-esteem and reduce anxiety, explain to the person that her phobia is a way of coping with anxiety, especially if she perceives her behaviour as silly or unreasonable.
- If the person's taking an antidepressant or anxiolytic medication, then stress the importance of complying with prescribed therapy. Teach her about adverse reactions and advise her which ones to report.

Specific phobia

In specific phobia (also called *simple phobia*), a person experiences intense, irrational anxiety when exposed to anticipating a specific feared object (such as a snake) or situation (such as being in an enclosed space). The exposure can take place either in real life or through images from movies, television, photographs or the imagination.

For many, the anxiety leads to avoidance or disabling behaviour that interferes with activities or even confines them to the home. Anxiety may reach panic levels, especially if there's no apparent escape from the feared thing or situation.

Just can't help feeling that way

Although adults with specific phobias realise their fears are irrational and out of proportion to any actual danger, they still experience severe anxiety or panic attacks when facing (or perhaps even thinking about) the feared object or situation. Most try to avoid the stimulus, or endure exposure to it with great difficulty. Some even make important career or personal decisions to avoid the object of their fears.

Types of specific phobias
The *DSM-IV-TR* classifies specific phobias into five main groups:
- natural environment type
- animal type
- blood-injection-injury type
- situational type
- other type.

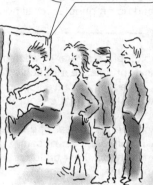

I'm terrified of enclosed spaces! Let me out of here!

Spiders, tight spaces and storms

Besides animals and enclosed spaces, common specific phobias include:
- insects
- heights
- lifts and escalators
- tunnels
- water
- storms
- blood or injections
- driving on motorways
- flying in aeroplanes.

Many people have multiple specific phobias. (See *The phobia file*, pages 210 and 211.)

Phobia figures

Specific phobias affect about 10% of the population. They're more common in women than men. Onset occurs in childhood to early adulthood (usually the mid-20s).

Most specific phobias persist for years or even decades. Only about 20% remit spontaneously without treatment.

Adult phobias are more persistent than childhood phobias. Childhood phobias usually disappear over time, although some continue into adulthood.

Phobias involving blood tend to run in families.

Causes

No one knows what causes specific phobias. Because they seem to run in families (especially those involving blood or injury), researchers suspect that genetic predisposition plays a role.

Other factors that may predispose a person to a specific phobia include:
- experiencing or observing a trauma
- repeated warnings of danger about the feared object or situation
- panic attacks when exposed to the feared object or situation.

The phobia file

You name it, and somebody somewhere is afraid of it. In the list here (which is by no means all-inclusive), you can read up on phobias for almost every letter of the alphabet.

A

Ablutophobia: Fear of washing
Acarophobia: Fear of itching or insects that cause itching
Acerophobia: Fear of sourness
Aerophobia: Fear of drafts
Achluophobia: Fear of darkness
Ailurophobia: Fear of cats
Antlophobia: Fear of floods
Apiphobia: Fear of bees
Arachnophobia: Fear of spiders
Astrapophobia: Fear of lightning

B

Bacteriophobia: Fear of bacteria
Bathmophobia: Fear of stairs or steep slopes
Bathophobia: Fear of depth
Blennophobia: Fear of slime
Bogyphobia: Fear of the bogeyman
Botanophobia: Fear of plants
Bromidrosiphobia or bromidrophobia: Fear of body smells

C

Cacophobia: Fear of ugliness
Cancerophobia: Fear of cancer
Carnophobia: Fear of meat
Catagelophobia: Fear of being ridiculed
Catapedaphobia: Fear of jumping from high or low places
Cathisophobia: Fear of sitting
Chaetophobia: Fear of hair
Coprastasophobia: Fear of constipation

D

Demophobia: Fear of crowds
Didaskaleinophobia: Fear of going to school

Dikephobia: Fear of justice
Dishabiliophobia: Fear of undressing in front of someone
Domatophobia or oikophobia: Fear of houses
Dysmorphophobia: Fear of deformity
Dystychiphobia: Fear of accidents

E

Ecclesiophobia: Fear of church
Ecophobia: Fear of home
Eisoptrophobia: Fear of mirrors or seeing oneself in a mirror
Emetophobia: Fear of vomiting
Enochlophobia: Fear of crowds

F

Febriphobia: Fear of fever
Frigophobia: Fear of cold or cold things

G

Gamophobia: Fear of marriage
Gerascophobia: Fear of growing old
Geumaphobia or geumophobia: Fear of taste
Glossophobia: Fear of speaking in public
Gynephobia or gynophobia: Fear of women

H

Heliophobia: Fear of the sun
Herpetophobia: Fear of reptiles or creepy, crawly things
Heterophobia: Fear of the opposite sex
Hierophobia: Fear of religious or sacred things

Hippophobia: Fear of horses
Hippopotomonstrosesquippedaliophobia: Fear of long words
Hypsiphobia: Fear of height

I

Iatrophobia: Fear of doctors
Ichthyophobia: Fear of fish
Ideophobia: Fear of ideas
Illyngophobia: Fear of vertigo or feeling dizzy when looking down
Iophobia: Fear of poison
Insectophobia: Fear of insects
Isolophobia: Fear of solitude

K

Kainolophobia: Fear of novelty
Kainophobia: Fear of anything new, novelty
Kakorrhaphiophobia: Fear of failure or defeat
Katagelophobia: Fear of ridicule
Kathisophobia: Fear of sitting down
Kopophobia: Fear of fatigue

L

Levophobia: Fear of objects to the left
Ligyrophobia: Fear of loud noises
Lilapsophobia: Fear of tornadoes and hurricanes
Logophobia: Fear of words

M

Macrophobia: Fear of long waits
Mageirocophobia: Fear of cooking
Maieusiophobia: Fear of childbirth
Medomalacuphobia: Fear of losing an erection
Menophobia: Fear of menstruation

The phobia file (continued)

Metallophobia: Fear of metal
Microbiophobia: Fear of microbes
Myctophobia: Fear of darkness
Myrmecophobia: Fear of ants

N

Neopharmaphobia: Fear of
new drugs
Neophobia: Fear of anything new
Nephophobia: Fear of clouds
Noctiphobia: Fear of the night
Nostophobia: Fear of returning
home
Novercaphobia: Fear of one's
stepmother

O

Ochlophobia: Fear of crowds
or mobs
Ochophobia: Fear of vehicles
Oenophobia: Fear of wines
Olfactophobia: Fear of smells
Ombrophobia: Fear of rain
Optophobia: Fear of opening
one's eyes
Ornithophobia: Fear of birds

P

Pagophobia: Fear of ice or frost
Panphobia: Fear of everything
Panthophobia: Fear of suffering and
disease
Pediculophobia: Fear of lice
Pedophobia: Fear of children
Phalacrophobia: Fear of becoming
bald

Photophobia: Fear of light
Pogonophobia: Fear of beards
Potamophobia: Fear of rivers
Prosophobia: Fear of progress
Psellismophobia: Fear of stuttering
Pyrophobia: Fear of fire

R

Ranidaphobia: Fear of frogs
Rhypophobia: Fear of defecation
Rhytiphobia: Fear of getting
wrinkles
Rupophobia: Fear of dirt

S

Sciophobia: Fear of shadows
Scoleciphobia: Fear of worms
Scolionophobia: Fear of school
Scotophobia: Fear of darkness
Scriptophobia: Fear of writing
in public
Selachophobia: Fear of sharks
Selaphobia: Fear of light flashes
Sesquipedalophobia: Fear of long
words
Siderodromophobia: Fear of trains
Syngenesophobia: Fear of relatives

T

Thaasophobia: Fear of sitting
Thanatophobia: Fear of death
Thalassophobia: Fear of the sea
Thermophobia: Fear of heat
Tocophobia: Fear of pregnancy or
childbirth

Triskaidekaphobia: Fear of the
number 13
Trypanophobia: Fear of injections

U

Uranophobia: Fear of heaven
Urophobia: Fear of urine or
urinating

V

Vaccinophobia: Fear of inoculations
Verbophobia: Fear of words
Verminophobia: Fear of germs
Vestiphobia: Fear of clothing

W

Wiccaphobia: Fear of witches and
witchcraft

X

Xanthophobia: Fear of the colour
yellow or the word yellow
Xenophobia: Fear of strangers or
foreigners
Xerophobia: Fear of dryness
Xylophobia: Fear of wooden
objects; fear of forests
Xyrophobia: Fear of razors

Z

Zelophobia: Fear of jealousy
Zoophobia: Fear of animals

Role models in fear

Generally, specific phobias don't result from exposure to a single traumatic
event, such as being bitten by a dog. Instead, other family members have phobias
and the person may have learned to adopt them. Spontaneous, unexpected panic
attacks also appear to play a role in development of specific phobia.

Signs and symptoms

The person experiences severe anxiety when confronted with the feared thing or situation, or even the threat of it. If she routinely avoids the object of her phobia, she may have low self-esteem, depression and feelings of weakness, cowardice or ineffectiveness.

Diagnosis

The person has a history of anxiety when exposed to or anticipating a specific object or situation. Official diagnosis hinges on the person meeting the criteria in the *DSM-IV-TR*. (See *Diagnostic criteria: Specific phobia*.)

Treatment

Successful treatment usually involves desensitisation or exposure therapy, in which a mental health professional or a trusted companion gradually exposes the person to what frightens her until the fear begins to fade. About 75% of

---

Diagnostic criteria: Specific phobia

The diagnosis of specific phobia is made when the person's signs and symptoms meet these criteria from the *Diagnostic and Statistical Manual of Mental Disorders*, Fourth Edition, Text Revision.

Irrational fear

- The person has a marked and persistent fear that's unreasonable or excessive. The fear is cued by confronting or anticipating a specific object or situation (such as animals, flying, heights, injections or seeing blood).
- Exposure to the phobic stimulus almost always causes an immediate anxiety response, which may take the form of a panic attack.
- The person realises the fear is unreasonable or excessive.
- The person avoids the phobic situation or endures it with intense anxiety or distress.
- The avoidance, anxious anticipation or distress aroused by the feared object or situation interferes significantly with the person's routine, occupational or academic functioning, social activities or relationships – or the person has marked distress about having the phobia.

Other features

- Anxiety, panic attacks or phobic avoidance aren't better explained by another mental disorder, such as obsessive–compulsive disorder, post-traumatic stress disorder, social phobia, separation anxiety disorder, panic disorder or agoraphobia.

Specific type

Specific phobia is categorised into five main types:

- animal type
- natural environment type (such as height or water)
- blood-injection-injury type
- situational type (such as flying in an aeroplane or being in an enclosed space)
- other type (for instance, situations that may lead to choking, vomiting or contracting an illness).

people benefit significantly from such treatment. It can be especially helpful for phobias involving driving, flying, heights, bridges or lifts.

Other techniques

Relaxation, breathing exercises and thought stopping can reduce anxiety symptoms. Role-playing in guided imagery teaches the person to relax while confronting a feared object or situation.

Pharmacological therapy

No proven drug treatment for specific phobias exist, but the doctor may prescribe medications to reduce anxiety symptoms in advance of a phobic situation, such as flying in an aeroplane.

Anxiolytic drugs may be used to manage short-term anxiety but aren't useful as long-term treatment. (See *Pharmacological therapy for anxiety disorders*, pages 214, 215 and 216.)

Nursing interventions

These nursing interventions may be appropriate for people with specific phobia.
• Encourage the person to discuss the feared object or situation.
• Collaborate with the person and the multidisciplinary team to develop and implement a systematic desensitisation programme in which the person is systematically exposed to the feared object or situation in a controlled environment.
• Teach assertiveness skills to help reduce submissive, fearful responses. Such strategies enable the person to experiment with new coping skills and discard coping skills that haven't worked in the past.
• Instruct the person in relaxation and thought-stopping techniques as appropriate.
• Administer antiphobic or antipanic medications as prescribed. These agents have a significant calming effect and may help the person change her behaviour by reducing anxiety during desensitisation sessions.

Obsessive–compulsive disorder

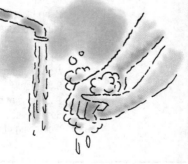

OCD is characterised by unwanted, recurrent, intrusive thoughts or images (obsessions), which the person tries to alleviate through repetitive behaviours or mental acts (compulsions). The compulsions are meant to reduce the anxiety or prevent some dreaded event from happening.

Obsessions and compulsions may be simple or complex and ritualised. Compulsions include both overt behaviours, such as hand washing or checking, and mental acts, such as praying or counting.

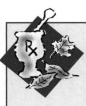

Meds matters

Pharmacological therapy for anxiety disorders

This chart highlights several drugs used to treat anxiety disorders.

Drug	Side effects	Contraindications	Nursing considerations
Benzodiazepines			
Alprazolam Diazepam	• Ataxia • Confusion • Constipation • Double or blurred vision • Dry mouth • Sedation • Skin reactions (rash, urticaria, photosensitivity) • Vertigo • Weight change	• Acute alcohol intoxication • Acute angle-closure glaucoma or untreated open-angle glaucoma • Coma • Depression or psychosis without anxiety • Pregnancy or breast-feeding • Shock • Within 14 days of taking a monoamine oxidase inhibitor (MAOI)	• Monitor closely after giving each dose because disinhibitory effect (excitement) rather than calming effect is possible. • Administer cautiously in the elderly and in people with epilepsy, myasthenia gravis, impaired hepatic or renal function, history of substance abuse or other central nervous system (CNS) depressant use. • Assess person for unexplained bleeding. • Monitor liver function and blood counts. • Instruct person to avoid alcohol, antidepressants and anticonvulsants. • Caution person not to drive or operate hazardous machinery until drowsiness subsides. • Stress the importance of avoiding abrupt drug withdrawal.
Beta-adrenergic blocking agent			
Propranolol	• Bradycardia • Dizziness • Emotional lability • Fatigue • Fever • GI disturbances • Heart block • Impaired concentration • Impotence and decreased libido • Mental depression • Skin rash • Shortness of breath • Sore throat • Worsening of angina	• Concomitant use of reserpine, MAOIs, digoxin, calcium channel blockers, theophylline, norepinephrine or dopamine • Compromised cardiac function • Diabetes • Respiratory disease	• Take person's apical pulse for 1 full minute after giving dose. • Monitor cardiac function (fluid intake and output, daily weight, serum electrolytes) • Assess person for signs and symptoms of depression. • Advise person not to change dose or stop drug intake without doctor's approval. • Instruct person to report weight gain of more than 2 lb per week. • Inform diabetic people that drug may mask hypoglycaemia symptoms. • Instruct person to take drug with food to minimise GI disturbance. • Teach person which side effects to report.

Pharmacological therapy for anxiety disorders (continued)

Drug	Side effects	Contraindications	Nursing considerations
Monoamine oxidase inhibitors			
Phenelzine sulphate Tranylcypromine sulphate	• Blurred vision • Constipation • Drowsiness or insomnia • Dry mouth • Fatigue • Hepatic dysfunction (jaundice, malaise, right upper abdominal quadrant pain, change in stool colour or consistency) • Hypertensive crisis • Hypomania • Muscle twitching • Orthostatic hypotension • Skin rash • Vertigo • Weakness • Weight gain	• Cardiovascular or cerebrovascular disease • Confusion or un-cooperativeness • Elderly or debilitated people • Glaucoma • Heart failure • History of severe headache • Impaired renal function • Liver disease • Pregnancy • Paranoid schizophrenia	• Use with caution in elderly people. • Monitor person's blood pressure every 2–4 hours during initial therapy. Instruct person to change positions slowly. • Assess person for signs and symptoms of hypertensive crisis. • Monitor fluid intake and output. • Monitor person for suicidal risk. • Caution person not to ingest foods and beverages containing tyramine, caffeine or tryptophan. Warn her that ingesting tyramine can cause a hypertensive crisis. Give her a list of foods and beverages that contain such substances, which include aged cheeses, sour cream, beer, Chianti, aged sherry, pickled herring, liver, canned figs, raisins, bananas, avocados, chocolate, soy, smoked fish, sausage, liver, bologna, fava beans, yeast extracts, meat tenderisers, coffee and colas. • Instruct person to avoid meperidine, epinephrine, local anaesthetics, decongestants, cough medicines, diet pills and most over-the-counter (OTC) agents. • Advise person to go to the emergency department if hypertensive crisis develops. • Instruct person to wear medical identification jewellery.
Selective serotonin reuptake inhibitors			
Fluoxetine Paroxetine	• Insomnia • Nausea • Nervousness • Vertigo	• Within 14 days of taking an MAOI	• Give in morning with or without food. • Monitor for weight loss if nausea occurs. • Instruct person to avoid alcoholic beverages. • Tell person to report side effects, especially rash or itching.
Tricyclic antidepressants			
Amitriptyline Imipramine	• Agranulocytosis • Arrhythmias • Blurred vision • Bone marrow depression • Constipation • Dry mouth • Oesophageal reflux • Galactorrhoea	• Concomitant use of MAOIs • Recent myocardial infarction • Renal or hepatic disease	• Monitor blood pressure and pulse for signs of orthostatic hypotension. • Monitor person for suicidal thoughts and behaviours. • Supervise drug ingestion. • Know that special monitoring is required if person has a history of angle-closure glaucoma or seizure disorder. • Monitor for side effects. • Monitor liver function and complete blood counts. • Tell person to change positions slowly.

(continued)

Pharmacological therapy for anxiety disorders (continued)

Drug	Side effects	Contraindications	Nursing considerations
Tricyclic antidepressants (continued)			
	• Hallucinations • Heart failure • Increased or decreased libido • Jaundice and fatigue • Mania • Myocardial infarction • Orthostatic hypotension or hypertension • Palpitations • Shock • Slowing of intracardiac conduction • Urinary hesitancy • Weight gain		• Instruct person to avoid driving or hazardous machinery if drowsiness occurs. • Teach person to avoid alcohol and OTC agents unless the doctor approves. • Inform person that desired drug effects may take up to 4 weeks to appear.
Another anxiolytic agent			
Buspirone	• Dizziness • Excitement • Headache • Light-headedness • Nausea • Nervousness	• Concomitant MAOI therapy • Renal or hepatic impairment	• Assist with ambulation if needed. • Instruct person to inform all health care providers of all prescription, OTC and recreational drug use. • Caution person against driving or operating machinery until drowsiness subsides. • Instruct person to report side effects. • Inform person that improvement may take 3–4 weeks. • Advise person to have liver and kidney tests periodically.

Run-on rituals

Obsessive–compulsive behaviours and activities take up more than 1 hour per day. For some people, compulsive rituals take hours to complete and become the major life activity.

Not surprisingly, OCD causes significant distress and may severely impair occupational and social functioning. Compulsive behaviours also can endanger health and safety. For example, severe dermatitis or a skin infection may result from compulsive hand washing.

But then, who's counting?

OCD affects about 2% of the general population, striking men and women equally. In males, it typically begins in adolescence to young adulthood; in females, in young adulthood. The onset usually is gradual – over months or years.

For most people, the disorder takes a fluctuating course, with exacerbations linked to stressful events. In some cases, psychosocial functioning steadily deteriorates.

To make matters worse . . .

Many OCD sufferers also have major depressive disorder, panic disorder, social phobia, specific phobia, eating disorders, substance abuse or personality disorders.

In clinical samples, approximately 20–30% of people with OCD report a past history of tics; about one-quarter meet the full criteria for Tourette's syndrome (a neurobehavioural disorder characterised by sudden, involuntary motor and vocal tics). Conversely, up to 50% of people with Tourette's syndrome develop OCD.

Causes

Genetic, biological and psychological factors may be involved in OCD development. (See *The strep connection*.)

Genetic factors

OCD tends to run in families. Also, the risk of OCD is higher among first-degree relatives with Tourette's syndrome.

The strep connection

Researchers have found an association between obsessive–compulsive disorder (OCD) and beta-haemolytic streptococci infection. Studies of children have linked the sudden appearance of obsessions, compulsions and motor or vocal tics with streptococcal throat infection.

Possibly, an autoimmune response to the infection occurs, in which antibodies attack both healthy and infected cells. This could cause inflammation of the basal ganglia, a brain region involved in movement and motor control.

Sad syndrome, cute name

The syndrome, called paediatric autoimmune neuropsychiatric disorders associated with streptococcal infections (PANDAS), typically affects children aged 5–11 and has a dramatic, sudden onset. In some of these children, OCD symptoms respond to prompt antibiotic treatment.

Biological aspects

Biological evidence is strong, too. MRI and computed tomography scans show enlarged basal ganglia in some people with OCD. Positron-emission tomography (PET) scans found increased glucose metabolism in a particular part of the basal ganglia.

Anatomic–physiological disturbances in brain areas involved in learning or acquiring and maintaining habits and skills may also be involved in OCD.

Psychological factors

Freudian psychoanalysts view OCD as the result of conflict between the ego and the id (the unconscious part of the psyche that gives rise to instinctual impulses): Impulses that are repugnant to the ego are controlled by unconscious defence mechanisms.

Behaviourists, on the other hand, see OCD as a conditioned response to anxiety-provoking events. In their view, linking anxiety with a neutral object or event causes obsessional preoccupation. Compulsive behaviour also is learned and reinforced. In the past, such behaviour helped control the person's anxiety, so she practises it again – even though it's no longer helpful.

Risk factors

For reasons not fully understood, such sociological factors as being young, divorced, separated or unemployed increase the risk for OCD.

Signs and symptoms

A person with OCD may exhibit or report:
• repetitive thoughts that cause stress (obsessions)
• repetitive behaviours (compulsions), such as hand washing, counting or checking and rechecking whether a door is locked
• social impairment caused by preoccupation with obsessions and compulsions
• perceived need to achieve perfection.

They know it's weird

Most people are aware that their obsessions are excessive or irrational and interfere with normal daily activities. In fact, many hide their symptoms out of embarrassment. However, a minority don't perceive their obsessions and compulsions as irrational. (See *Cultural practices and OCD*, page 219.)

Diagnosis

The diagnosis of OCD is confirmed if the person meets the criteria listed in the *DSM-IV-TR*. (See *Diagnostic criteria: Obsessive–compulsive disorder*, page 220.)

Bridging the gap

Cultural practices and OCD

Don't mistake certain cultural or religious practices for obsessive–compulsive disorder (OCD). In some cultures, for instance, people pray repetitively or mourn a loved one's death with intensely ritualised behaviour that seems obsessive or compulsive to an observer. For this reason, always assess the person within the context of cultural and religious background.

Crucial criteria

Remember – culturally prescribed ritual behaviour in itself doesn't signal OCD unless it:

- exceeds cultural norms
- occurs at times and places that others in the culture would judge inappropriate
- interferes with the person's social role functioning.

Treatment

Treatment options for OCD include:
- behavioural techniques
- relaxation techniques, such as deep breathing, progressive muscle relaxation, meditation, imagery or music
- support groups, which decrease the person's isolation
- partial hospitalisation and day treatment programmes
- medication.

Exposing themselves

The behavioural technique of exposure and response prevention may be used to treat people with OCD. This method exposes the person to the object or situation that triggers her obsessions – but then asks her to refrain from engaging in her usual compulsive response. The person writes down what happens as a result of the behavioural restraint, and comes to realise that not performing the ritual doesn't bring distressing outcomes. Eventually, she learns to manage her intense anxiety until it subsides.

For example, a person who obsesses about contamination and germs stops herself from washing after shaking hands or coming into contact with public surfaces. Ultimately, the anxiety and obsessions disappear.

Diagnostic criteria: Obsessive–compulsive disorder

Obsessive–compulsive disorder is diagnosed when the person's signs and symptoms meet these criteria from the *Diagnostic and Statistical Manual of Mental Disorders*, Fourth Edition, Text Revision.

Either obsessions or compulsions

Obsessions are defined as all of these examples:

- Recurrent and persistent thoughts, impulses or images that are experienced at some time during the disturbance as intrusive and inappropriate and that cause marked anxiety or distress.
- The thoughts, impulses or images aren't simply excessive worries about real-life problems.
- The person tries to ignore or suppress such thoughts or impulses, or to neutralise them with some other thought or action.
- The person recognises that the obsessions are the products of her mind and not externally imposed.

Compulsions are defined as all of these examples:

- Repetitive behaviours or mental acts performed by the person, who feels drive to perform them in response to an obsession or according to rules that must be applied rigidly.
- The behaviour or mental acts are aimed at preventing or reducing distress or preventing some dreaded event or situation. However, either the activity isn't connected in a realistic way with what it's designed to neutralise or prevent, or it's clearly excessive.

- The person recognises that her behaviour is excessive or unreasonable. (This may not be true for young children or people whose obsessions have evolved into overvalued ideas.)

Other features

- At some point, the person recognises that the obsessions or compulsions are excessive or unreasonable.
- The obsessions or compulsions cause marked distress, are time-consuming (take more than 1 hour a day) or significantly interfere with the person's normal routine, occupational functioning or usual social activities or relationships.
- If another Axis I disorder (a major mental disorder) is present, the content of the obsession isn't related to it. For example, the ideas, thoughts or images aren't about food if the person has an eating disorder, about drugs if she has a psychoactive substance use disorder or about guilt thoughts if she has major depressive disorder.
- The disturbance isn't caused by the direct physiological effects of a substance or a general medical condition.

Could it have helped Lady Macbeth?

Exposure and response-prevention therapy proves effective in about 80% of people. Its success rate has led to its use in telephone-access therapy, in which people with OCD call in and get computer-generated response-prevention therapy.

Pharmacological therapy

Pharmacological interventions may include benzodiazepines, MAOIs, SSRIs and TCAs. MAOIs and at times benzodiazepines should be avoided if possible due to psychological addiction.

Nursing interventions

These nursing interventions may be appropriate for people with OCD.
• Approach the person unhurriedly. Ask specific questions about her thoughts and behaviours, especially if you note physical cues, such as chafed or reddened hands or hair loss due to compulsive pulling.
• Identify disturbing topics of conversation that reflect underlying anxiety or terror.
• Keep the person's physical health in mind. For example, compulsive hand washing may cause skin breakdown; rituals or preoccupations may cause inadequate food and fluid intake and exhaustion. Provide for basic needs, such as rest, nutrition and grooming, if the person becomes involved in ritualistic thoughts and behaviours to the point of self-neglect.

Isn't it tiring?

• Let the person know you're aware of her behaviour. For example, you might say, 'I noticed you've made your bed three times today. That must be very tiring for you.'
• Help her to explore feelings associated with the behaviour. For example, ask, 'What do you think about while you perform your chores?' Listen attentively, offering feedback.
• Explore patterns leading to the behaviour or recurring problems.

Don't be shocked

• Maintain an accepting attitude.
• Don't show shock, amusement or criticism of the ritualistic behaviour.

Don't try to block

• Give the person time to carry out the ritualistic behaviour (unless it's dangerous) until she can be distracted by some other activity. Be aware that blocking such behaviour could increase her anxiety to an intolerable level.
• Make reasonable demands and set reasonable limits – and make their purpose clear. Avoid creating situations that increase frustration and provoke anger, which may interfere with treatment.

Diversionary tactics

• Encourage active diversions, such as whistling or humming a tune, to divert attention from the unwanted thoughts and promote a pleasurable experience.
• Explain how to channel emotional energy to relieve stress (for example, through creative endeavours).
• Engage the person in activities that create positive accomplishments and raise self-esteem and confidence.

Memory jogger

To help the person cope with OCD, remember the word COPING.

C Concerns and feelings are discussed

O Offer a structured routine that allows time for rituals

P Practice thought-stopping skills

I Initiate a behavioural contract to decrease rituals and reward non-ritualistic behaviours

N Nurture effective ways to problem-solve stressful situations

G Get the person to perform relaxation techniques

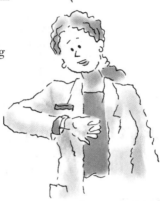

In one OCD intervention, you shorten the time that the person may engage in compulsive behaviour.

Time's up!

• Assist the person in exploring new ways to solve problems and developing more effective coping skills by setting limits on unacceptable behaviour (for example, by limiting the number of times per day she may indulge in compulsive behaviour). Gradually shorten the time allowed. For the remainder of the time, help her focus on other feelings or problems.

• Identify insight and improved behaviour (reduced compulsive behaviour and fewer obsessive thoughts). Evaluate behavioural changes by your own and the person's reports.

• Observe when interventions don't work; reevaluate and recommend alternative strategies.

What did you expect?

• Help the person identify progress and set realistic expectations for herself.

• Encourage the use of appropriate coping mechanisms to relieve loneliness and isolation.

• Monitor the person for suicidal behaviours and thoughts. Hopelessness and helplessness may overwhelm her as she realises the absurdity of her behaviour but feels powerless to control it.

• Monitor for desired and side effects of prescribed drugs.

Quick quiz

1. Signs and symptoms of acute stress disorder may occur:
   A. immediately after a trauma.
   B. as early as 2 days after a trauma.
   C. about 1 month after a trauma.
   D. several months after a trauma.

Answer: B. Acute distress disorder may cause symptoms as soon as 2 days after a trauma.

2. Fear of situations or places that may be difficult or embarrassing to leave describes:
  A. social phobia.
  B. panic disorder.
  C. agoraphobia.
  D. generalised anxiety disorder.

Answer: C. Agoraphobia is the fear and avoidance of situations or places that may be difficult or embarrassing to leave.

3. Unresolved conflicts, a tendency to misinterpret events and avoidance of new situations may be risk factors for:
  A. panic disorder.
  B. GAD.
  C. social phobia.
  D. cacophobia.

Answer: B. The risk for GAD is higher in people with unresolved conflicts, a tendency to misinterpret events and avoidance of new situations. Panic disorder, social phobia and cacophobia share some but not all of these risk factors.

4. The fear of losing one's mind or having a heart attack is most likely to occur in:
  A. social phobia.
  B. panic disorder.
  C. GAD.
  D. myctophobia.

Answer: B. Anxiety severe enough to cause the person to fear she's losing her mind or having a heart attack occurs with panic disorder. Social phobia, GAD and myctophobia may have a panic component to them, but the anxiety is less severe.

5. Flashbacks of an unpleasant, terrifying or painful experience may occur in:
  A. PTSD.
  B. panic disorder.
  C. agoraphobia.
  D. obsessive–compulsive disorder.

Answer: A. Flashbacks are characteristic of PTSD. They aren't major components of panic disorder, agoraphobia or OCD.

6. Fear of embarrassing oneself in public characterises:
  A. generalised anxiety disorder.
  B. panic disorder.
  C. specific phobia.
  D. social phobia.

Answer: D. Social phobia is characterised by a dread of being scrutinised and subsequently being embarrassed in public.

7. A person with a history of panic attacks says he feels trapped after an attack. He most likely fears:

    A.   loss of maturity.
    B.   loss of control.
    C.   loss of memory.
    D.   loss of identity.

Answer: B. People who fear loss of control during a panic attack commonly make statements about feeling trapped, getting hurt or having little or no personal control over their situations.

Scoring

☆☆☆   If you answered all seven items correctly, terrific! We're sending you on a worry-free vacation to the Sea of Tranquillity.

☆☆   If you answered five or six items correctly, relax. You have nothing to be anxious about when it comes to understanding anxiety disorders.

☆   If you answered fewer than five items correctly, no need to panic. Just breathe deeply, relax, stop those negative thoughts – and then reexpose yourself to the chapter for further study.

7 Psychosomatic disorders

Just the facts

In this chapter, you'll learn:

♦ how stress can be converted to physical symptoms

♦ differences between conversion disorder and pseudo disorders

♦ proposed causes of somatisation and psychosomatic disorders

♦ signs and symptoms of psychosomatic disorders

♦ assessment and interventions for people with psychosomatic disorders.

A look at psychosomatic disorders

Psychosomatic disorders are a group of psychiatric disorders in which the person has persistent physical (bodily) complaints that can't be explained by a physical disorder, substance use or another mental disorder. Instead, the symptoms are linked to psychological factors. Distress and preoccupation with the symptoms can lead to occupational, academic, social and other impairments.

This chapter discusses the major psychosomatic disorders – body dysmorphic disorder (BDD), hypochondriasis, pain disorder, conversion disorder and somatisation disorder.

They're not faking it

People with psychosomatic disorders don't feign their symptoms (as in malingering, or conscious 'faking'). Instead, they believe their symptoms indicate a real physical disorder. Because they don't produce the symptoms intentionally or feel a sense of control over them, they have trouble accepting that the symptoms have a psychological origin.

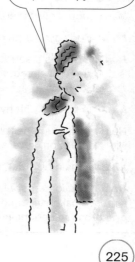

I seem to be disappearing, but I'm trying not to let it preoccupy me.

Most types of psychosomatic disorder affect more females than males. Also, somatic complaints without a physical basis are common in the elderly.

Converting stress into symptoms

Somatisation refers to the conversion of emotional or mental states into bodily symptoms. According to experts, people with psychosomatic disorders internalise their anxiety, stress and frustration. Instead of confronting these feelings directly, they express them through physical symptoms.

Although relatively few people meet the criteria for a psychosomatic *disorder*, psychosomatic *symptoms* are extremely common. One study found no organic cause in more than 80% of primary care person visits for the evaluation of such symptoms as chest pain, dizziness or fatigue. (See *The scoop on psychosomatic disorders*.)

All in her head – not!

Health care professionals who can't find a physical basis for a person's symptoms may tell them that the illness is 'all in your head'. Failure to recognise somatisation and manage it appropriately, however, can lead to frustrating, costly and potentially dangerous tests and treatments.

Many people go from doctor to doctor in search of a diagnosis and treatment. Generally, tests fail to identify organic disease, and treatments (if prescribed) don't ease the person's suffering. What's more, some people are misdiagnosed with organic conditions and may experience complications from diagnostic, medical or surgical procedures.

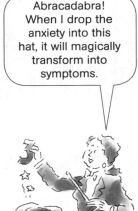

Abracadabra! When I drop the anxiety into this hat, it will magically transform into symptoms.

Myth busters

The scoop on psychosomatic disorders

Many people misunderstand the nature of psychosomatic disorders. To separate yourself from the masses, read on.

Myth: Body dysmorphic disorder (BDD) is a simple disturbance in a person's body image.

Reality: BDD is a serious disorder characterised by preoccupation with the exaggerated belief that one's body is deformed or defective. The person may spend hours in checking and grooming behaviours and may undergo various dermatologic treatments or cosmetic surgeries.

Myth: In people with hypochondriasis, the primary emotional feature is fear.

Reality: Although people with hypochondriasis may fear they have a life-threatening disease, many also struggle with depression, severe anxiety and obsessive–compulsive symptoms.

Myth: In pain disorder, no medical evidence of a pathological process exists.

Reality: In some people with pain disorder, diagnostic tests identify evidence of a pathological process, such as a musculoskeletal condition or cancer. Nonetheless, psychological factors play a predominant role in the severity, exacerbation and maintenance of the pain.

Coexisting disorders

Many people with psychosomatic disorders also have personality disorders – probably because of the inherent relationship between physical illness and certain personality traits or types of character structure.

Dual diagnoses

Some people also have coexisting depressive disorders or anxiety disorders – for instance:
• people with psychosomatic disorder often develop panic attacks or agoraphobia
• pain disorder often exists concomitantly with depression
• BDD commonly overlaps with obsessive–compulsive disorder (OCD).

Cultural and ethnic factors

Culture and ethnicity may affect the prevalence of psychosomatic symptoms and psychosomatic disorders. Here are some examples:
• Compared to Westerners, Asians and Africans more often express their mental distress as physical complaints such as tiredness, headaches, palpitations, weight loss and vague aches and pains.
• Culture and ethnicity also can determine the types of treatment a person will consider. (See *How culture influences treatment choices*.)

Causes

The precise causes of psychosomatic disorders remain mostly a mystery. In the view of psychodynamic theorists, these conditions result from repression of emotions, such as after a traumatic event. The symptoms are manifestations of the person's repressed emotions.

Family stress

Among children and adolescents, family stress is thought to be a common cause of psychosomatic disorders. For instance, in hypochondriasis and somatisation disorder, a child may unconsciously reflect or imitate a parent's behaviour – especially if the parent reaped considerable secondary gain (such as attention) from the symptoms. (See *Primary and secondary gain*, page 228.)

Learned responses

Behavioural theorists view psychosomatic symptoms as responses that the person has consciously learned and subsequently maintains because they bring some type of reward. The symptoms, for instance, may allow the person to:
• gain concern or sympathy
• avoid unpleasant tasks
• explain or justify failures.

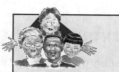

Bridging the gap

How culture influences treatment choices

A person's cultural or ethnic background may influence her treatment preferences and choices. People from some cultures may be suspicious of alternative medicine, whereas those from other cultures may often use alternative techniques – but hesitate to disclose this. Their hesitancy may arise from previous experiences with sceptical health care professionals.

Primary and secondary gain

Primary gain refers to relief of the unconscious psychological conflict, wish or need that's causing the physical symptom. As the person's anxiety increases and threatens to emerge into consciousness, she 'converts' it to physical symptoms. This relieves the pressure to deal with it directly.

Secondary gain, in contrast, refers to the benefit, resources or advantages that come from having the symptom – such as avoiding difficult situations or getting emotional support or sympathy that the person might not otherwise receive.

Psychobiological mechanisms

Some experts describe four independent psychobiological mechanisms at work in somatisation:

- heightened body sensations
- increased autonomic arousal
- identification of the 'patient' within a family
- perceived need to be sick.

A person may show evidence of a single mechanism or any combination of the four.

Heightened body sensations

Psychosomatic disorders may be linked to a heightened awareness of normal body sensations. Paired with a cognitive bias, this heightened awareness may predispose the person to interpret any physical symptom as a sign of physical illness.

A person who's worried about physical disease may focus attention on common variations in bodily sensations – to the point that these sensations become disturbing and unpleasant. The person thinks the sensations confirm the suspected presence of physical disease. The perception of such altered sensations exacerbates their concerns, further increasing their anxiety and amplifying the sensations.

Increased autonomic arousal

Some people with psychosomatic disorders may have heightened autonomic arousal. Such arousal may be associated with the effects of body chemicals that cause norepinephrine release, resulting in such symptoms as tachycardia or gastric hypermotility.

Heightened autonomic arousal also may cause pain and muscle tension associated with muscular hyperactivity, as in muscle-tension headache.

Identification of the 'patient' within a family

In a family under stress, identifying one member as the 'patient' may provide a focus that relieves anxiety. With a single member taking on the 'sick' role,

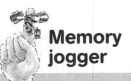

Memory jogger

SIGNS of psychosomatic disorders

S Sexual or reproductive symptoms

I Intense pain (in pain disorder)

G GI problems

N Neurological symptoms

S Symptoms of anxiety and depression

family behaviour patterns may become dysfunctional. Health care providers may reinforce this dynamic by focusing medical attention on the 'sick' family member's disability and illness.

Perceived need to be sick

People with psychosomatic disorders may seek the 'sick' role because it provides relief from stressful interpersonal expectations and, in most societies, offers attention and caring.

Evaluation and treatment

Accurate diagnosis of psychosomatic disorders can prevent unnecessary laboratory tests, surgery and other procedures. The person should undergo a thorough physical assessment to rule out medical and neurological conditions and, in people with pain, to assess pain severity. Other psychiatric disorders that resemble psychosomatic disorder must be ruled out, too.

One-stop shopping

Ideally, a person with a psychosomatic disorder should develop a long-term relationship with a single, trusted primary health care provider. This helps guard against unnecessary tests and treatments.

Specialist referrals should be minimised to help ensure continuity of care and effective person monitoring – and to avoid the perception that the health care provider is 'abandoning' the person. Referrals to mental health professionals should be handled with great sensitivity.

Service user's role

The person should take an active role in treatment and be willing to take responsibility for moving forwards with the treatment plan (such as by keeping a diary of symptoms and activities). Also, they should be encouraged to get regular exercise because self-initiated physical activity fosters responsibility and a sense of control. Periodic conferences should be scheduled with the person and their family to provide a forum for communication and education.

A little bit of knowledge . . .

Teaching people about signs and symptoms of disorders linked to anxiety or depression may decrease their stress and ease their symptoms. Many people improve just by learning about the mind–body connection (the effects of the mind and emotions on physical symptoms and disease).

Parents and childcare providers need to be taught about the symptoms of stress in children, which can manifest as physical disorders. (See *Stress-related disorders in children*, page 230.)

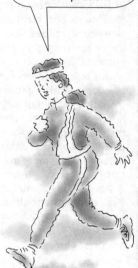

I tell service users that regular exercise gives them a sense of control – and I like to practise what I preach.

Stress-related disorders in children

Stress can produce certain disorders in children. These include stuttering, sleepwalking, sleep terrors, functional enuresis and functional encopresis.

Stuttering

In *stuttering*, speech rhythms are abnormal, with repetitions and hesitations at the beginning of words. Sometimes, these abnormalities are accompanied by movements of the face, shoulders and respiratory muscles.

Stuttering is most common in children of average or superior intelligence who fear they can't meet the expectations of socially striving, success-oriented families. Sometimes, however, it's associated with mental dullness, poor social background and a history of birth trauma. Stuttering can lower the child's self-esteem and cause anxiety, humiliation and withdrawal from social situations.

About 80% of stutterers recover after age 16. Evaluation and treatment by a speech and language therapist teaches the stutterer to place equal weight on each syllable in a sentence, to breathe properly and to control anxiety.

Sleepwalking and sleep terrors

In *sleepwalking*, the child calmly rises from bed in an altered state of consciousness and walks about, with no subsequent recollection of dream content.

In *sleep terrors*, he awakes terrified, in a state of clouded consciousness, often unable to recognise parents and familiar surroundings. Visual hallucinations may occur, too.

Sleep terrors are a normal developmental occurrence in children aged 2 or 3. They most often arise within 30 minutes to 3½ hours of sleep onset. Associated signs include tachycardia, tachypnoea, diaphoresis, dilated pupils and piloerection. Usually, sleep terrors are self-limiting and subside within a few weeks.

Nocturnal enuresis

Nocturnal enuresis (bed-wetting) is characterised by intentional or involuntary voiding of urine, usually at night. Considered normal in children up to age 3 or 4, functional enuresis persists in 10% of children to age 5, in 5% to age 10 and in 1% of males to age 18.

The condition may be linked to stress, as from the birth of a sibling, a move to a new home, parental divorce or separation, hospitalisation, faulty toilet training or unrealistic, age-inappropriate responsibilities. Associated problems include low self-esteem, social withdrawal from peers because of ostracism and ridicule, and anger, rejection and punishment by caregivers.

Dry-bed therapy may include the use of an alarm apparatus (wet bell pad), social motivation, self-correction of accidents and positive reinforcement.

Functional encopresis

Functional encopresis is the evacuation of faeces into the child's clothes or inappropriate receptacles. It's associated with low intelligence, cerebral dysfunction or other developmental symptoms, such as a lag in language development.

Predisposing factors may include psychosocial stress and inadequate or inconsistent toilet training. Related problems include repressed anger, withdrawal from peers and low self-esteem.

The child should undergo a medical examination to rule out physical disorders. Child, adult and family therapy may be needed to reduce anger and disappointment over the child's development and to improve parenting techniques.

Therapeutic approaches

The most effective treatments for psychosomatic disorders are cognitive and behavioural therapies and similar approaches that aim to reduce symptoms. On the other hand, psychoanalysis and other forms of insight-oriented psychotherapy are less effective, although some people may benefit from group therapy or support groups.

Family therapy

Family therapy may be recommended for children or adolescents with psychosomatic disorders, particularly if the parents seem to be using the child to divert attention from other difficulties.

For people with pain disorder, family therapy can help avoid reinforcement of dependency among family members.

Alternative therapies

Alternative therapies may relieve stress, pain and other symptoms, not just on a physical level but also on a mental, emotional and spiritual level. These therapies include:
- acupuncture
- hydrotherapy
- therapeutic massage
- meditation
- aromatherapy
- reflexology
- homoeopathic treatment.

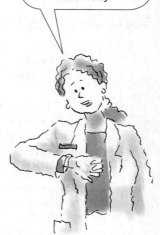

A person with BDD thinks about the perceived flaw for at least an hour each day.

Body dysmorphic disorder

In BDD, the person is preoccupied with an imagined or slight defect in physical appearance. She thinks she's hideous or grotesque, even though others reassure her that she looks fine. She can't be convinced that the flaw is minimal or, in many cases, nonexistent. She thinks about the perceived defect for at least an hour each day.

This preoccupation can lead to severe distress and impaired functioning. In extreme cases, it results in psychiatric hospitalisation, suicidal ideation or suicide attempts.

Facial focus

Most often, BDD people perceive a flaw of the face or head – especially the skin, nose, hair or ears. Some worry that they have acne or scarring. Others think they have a big nose or asymmetrical facial features.

Still others focus on the shape or size of a particular body part, such as the breasts, genitals, muscles or buttocks. Young men may believe they're puny, and obsessively try to gain weight and add muscle. Many people are preoccupied with several body parts at a time.

Mirror, mirror, see my flaw

To confirm or avoid the perceived defect, the person engages in ritualistic, compulsive behaviours such as:
- frequently checking her appearance in mirrors (or, conversely, avoiding mirrors)

- comparing her perceived defect with others' defects
- grooming excessively (combing hair, applying make-up or picking skin)
- seeking constant reassurance from others that her defect is 'not that bad'.
  Although the person thinks that doing these things will reduce her anxiety, they only intensify it.

Cosmetic surgery sign-up sheet

Many people consult cosmetic specialists, such as plastic surgeons and dermatologists. Some even stay in hiding, convinced that they're hideous.

Prevalence and onset

BDD affects a large proportion of the population; research shows that it affects 1% of the population in the UK, both men and women equally. This figure may be an underestimate because BDD frequently goes undiagnosed. One in four people affected by BDD attempt suicide.

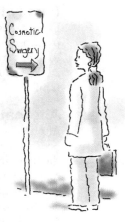

Teenagers in torment

A chronic condition, BDD usually begins during the late teens. The average age of onset is 17.

The disorder may come on gradually or abruptly. It takes a fluctuating course.

A person who receives appropriate treatment has a good prognosis. Without treatment, the person may become delusional or grow increasingly depressed – perhaps even suicidal.

To complicate matters . . .

Many people with BDD have additional psychiatric disorders, including:
- depression
- OCD
- eating disorders
- anxiety disorders
- agoraphobia
- trichotillomania (hair pulling).

BDD may predispose the person to major depressive disorder. In clinical settings, about 60% of people with BDD have major depression; their lifetime risk of major depression is 80%. The combination of BDD and major depression puts them at high risk for suicide (especially in females with perceived facial defects).

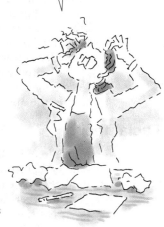

If I did this all the time, a psychiatrist would call it trichotillomania.

Not a trivia question

BDD may be misdiagnosed or trivialised. Many sufferers are too embarrassed to reveal their distress to others (including health care professionals). Some downplay the problem; others don't even realise they need help.

Family members may trivialise the problem, too, not realising that BDD is an extreme distortion that the sufferer can't simply 'get over' or 'grow out of'.

Even some health care professionals may be unaware that BDD is a known psychiatric disorder that responds to appropriate treatment.

Causes

No one knows what causes BDD. Generally, two different explanations exist – one biological and the other psychological. Both may be correct.

Biological theory

Some people may have a genetic predisposition to psychiatric disorders, making them more likely to develop BDD. Certain stresses or life events, especially during adolescence, may precipitate onset of the disorder.

BDD also may be associated with an imbalance of serotonin or other brain chemicals.

Psychological theory

Low self-esteem and a tendency to judge oneself almost exclusively by appearance may contribute to BDD. Sufferers may be perfectionists striving for an impossible ideal – and not liking what they see in the mirror.

So self-absorbed

As they pay excessive attention to their appearance, they develop a heightened perception of it, increasingly focusing on every imperfection or slight abnormality. Avoiding certain situations or using safety behaviours perpetuates their fear that others will judge them – which only intensifies their excessive attention on themselves.

Beauty-obsessed culture

Societal values play a large role, too. In Western culture, certain standards of beauty are idealised. Many people compare themselves to so-called 'beautiful' celebrities, actors and models – and find themselves lacking. Adolescents are especially vulnerable to this type of pressure.

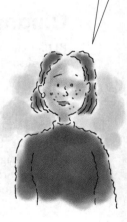

No wonder I have BDD. I see gorgeous people on TV all the time, and then I look in the mirror and see this!

Signs and symptoms

Suspect BDD if the person reports or exhibits these behaviours:
- often checks her reflection in the mirror, or avoids mirrors
- frequently compares her appearance with others' or examines others' appearance
- tries to cover the perceived defect with clothing, make-up or a hat or by changing her posture
- seeks corrective treatment, such as surgery or dermatological therapy, to eradicate the perceived defect (even though doctors, family and friends think such measures aren't necessary)
- constantly seeks reassurance from others about the perceived flaw or, conversely, tries to convince others of its repulsiveness

- performs long grooming rituals, such as repeatedly combing or cutting the hair or applying make-up or cover-up creams
- picks at her skin or squeezes pimples or blackheads for hours
- frequently touches the perceived problem area
- measures the body part she thinks is repulsive
- is anxious and self-conscious around peers
- feels acute distress over her appearance, causing functional impairment
- avoids social situations where the perceived defect may be exposed
- has difficulty maintaining relationships with peers, family and spouses
- performs poorly in school or work, or takes frequent sick days
- has low self-esteem
- has suicidal thoughts or behaviours.

The reclusive solution

Symptom severity varies. For some people, distress is manageable and they're able to function on a day-to-day basis (although not to their full potential). Others have severe functional impairment, and some are so embarrassed by their appearance that they become recluses.

Diagnosis

BDD may be misdiagnosed as anorexia nervosa, social phobia, agoraphobia, panic disorder, trichotillomania, OCD or depression.

The OCD link

OCD in particular shares many features with BDD. Some experts believe BDD is an OCD 'spectrum' disorder – meaning it has the same core symptoms, but focuses on just one aspect of appearance.

The diagnosis of BDD is confirmed if the person meets the criteria in the *Diagnostic and Statistical Manual of Mental Disorders*, Fourth Edition, Text Revision *(DSM-IV-TR)*. (See *Diagnostic criteria: Body dysmorphic disorder*.)

Memory jogger

Each letter of BODY stands for a major feature of body dysmorphic disorder.

B Body image disturbance

O Obsession over a perceived physical defect

D 'Defect' in appearance leads to preoccupation and compulsive behaviours

Y Yearns and 'doctor shops' to correct the perceived defect

Diagnostic criteria: Body dysmorphic disorder

The diagnosis of body dysmorphic disorder is confirmed when the person meets these criteria from the *Diagnostic and Statistical Manual of Mental Disorders*, Fourth Edition, Text Revision.

- The person is preoccupied with an imagined defect in appearance. If a slight physical abnormality actually is present, her concern over it is markedly excessive.
- The preoccupation causes clinically significant distress or impairment in social, occupational or other important areas of functioning.
- The preoccupation isn't better explained by another mental disorder (such as anorexia nervosa).

Assessment by multidisciplinary teams

Assessment by multidisciplinary teams with specific expertise in BDD should include:

- comprehensive assessment of symptom profile
- previous psychological and pharmacological treatments
- adherence to prescribed medication
- history of side effects
- comorbid conditions such as depression
- suicide risk
- psychosocial stressors
- relationship with family/carers
- personality factors.

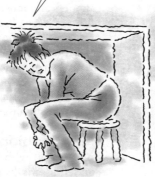

I feel too ugly to leave my room.

Treatment

Treatment for BDD seeks to:

- enhance the person's self-esteem
- reduce her preoccupation with the perceived flaw and decrease the time spent on compulsive behaviour
- eliminate harmful effects of compulsive behaviours
- improve functional abilities
- encourage the person to express, and cope with, feelings of anxiety as they arise without resorting to excessive behaviours.

Group therapy may reduce the person's sense of helplessness and help her to communicate her thoughts, feelings and desires directly.

Psychological treatments

In the initial treatment of adults with BDD, low-intensity psychological treatments (including exposure and response prevention [ERP]) should be offered if the person's degree of functional impairment is mild and/or the person expresses a preference for a low-intensity approach. Low-intensity treatments include brief individual cognitive behavioural therapy (CBT) including ERP using structured self-help materials and group CBT including ERP.

Adults with BDD with moderate functional impairment should be offered the choice of either a course of selective serotonin reuptake inhibitor (SSRI) or more intensive individual CBT including ERP that addresses key features of BDD.

All children and young people with BDD should be offered CBT, including ERP that involves family and carers, and that is adapted to suit the developmental age of the child or young person as first-line treatment.

Cognitive behavioural therapy

Many people with BDD benefit from CBT. Specific techniques include:

- teaching the person to resist compulsive behaviours
- decreasing the time she spends on obsessive thoughts and compulsive behaviour
- helping her to face the situations she's been avoiding.

Hold that thought!

Thought stopping breaks the habit of thinking disturbing thoughts by interrupting them and substituting competing ones. The person is taught to use an intense distracting stimulus (such as snapping a rubber band around the wrist) to stop the offending thought. Then she focuses on achieving calmness and muscle relaxation.

To replace obsessive thoughts, the person may be taught the technique of *thought replacement* or *thought switching*. In these methods, she practises replacing negative thoughts with positive ones until the positive thoughts become strong enough to overcome the negative ones.

Response prevention aims to prevent compulsive behaviour through distraction, persuasion or redirection of activity. To be effective, it may require hospitalisation or family involvement.

Pharmacological treatments

Some people with BDD have been treated successfully with the antidepressant drugs called selective serotonin reuptake inhibitors (SSRIs), including fluoxetine. These drugs effectively diminish preoccupation, distress, depression and anxiety. The tricyclic antidepressant clomipramine also has proven effective.

Nursing interventions

These nursing interventions may be appropriate for a person with BDD.
- Approach the person unhurriedly. Provide an accepting, nonjudgemental atmosphere. Don't express shock, amusement or criticism of her behaviour.
- Keep the person's physical health in mind. (For example, constantly picking at the skin may cause infection or skin breakdown.) If she becomes involved in ritualistic thoughts and behaviours to the point of self-neglect, provide for basic needs, such as rest, nutrition and grooming.
- Let the person know you're aware of her behaviour. Help her explore feelings associated with the behaviour. You might ask her, 'What do you think about while you perform this behaviour?'

> I'll let her carry out her rituals, but I won't let her neglect her basic needs.

Blocking ban

- Give the person time to carry out compulsive or ritualistic behaviour (unless it's dangerous), until she can be distracted into some other activity. Don't block ritualistic behaviour; doing so could raise her anxiety to an intolerable level.
- Impose reasonable demands and set reasonable limits; be sure to make their purpose clear.
- Avoid creating situations that increase frustration and provoke anger, which may interfere with treatment.

- Identify insight and improved behaviour, such as fewer obsessive thoughts and reduced time spent on ritualistic behaviour. Evaluate behavioural changes by your own and the person's reports.

Diversion tactics

- Engage the person in activities that create positive accomplishments and raise her self-esteem and confidence.
- Suggest active diversions, such as whistling or humming, to divert the person's attention away from unwanted thoughts.

Compulsion cutbacks

- Help the person devise new ways to solve problems and develop more effective coping skills by setting limits on unacceptable behaviour. For instance, gradually shorten the time allowed for engaging in the behaviour. Help her focus on other feelings or problems for the remainder of the time.
- Note when interventions don't work. Reevaluate and recommend alternative strategies.

Terrifying topics

- Identify disturbing topics of conversation that reflect underlying anxiety or terror.
- Listen attentively, offering feedback.
- Encourage the person to use appropriate techniques to relieve stress, loneliness and isolation.
- Monitor for desired and side effects of drug therapy, as appropriate.

Hypochondriasis

Hypochondriasis is marked by the persistent conviction that one has or is likely to get a serious disease – despite medical evidence and reassurance to the contrary. The person bases her conviction on bodily sensations or symptoms that she has misinterpreted. For instance, she might misinterpret a feeling of abdominal pressure as abdominal pain.

She doesn't consciously cause her symptoms and isn't consciously aware of the benefits they bring (such as increased attention). Her thinking pattern, though, stops short of delusional.

Hypochondriacs sometimes do get sick

Hypochondriasis can lead to significant psychological distress or impairment in social and occupational functioning. What's more, a long history of previously unfounded complaints may contribute to the doctor overlooking a serious organic disease. The person is also at risk for complications from multiple evaluations, tests and invasive procedures.

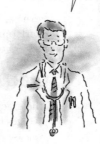

Have I ever overlooked organic disease in a person with hypochondriasis? I hope not, but I can't be sure.

Advice from the experts

Assessing older adults for psychosomatic disorders

Older adults may perceive themselves to be in poor health even if they have no significant physical impairments. Their tendency to present with psychosomatic complaints poses a challenge to assessment and management.

As a first step, the person should undergo a comprehensive medical assessment (and laboratory tests, as needed) to check for a physical basis for complaints. Cognitive and psychiatric examinations may be warranted, too.

Essential assessment data

When assessing an older adult for a psychosomatic disorder, always gather a complete history. Be sure to obtain:

- past level of functioning
- extent of current disabilities
- cognitive deficits
- manifestations of emotional distress.

Also assess the person's psychosocial status, including:

- living situation
- social supports

- role within the family
- key support people outside the family.

To verify the person's information, obtain a collaborative history from family members, if possible.

Family stress and abuse

Be aware that the family may respond to the person's psychosomatic symptoms by giving her more time and attention. In some cases, however, family members become angry and frustrated as conflicts arise and escalate. The person may even suffer neglect and abuse. If you suspect this is happening, make sure it's reported to the proper authorities.

Prevalence and onset

In general medical clinic populations, the prevalence of hypochondriasis may approach 6%. The disorder accounts for about 5% of psychiatric people.

Hypochondriasis affects as many men as women. It's most common between ages 20 and 30, although it's seen increasingly in children and adolescents. It may also develop in elderly people without previous histories of health-related fears. (See *Assessing older adults for psychosomatic disorders*.)

Hypochondriasis may persist for years, but usually occurs as a series of episodes rather than continuous treatment seeking. Flare-ups often follow stressful events.

What the future holds

Perhaps 5% of people with hypochondriasis recover permanently. Those with overlapping depression usually have a poor prognosis for recovery from the depression.

Causes

The exact cause of hypochondriasis isn't known, but some experts believe it involves biologically based hypersensitivity to internal stimuli.

Also, the disorder is more common in people who have experienced an organic disease, as well as their relatives. It has been found in nearly 8% of first-degree relatives of people with hypochondriasis. These relatives have a high rate of other psychosomatic disorders as well as anxiety and depressive disorders.

Just like Mummy or Daddy

Most likely, psychological factors play a role. For instance, children may complain of physical symptoms that resemble those of other family members.

Sick excuse

In adults, hypochondriasis may reflect self-centredness or a wish to be taken care of. The condition enables the person to take on a dependent sick role and thereby escape responsibilities or postpone unwelcome challenges.

Angry, then ill

Emotionally, the person's symptoms may be linked to – or may be an expression of – anger or guilt. Many people with hypochondriasis also suffer from anxiety and depression.

Contributing factors

Factors that may contribute to hypochondriasis include:
- death of a loved one
- family member or friend with a serious illness
- a history of serious illness.

In older adults, hypochondriasis may be associated with depression or grief.

Signs and symptoms

Signs and symptoms of hypochondriasis range from specific to general complaints. Usually, the person has multiple complaints that involve a single body system and reflect a preoccupation with normal body functions.

Mountains from molehills

Physical sensations and symptoms commonly misinterpreted as signs of organic disease include:
- borborygmi (rumbling sounds caused by gas and fluids moving through the intestines)
- abdominal bloating
- crampy discomfort
- cardiac awareness
- sweating.

Doting on details

Typically, the person describes the symptom's location, quality and duration in minute detail. Yet these symptoms rarely follow a recognisable pattern of organic dysfunction and usually aren't associated with abnormal physical findings. As medical evaluation proceeds, the person's complaints may change.

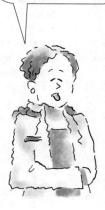

They want me to work a double shift tomorrow – but I think I feel the flu coming on.

Don't confuse me with the facts

Examination and reassurance by a doctor don't relieve her concerns. Instead, she tends to believe the doctor has failed to find the real cause of the disorder.

Sensory symptoms

Sensory symptoms often reported by people with hypochondriasis include:
- anaesthesia
- paraesthesia
- deafness
- blindness
- tunnel vision.

Motor symptoms

Common motor complaints include:
- abnormal movements
- gait disturbances
- weakness
- paralysis
- tremors
- tics
- jerks.

Neurological symptoms

Some people have neurological complaints, including seizure-like symptoms and symptoms that mimic those of degenerative neurological disorders.

Other findings

Other assessment findings in people with hypochondriasis may include:
- abnormal focus on bodily functions and sensations
- anger, frustration and depression
- frequent doctor visits despite assurance from health care providers that the person is healthy
- intensified symptoms when around sympathetic people
- rejection of the notion that symptoms are stress related
- use of symptoms to avoid difficult situations.

Diagnosis

Projective psychological tests (such as inkblot interpretation and sentence completion tests) may show a preoccupation with somatic concerns. A complete patient history, with an emphasis on current psychological stressors, is helpful.

The doctor may perform tests to rule out underlying organic disease, although invasive procedures should be minimised. Typically, test results are inconsistent with the person's complaints and physical findings.

> Sensory loss, abnormal movements and gait disturbances are common complaints in people with hypochondriasis.

Diagnostic criteria: Hypochondriasis

The diagnosis of hypochondriasis is confirmed when the person meets these criteria from the *Diagnostic and Statistical Manual of Mental Disorders*, Fourth Edition, Text Revision.

- The person is preoccupied with fears of having a serious disease based on misinterpretation of signs or symptoms.
- The preoccupation persists despite appropriate medical evaluation and reassurance.
- The person's belief lacks delusional intensity and isn't restricted to a circumscribed concern about appearance (as in body dysmorphic disorder).
- The preoccupation causes clinically significant distress or impairment in social, occupational or other important areas of functioning.
- The disturbance lasts at least 6 months.

- The preoccupation isn't better explained by generalised anxiety disorder, obsessive–compulsive disorder, panic disorder, a major depressive episode, separation anxiety or another psychosomatic disorder.

Other features

The person is deemed to have poor insight if, for most of the time during the current episode, she doesn't recognise that the concern about having a serious illness is excessive or unreasonable.

Let's make it official

Although history and physical findings may suggest hypochondriasis, the diagnosis is official only if the person meets the criteria in the *DSM-IV-TR*. (See *Diagnostic criteria: Hypochondriasis*.)

Treatment

The goal of treatment is to help the person lead a productive life despite distressing symptoms and fears. Appropriate teaching and a supportive relationship with a single competent, trusted health care professional are crucial.

Breaking the not-so-awful news

After medical evaluation is complete, the person should be told that she doesn't have a serious disease but that continued medical follow-up will help control her symptoms. Although providing a diagnosis may not make hypochondriasis disappear, it may ease some of her anxiety.

Linking the diagnosis to psychological stressors can also prove therapeutic. On the other hand, telling the person her symptoms are imaginary could be counterproductive.

Follow-up care

Besides aiding detection of organic illness, regular outpatient follow-up care can help the person deal with symptoms. That's important because up to 30% of people with hypochondriasis later develop organic disease.

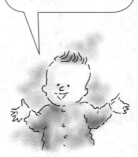

I feel so much calmer since Dr. Welby told me my drooling was perfectly normal.

Psychotherapy

Most people with hypochondriasis don't acknowledge any psychological influence on their symptoms, and resist psychiatric treatment. However, a person who's willing to try psychotherapy may be treated individually, in a group or as part of a family.

• *Individual* psychotherapy uses psychodynamic principles to help the person understand unconscious conflicts.

• *Group* therapy provides support to help her learn to cope with symptoms and to improve her social skills.

• *Family* therapy focuses on improving family members' awareness of their interaction patterns and on enhancing their communication with each other.

Cognitive behavioural therapy

Other therapeutic approaches to hypochondriasis include cognitive and behavioural techniques.

Nursing interventions

These nursing interventions may be appropriate for a person with hypochondriasis.

• Help the person deal with ineffective individual coping and altered health maintenance.

• Assess her level of knowledge about the effects of emotions and stress on physiological functioning. Provide appropriate teaching.

• Encourage her to express her feelings to deter emotional repression, which can have physical consequences.

Change the subject

• Respond to the person's symptoms in a matter-of-fact way to reduce the secondary gain she gets from talking about them.

• Engage the person in conversations that focus on something other than her physical maladies.

• Create a supportive relationship that helps her feel cared for and understood.

• Keep in mind that the person with hypochondriasis feels real pain and distress. Don't deny her symptoms or challenge her behaviour. Instead, help her find new ways to deal with stress other than developing physical symptoms.

Don't get mad

• Recognise that the person will probably never be symptom-free, and don't get angry when she doesn't give up her symptoms. Such anger can drive her away to yet another unnecessary medical evaluation.

• Help the person learn strategies to reduce distress, such as imagery, relaxation, hypnosis, biofeedback and massage. (See *Relaxation techniques*, page 243.) Also teach her assertiveness techniques, if appropriate.

Relaxation techniques

If the person has symptoms related to stress or anxiety, relaxation techniques may help. Simple relaxation techniques include:

- deep breathing, in which the person takes a series of slow, deep breaths and releases each breath slowly
- meditation, in which the person either clears her mind or focuses on a single soothing thought, image or sound.

Deep breathing

To teach the person how to perform deep breathing, first instruct her to sit in a comfortable position with her eyes closed. Next, tell her to focus on a peaceful sound or image, and then breathe in through her nose to a count of 4.

Have her hold her breath for a count of 2. Then instruct her to breathe out through her mouth for a count of 6. She should repeat this cycle for 30 seconds to 5 minutes.

Meditation

Meditation may offset some of the negative physiological effects of stress through a mechanism called the *relaxation response*. Meditating takes about 20 minutes and can be done anywhere at any time – or it may be done as a scheduled activity. Tell the person that learning to meditate takes some practice – ideally, she should practise it daily.

Techniques include concentrative and mindful meditation. For *concentrative* meditation, instruct the person to focus on a peaceful image, thought, sound or her own breathing.

For *mindful* meditation, instruct her to remain aware of all sensations, feelings, images, thoughts, sounds and smells that pass through her mind – without actually thinking about them.

Whichever technique the person uses, encourage her to make a conscious effort to relax her muscles and maintain a comfortable posture as she meditates. Closing her eyes can help her focus on inner peace.

Pain disorder

In pain disorder, the person complains of persistent pain, which results predominantly or exclusively from psychological factors. The pain becomes the person's main focus of attention and causes significant distress.

The pain may be acute or chronic. In some cases, the person has an underlying physical disorder that explains the pain – but not its severity, duration or the resulting disability. The pain is severe enough to warrant clinical attention and to impair social, occupational or other important areas of functioning.

Much pain, nothing feigned

Although the pain isn't feigned or intentionally produced, psychological factors play a key role in its onset, severity or maintenance.

Pain associated with psychological factors is common in many psychiatric conditions, especially mood and anxiety disorders. In pain disorder, however, the predominant feature is the pain itself.

Prevalence and onset

The prevalence of pain disorder is unknown. However, roughly 10–15% of adults have some form of work disability due to back pain alone. Pain disorder is more common in blue-collar workers – possibly because of their increased risk of job-related injuries.

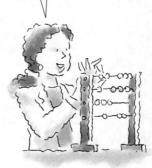

There are no hard statistics on the prevalence of pain disorder, but I'm keeping an informal count of the people I see.

Females with pain disorder outnumber males by about two to one. They also experience certain forms of pain, such as chronic headache, more often.

The peak of pain

The 30s and 40s are the peak age of onset for pain disorder. Remissions and exacerbations may occur.

Pain disorder can cause such complications as psychoactive substance dependence, multiple surgical interventions and complications of extensive diagnostic evaluations.

Disorders that commonly overlap with pain disorder include substance dependence, anxiety and depression.

Causes

No specific cause for pain disorder exists, although stress or conflict may underlie the problem. Also, chronic anxiety and depression may predispose the person to pain disorder by decreasing her pain threshold.

Real pain, real gain

For some people, the pain may have special significance or serve as a way to get attention, sympathy or relief from responsibilities or to manipulate others and gain advantage in interpersonal relationships.

Psychological theories

According to one psychological theory, a person with pain disorder converts unconscious conflicts to pain symptoms or expresses an intrapsychic conflict through pain. Unable to articulate her feelings in words, she expresses them through her body.

Behaviourally, pain behaviours are reinforced when they are rewarded and inhibited when they are ignored or punished.

Life events

A recent history of a traumatic, stressful or humiliating experience may be a contributing factor for pain disorder.

Signs and symptoms

Key assessment findings in pain disorder include:
- acute or chronic pain not explained by a physiological cause
- pain whose severity, duration or resulting disability isn't explained by an underlying physical disorder
- insomnia
- anger, frustration and depression
- anger directed at health care professionals (because they have failed to relieve her pain)
- drug-seeking behaviour in an attempt to relieve pain
- frequent visits to multiple doctors to seek pain relief.

Although the pain may involve any part of the body, it most often involves the back, head, abdomen and chest.

If a medical condition contributes to the pain, physical findings are consistent with that condition.

It's a long story

The person may relate a long history of medical assessments and procedures in multiple settings, without much noticeable pain relief. Because of frequent medical care or hospitalisations, she may be familiar with pain medications and tranquillisers. She may even ask for a specific drug and know its correct dosage and administration route.

Diagnosis

Diagnosing a person with suspected pain disorder may be challenging because the perception of pain is subjective. The doctor must rule out physical and neurological conditions, as well as other psychiatric disorders (especially other psychosomatic disorders and malingering).

If the person undergoes diagnostic tests, they fail to find an organic cause of the pain (or its severity or duration).

The diagnosis is confirmed if the person meets the criteria for pain disorder in the *DSM-IV-TR*. (See *Diagnostic criteria: Pain disorder*.)

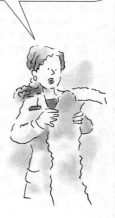

Yikes! This service user's history is as long as Billy the Kid's rap sheet!

Diagnostic criteria: Pain disorder

The diagnosis of pain disorder is confirmed when the person meets these criteria from the *Diagnostic and Statistical Manual of Mental Disorders*, Fourth Edition, Text Revision.

Pain features

- The person's chief complaint is pain in one or more anatomic sites that's severe enough to warrant clinical attention.
- The pain causes clinically significant distress or impairment in social, occupational or other important areas of functioning.
- Psychological factors are judged to play an important part in the onset, severity, exacerbation or maintenance of the pain.
- The person doesn't intentionally produce or feign the pain.
- The pain isn't better explained by a mood, anxiety or psychotic disorder and doesn't meet the criteria for dyspareunia (painful sexual intercourse).

Subtypes of pain disorder

- In pain disorder associated with *psychological factors*, psychological factors are judged to play a major role in pain onset, severity, exacerbation or maintenance. (However, this type of pain disorder isn't diagnosed if the person also meets the criteria for somatisation disorder.)
- In pain disorder associated with a *general medical condition*, a general medical condition plays a major role in the onset, severity, exacerbation or maintenance of the pain.
- In pain disorder associated with both psychological factors and a general medical condition, psychological factors and a general medical condition are both judged to play important roles in pain onset, severity, exacerbation or maintenance.

Common alternative therapies

A person with pain disorder or other psychosomatic disorders may consider trying one of these alternative therapies.

- *Nutritional therapy.* Nutritional therapy uses whole foods, nutritional supplements, if needed, and controlled fasting to treat disease and maintain health.
- *Herbal therapy.* Herbal remedies may be taken internally or applied externally to treat the internal conditions that manifest as disease.
- *Homoeopathic remedies.* Homoeopathic solutions are dilute preparations of natural substances that, in large amounts, cause certain symptoms but, in small amounts, may relieve them.
- *Acupuncture.* Commonly used to relieve pain, acupuncture involves the insertion of very fine needles into designated points on the skin to stimulate the body's vital energy flow.
- *Hydrotherapy.* Hydrotherapy involves the use of special baths and other water-based treatments to cure disorders and maintain health.
- *Naturopathic manipulative therapy.* Physical treatments may include manipulation of the bones and spine (in a manner similar to chiropractic), as well as massage, heat, cold, touch, electricity and sound, ultrasound, diathermy and therapeutic exercises.

Treatment

Treatment aims to ease the person's pain and help her live with it. The doctor may recommend that she attend a comprehensive pain centre and receive treatment for any coexisting psychiatric disorders.

A continuing, supportive relationship with an understanding health care professional is essential, as are regularly scheduled follow-up appointments.

Supportive measures

Supportive measures for pain relief include hot or cold packs, physical therapy, distraction techniques, hypnotherapy and cutaneous stimulation with massage or transcutaneous electrical nerve stimulation. Measures to reduce anxiety also may help.

Some people with pain disorder use alternative therapies for relief. (See *Common alternative therapies*.)

Painful insights

Sometimes, emphatically pointing out the link between pain and an obvious psychosocial stressor helps the person gain insight. However, some people are unable or unwilling to associate their problem with a psychosocial stressor and will reject any form of psychotherapy.

Pharmacological therapy

The doctor is likely to prescribe analgesics for a person with pain disorder. Regularly scheduled analgesic doses control pain more effectively than those given on an as-needed schedule. They also reduce the person's anxiety about asking for pain medication and eliminate unnecessary confrontations.

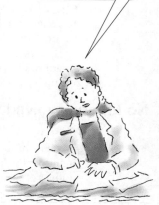

Be sure to assess and document the severity, duration and other features of the person's pain.

Other types of drugs may be prescribed as well, including: anxiolytics (benzodiazepines), such as lorazepam and alprazolam.

Placebo prohibition

Placebos shouldn't be used in an effort to 'prove' to the person that her pain is psychogenic. If she discovers the deceit, she'll become angry and distrustful.

Nursing interventions

These nursing interventions may be appropriate for a person with pain disorder.
- Assess and record characteristics of the person's pain, including its severity, duration, any precipitating or alleviating factors and any resulting disabilities.
- Provide assistance in relieving the person's pain and reducing her anxiety.
- Ensure a safe, accepting environment to promote therapeutic communication.

Caring collaboration

- Provide a caring atmosphere in which the person's complaints are taken seriously and every effort is made to provide relief. For example, tell her you'll collaborate with her on a treatment plan, and then clearly state the limitations. (You might say, 'I can stay with you now for 15 minutes, but you can't receive more pain medication until 2 p.m.')
- Don't tell the person she's imagining the pain or can wait longer for medication that's due.
- Acknowledge the person's pain to discourage her from trying to convince you that it's real.

Looking for linkage

- Help the person understand what's contributing to her pain. To elicit contributing perceptions and fears, you might say, 'I've noticed you complain of more pain after your doctor visits. What are those visits like for you?'
- Offer attention at times other than when the person complains of pain, to weaken the link to secondary gain.
- Encourage the person to recognise situations that precipitate her pain.
- Provide nonpharmacological comfort measures, such as repositioning, back massage or heat application, whenever possible.

Strategies for coping

- Teach the person coping strategies to help her deal with the pain – for example, progressive muscle relaxation or deep breathing exercises.
- Encourage her to remain independent despite her pain.
- Consider psychiatric referrals – but realise that the person may resist psychiatric intervention.

Conversion disorder

Conversion disorder is marked by the loss of or change in voluntary motor or sensory functioning (for instance, blindness, paralysis or anaesthesia) that suggests a physical illness but has no demonstrable physiological basis. Instead, the symptom has a psychological basis, as suggested by:

- exacerbation during times of emotional stress
- relief of stress or inner conflict provided by the symptom
- attention, support or avoidance of responsibilities provided by the symptom.

The conversion symptom itself isn't life threatening and usually has a short duration. However, it's clinically significant and distressing enough to disrupt social, occupational or other important areas of functioning.

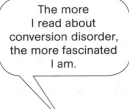

The more I read about conversion disorder, the more fascinated I am.

No fakery involved

The symptom isn't under the person's voluntary control. Unlike in factitious disorders or malingering, the person with a conversion disorder doesn't feign or intentionally produce the symptoms, although she probably has the unconscious motives of primary or secondary gain. (See *Facts about factitious disorders*.)

Facts about factitious disorders

Factitious disorders (FDs) are conditions in which a person deliberately produces or exaggerates symptoms of a physical or mental illness to assume the role of a sick person. These disorders aren't a form of malingering (pretending illness for a clear benefit, such as financial gain). Instead, the person has a deep-seated need to be seen as ill or injured.

People create their symptoms using various methods – injecting themselves with bacteria to produce infections, contaminating urine samples with blood, taking hallucinogens or other behaviours.

Except for FDs that occur by proxy, these disorders are more common in men than women. The *Diagnostic and Statistical Manual of Mental Disorders,* Fourth Edition, Text Revision *(DSM-IV-TR)* recognises four types of FDs:

- those with predominantly psychological symptoms
- those with predominantly physical symptoms
- those with combined psychological and physical symptoms
- those not otherwise specified.

Factitious disorder with physical symptoms

In FD with physical symptoms (also called Munchausen syndrome), the person convincingly presents with intentionally feigned physical symptoms. These symptoms may be:

- fabricated (as in acute abdominal pain without underlying disease)
- self-inflicted (as by deliberately infecting an open wound)
- an exacerbation or exaggeration of a preexisting disorder (as from taking penicillin despite a known allergy to it)
- a combination of the above.

Some people with this type of FD go so far as to have major surgery repeatedly.

History lessons

The typical person with Munchausen syndrome is an unmarried male who's estranged from his family. His history may include:

- multiple admissions to various hospitals, typically across a wide geographic area

Facts about factitious disorders (continued)

- extensive knowledge of medical terminology
- pathological lying
- shifting complaints, signs and symptoms
- poor interpersonal relationships
- refusal of psychiatric examination
- psychoactive substance or analgesic use
- eagerness to undergo hazardous, painful procedures
- evidence of previous treatments, such as surgery
- discharge against medical advice to avoid detection.

Factitious disorder with psychological symptoms

In FD with psychological symptoms, the person's symptoms suggest a mental disorder, such as schizophrenia. For instance, he may report hallucinations, seem confused or make absurd statements. However, the feigned symptoms represent how he views the mental disorder and seldom conform to those described in the *DSM-IV-TR*.

This disorder almost always coexists with a severe personality disorder. Most people have a history of psychoactive substance use – and may use such substances to try to elicit the desired symptoms.

Factitious disorder with combined psychological and physical symptoms

In the combined form of FD, both psychological and physical symptoms are present but neither predominates.

Factitious disorder not otherwise specified

A person whose factitious symptoms don't meet the criteria for a specific FD is diagnosed with FD not otherwise specified. An example is Munchausen syndrome by proxy (MBP), in which the person's goal is to assume the sick role indirectly.

In MBP, the person (typically, a parent) intentionally produces or causes a physical illness in another person (most often a child) through such actions as:

- falsifying the child's medical history
- tampering with laboratory tests to make the child appear sick
- injecting toxic substances into the child
- tampering with treatments (for instance, I.V. or ventilator settings)
- biting or mutilating the child.

Complications and consequences

Conversion symptoms can severely impede the person's normal activities. Prolonged loss of function may lead to serious complications, such as contractures, disuse atrophy and pressure ulcers. Curiously, such complications are rare.

Unnecessary diagnostic or therapeutic medical procedures increase the risk of complications. If the person has a dependent personality, conversion disorder may encourage her to take on the role of a chronic invalid.

Prevalence and onset

In the general population, conversion disorder is rare. In general hospitals, however, roughly 5–15% of psychiatric consultations are for conversion disorders.

Conversion disorder affects two to five times more females than males. It's more prevalent in rural populations and in people with less education and lower socioeconomic status. Males are more likely to develop conversion disorders in occupational settings or military service.

An early start

Conversion disorder usually begins in adolescence or early adulthood, although onset can occur at any age. It's the most common psychosomatic disorder in children and adolescents. (See *Conversion disorders in children*.)

Conversion disorder is rarely chronic. In hospitalised people, symptoms generally improve within 2 weeks. About 90% of people recover within 1 month.

However, about 20–25% of people have recurrent symptoms within 1 year. In a few, symptoms become chronic.

A little extra something

About one-third of people with conversion disorder also have somatisation disorder. (See 'Somatisation disorder', page 254.)

Causes

Conversion disorder may have both biological and psychological components.

Biological factors

More conversion symptoms occur on the left side of the body than the right. This finding suggests that the brain's left hemisphere, where verbal capacities are centralised, somehow blocks impulses carrying painful emotional content from the right hemisphere.

Psychological factors

Psychodynamic theory explains conversion disorder as a defence mechanism that absorbs and neutralises the anxiety evoked by an unacceptable impulse or wish. The person represses unconscious intrapsychic conflicts and converts her anxiety into a physical symptom. For example, she may lose her voice in a circumstance in which she's afraid to speak. Thus, the symptom gets her out of an unpleasant situation.

Seeing no evil

Often, conversion symptoms arise suddenly – soon after the person experiences a traumatic conflict she feels she can't cope with. Two theories may explain why this occurs:

The person achieves a primary gain as the symptom keeps her psychological distress out of conscious awareness. For example, she may experience blindness after witnessing a violent crime.

The person achieves a secondary gain by avoiding a traumatic activity. For example, a soldier may develop a 'paralysed' hand that prevents entry into combat.

Conversion disorders in children

Among children and adolescents, conversion disorder often reflects stress in the family or in school rather than a long-term psychiatric problem.

According to some experts, children and adolescents with conversion disorders have an overprotective or over-involved parent with a subconscious need to see their child as sick. The child's symptoms then become the centre of attention in the family.

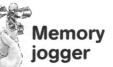

Memory jogger

The word *convert* is your clue to what happens in conversion disorder. Convert means to change from one form or function to another. People with conversion disorder convert stress into physical symptoms.

Risk factors

Risk factors for conversion disorder include a history of histrionic personality disorder (marked by excessive emotionality and attention seeking). Also, children are more likely to have conversion disorder if their family members have a history of the disorder or are seriously ill or in chronic pain.

In some children and adolescents, conversion disorder is linked to physical or sexual abuse within the family.

Signs and symptoms

The person's history may reveal the sudden onset of a single, debilitating sign or symptom that prevents normal function of the affected body part, such as weakness, paralysis or sensation loss in a specific body part.

Other common conversion symptoms include:
- pseudoseizures (seizure-like attacks that are thought to be psychogenically produced)
- loss of a special sense, such as vision (blindness or double vision), hearing (deafness) or touch
- aphonia (inability to use the voice)
- dysphagia (difficulty swallowing)
- impaired balance or coordination
- sensation of a lump in the throat
- urinary retention.

The person may report that the symptom began after a traumatic event.

> Aphonia means loss of the voice. If only my dog would come down with it right now!

La belle indifférence

Oddly, many people with conversion disorder don't show concern over the symptoms or their functional limitations. Called la belle indifférence (French for 'the beautiful indifference'), this apathy is a hallmark of the disorder.

Things just don't add up

Conversion symptoms rarely conform fully to the known anatomic and physiological mechanisms underlying a true physical disorder. Here are three examples:

 Tendon reflexes may be normal in a 'paralysed' body part.

Reported loss of function fails to follow anatomical patterns of innervation.

Normal pupillary responses and evoked potentials are present in a person who complains of blindness.

Diagnosis

With many people, the diagnosis of conversion disorder is considered only after extensive physical examination and laboratory tests fail to reveal a physical disorder that fully accounts for their symptoms. Nonetheless, early consideration of the disorder may avoid tests that increase person costs and risks. What's more, unnecessary, painful or invasive testing may reinforce and cause fixation of the person's symptoms.

Process of elimination

Depending on the person's symptoms, she may undergo a neurological evaluation to rule out physical illnesses that affect sensory function (for instance, blindness or anaesthesia) or voluntary motor function (such as paralysis or the inability to walk or stand). The doctor also must exclude diseases with a vague onset (such as multiple sclerosis or systemic lupus erythematosus).

Laboratory tests can eliminate such conditions as:
- hypoglycaemia or hyperglycaemia
- electrolyte disturbances
- renal failure
- systemic infection
- toxins
- effects of prescribed, over-the-counter or illicit drugs.

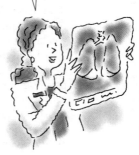

The doctor may order a chest X-ray to rule out neoplasms in a person with suspected conversion disorder.

Scans, X-rays and punctures

Some people may undergo diagnostic procedures, including:
- computed tomography or magnetic resonance imaging scans to exclude a space-occupying lesion in the brain or spinal cord
- chest X-ray to rule out neoplasms
- lumbar puncture for spinal fluid analysis, which can rule out infection and other causes of neurological symptoms
- EEG to help distinguish pseudoseizures from true seizures.

Inconsistency's the key

In conversion disorder, physical and diagnostic findings are inconsistent with the person's complaints. The diagnosis is confirmed if the person fulfills the criteria listed in the *DSM-IV-TR*. (See *Diagnostic criteria: Conversion disorder*, page 253.)

Treatment

A trusting clinician–service user relationship is essential. In many cases, simply reassuring the person that the symptom doesn't indicate a serious underlying disorder makes her feel better and leads to symptom disappearance.

Psychotherapy, family therapy, relaxation training, behaviour modification or hypnosis may be used alone or in combination to treat conversion disorder. However, none of these methods is uniformly effective. For a child or adolescent, family therapy is the treatment of choice.

Exploratory spell

In hypnosis, the hypnotist identifies and explores psychological issues with the hypnotised person. The discussion continues after hypnosis when the person is fully alert.

Diagnostic criteria: Conversion disorder

The diagnosis of conversion disorder is confirmed when the person meets these criteria from the *Diagnostic and Statistical Manual of Mental Disorders*, Fourth Edition, Text Revision.

Symptom or deficit features

- The person exhibits the loss of or a change in voluntary motor or sensory function that suggests a physical disorder.
- Psychological factors seem to be associated with the symptom or deficit, because its onset or exacerbation follows a psychological conflict or another stressor.
- The person isn't intentionally producing or feigning the symptom or deficit.
- The symptom or deficit can't be explained by a general medical condition, direct physiological effects of a substance or culturally sanctioned behaviour.
- The symptom or deficit causes clinically significant distress or impairment of social, occupational or other important areas of functioning.
- The symptom or deficit isn't limited to pain or sexual dysfunction.
- The symptom or deficit isn't better explained by another mental disorder.

Other features

The symptom or deficit is specified as a:

- motor symptom or deficit
- sensory symptom or deficit
- seizure or convulsion
- mixed presentation.

Using biofeedback

Biofeedback training promotes relaxation and may relieve conversion symptoms by teaching the person how to consciously control body functions – such as blood pressure, heart and respiratory rates, temperature and perspiration. It involves the use of an electronic device that informs the person when changes in these functions occur.

Biofeedback has more than 150 applications for prevention of disease and restoration of health. It's often used for stress-related disorders and has many applications in therapy.

In some cases, the person may undergo narcoanalysis, a type of psychotherapy that uses barbiturates to induce release of suppressed or repressed thoughts.

Pharmacological therapy

Benzodiazepines, such as lorazepam and alprazolam, have proven useful in treating some people with conversion disorder.

Nursing interventions

These nursing interventions may be appropriate for a person with conversion disorder.

- Establish a supportive relationship that communicates acceptance of the person but keeps the focus away from her symptoms. Doing this helps her learn to recognise and express anxiety.

- Don't force the person to talk, but convey a caring attitude that encourages her to share feelings.
- Encourage her to seek psychiatric care if she isn't already receiving it.

Hint at emotional links

- Help the person identify any emotional conflicts that preceded symptom onset, to help clarify the link between the conflict and the symptom. But don't imply that the symptoms are all in her head.
- Help the person increase her coping ability, reduce anxiety and enhance self-esteem.
- Use measures to maintain the integrity of the affected body system or part. For instance, regularly exercise a 'paralysed' limb to prevent muscle wasting and contractures. Frequently change a bedridden person's position to prevent pressure ulcers.

Ditch the insistence

- Don't insist that the person use the affected body part or body system. This would only anger her and impede a therapeutic relationship.
- Ensure adequate nutrition even if the person complains of GI distress.
- Promote social interaction to decrease the person's self-involvement.

Call for a casting change

- Identify constructive coping mechanisms to encourage the person to use practical coping skills and relinquish the 'sick' role.
- Include the person's family in her care. Not only may they be contributing to her stress, they're also essential in providing support for her and helping her regain normal function.

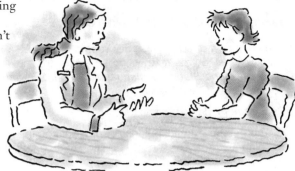

We need to rethink your role, darling. The invalid bit just isn't working for you!

Somatisation disorder

Somatisation disorder is characterised by multiple and often vague physical complaints that suggest a physical disorder but have no physical basis. Typically, the symptoms are recurrent.

Complaints may involve any body system and often persist for years. They may begin or get worse after a job loss, death of a close relative or friend or some other loss. Stress tends to intensify the symptoms.

Sickly life story

People with somatisation disorder may have impairments in occupational, social and other functioning and may become extremely dependent in their relationships. It isn't unusual for them to increasingly demand help and emotional support, and they may get enraged if they feel their needs are going unmet. Many have a lifelong history of sickliness and relate to others only through their symptoms.

Pleasure and punishment

The person may try to manipulate others, even going so far as to threaten or attempt suicide. She may wish to be cared for in every aspect of life.

Although her symptoms help her avoid responsibilities, they also prevent her from experiencing pleasure and can serve as punishment. This suggests underlying feelings of unworthiness and guilt.

Revolving clinic doors

Commonly, the person undergoes repeated medical assessments which (unlike the symptoms themselves) can be potentially damaging and debilitating. When she grows dissatisfied with the medical care she receives, she finds another doctor and presses for more tests and treatments. She may even undergo unnecessary surgery.

Even if she has a satisfactory relationship with one doctor, she continues to request specialist consultations and referrals. However, unlike a person with hypochondriasis, she isn't preoccupied with the belief that she has a specific disease.

Prevalence and onset

Somatisation disorder affects an estimated 0.2–2% of the general population. It's 10 times more common in females – possibly reflecting cultural pressures on women or greater social 'permission' for women to be physically weak or sickly. Symptoms begin before age 30, often in adolescence or early adulthood.

Somatisation disorder is a chronic condition of fluctuating course and a poor prognosis. Complete, spontaneous remission is rare.

Ever-present illness

Symptoms may be most obvious during early adulthood, but few people are entirely asymptomatic or go more than 1 or 2 years without seeking medical attention. In fact, most are disabled for much of their lives.

Somatisation disorder often coexists with other psychiatric conditions, including major depression and anxiety. Many people also have antisocial personality disorder, abuse alcohol or drugs or exhibit suicidal behaviour (although they rarely complete the suicide). They're at increased risk for substance-abuse disorders involving prescription medications, as well as drug interactions from prescriptions written by multiple doctors.

This is your third admission to the hospital this year, isn't it?

Causes

Somatisation disorder has no specific cause, but genetic, biological, environmental and psychological factors may contribute to its development.

Biological theories

People with somatisation disorder may perceive and process pain differently than others. They may also have a lower pain threshold, which increases their sensitivity to physical sensations.

Genetic factors

The disorder may run in families. It's seen in 10–20% of primary female relatives of people with somatisation disorder. Interestingly, primary male relatives of these people have an increased incidence of alcoholism, drug abuse and antisocial personality disorder.

Other factors

Many experts believe somatisation disorder involves underlying feelings of depression, anxiety or other distress, which the person doesn't recognise. Also, recent studies link somatisation with child abuse, particularly sexual abuse.

Signs and symptoms

Signs and symptoms may involve any body system but most commonly involve the GI, neurological, cardiopulmonary or reproductive systems. Many people complain of multiple symptoms at the same time. (See *Common assessment findings in somatisation disorder*, page 257.)

An important clue to this disorder is a history of multiple medical evaluations by different doctors at different health care facilities (sometimes simultaneously) – without significant findings.

Theatrical rendition

The person tends to report complaints and previous medical assessments in a dramatic, vague – or conversely, highly detailed – fashion. She may have a complicated medical history in which many physical diagnoses have been considered. She may seem quite knowledgeable about tests, procedures and medical jargon.

The person may complain that people think she's imagining her symptoms. She tends to disparage previous health care professionals and previous diagnoses and treatments.

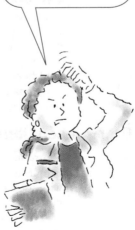

What a complicated medical history! It's typical for a person with psychosomatic disorder.

Diagnosis

Somatisation disorder can't be verified by specific tests. The person should undergo a physical examination and limited diagnostic tests to rule out physical conditions that may produce vague, confusing symptoms (such as

Advice from the experts

Common assessment findings in somatisation disorder

Signs and symptoms of somatisation disorder may mimic actual disorders and are just as real to the person as the physical disorders that can cause them. They most often involve a few key body systems.

Cardiopulmonary symptoms

- Chest pain
- Dizziness
- Palpitations
- Shortness of breath (without exertion)

Female reproductive signs and symptoms

- Excessive menstrual bleeding
- Irregular menses
- Vomiting throughout pregnancy

GI signs and symptoms

- Abdominal pain (excluding menstruation)
- Diarrhoea
- Flatulence
- Intolerance to foods
- Nausea and vomiting (excluding motion sickness)

Pain

- In extremities
- In the back
- During urination

Pseudoneurological signs and symptoms

- Amnesia
- Blindness
- Difficulty walking, paralysis or weakness
- Double or blurred vision
- Dysphagia
- Dysuria or urinary retention
- Fainting or loss of consciousness
- Loss of voice or hearing
- Seizures

Sexual signs and symptoms

- Burning sensation in sexual organs or rectum (except during intercourse)
- Dyspareunia or lack of pleasure during sex
- Impotence
- Sexual indifference

multiple sclerosis, hypothyroidism, hyperparathyroidism, systemic lupus erythematosus and porphyria).

A psychological evaluation can rule out related psychiatric disorders, including:

- depression
- schizophrenia with somatic delusions
- hypochondriasis
- malingering.

The diagnosis is confirmed if the person meets the criteria in the *DSM-IV-TR*. (See *Diagnostic criteria: Somatisation disorder*, page 258.)

Diagnostic criteria: Somatisation disorder

The diagnosis of somatisation disorder is confirmed when the person meets these criteria from the *Diagnostic and Statistical Manual of Mental Disorders*, Fourth Edition, Text Revision.

History of complaints

The person has a history of many physical complaints, beginning before age 30 and persisting for several years, that cause her to seek medical treatment or that impair important areas of functioning.

Symptom features

The person reports all of these symptoms at some time during the disturbance:

- two GI signs or symptoms: vomiting (other than during pregnancy), abdominal pain (other than during menstruation), nausea (other than motion sickness), bloating, diarrhoea or intolerance of different foods
- four pain symptoms: pain in the extremities, back, joints or rectum; menstrual pain; pain during urination; pain during sexual intercourse; or other pain (excluding headache)

- one conversion or pseudoneurological symptom: amnesia, difficulty swallowing, loss of voice, deafness, double or blurred vision, blindness, fainting or loss of consciousness, seizures, difficulty walking, paralysis or muscle weakness, urinary retention or difficulty urinating
- one sexual symptom: burning sensation in the sexual organs or rectum (other than during intercourse), sexual indifference, pain during intercourse, impotence, painful menstruation, irregular menstrual periods, excessive menstrual bleeding or vomiting throughout pregnancy.

Other features

- The person's symptoms aren't explained by a known general medical condition or the direct effects of a substance. Or, if a related general medical condition is present, the complaint or resulting social or occupational impairment exceeds what would be expected from the history, physical examination or laboratory findings.
- The symptoms aren't feigned or intentionally produced.

Treatment

No definitive therapy for somatisation disorder exists. The person isn't likely to acknowledge any psychological aspect of her symptoms or to consider psychiatric treatment.

The goal is control

The goal of treatment is to help her learn to control and cope with her symptoms, rather than eliminate them completely. Telling her that her symptoms are imaginary won't help. Instead, she should be told that although she doesn't have a serious illness, she'll continue to receive care to ease her symptoms.

A single gatekeeper

Management also focuses on preventing unnecessary medical and surgical interventions and turning the person's attention away from her symptoms. Ideally, she should have a continuing, supportive relationship with one empathetic health care provider, rather than multiple providers. (The more providers involved, the greater her opportunity for manipulation and unnecessary medical intervention.)

The health care provider should support healthy and adaptive behaviours, and encourage the person to move beyond her somatisation and manage her life effectively.

Pharmacological treatment

A person with a coexisting depressive or anxiety disorder may benefit from antidepressant drugs, such as SSRIs or monoamine oxidase inhibitors, to ease her preoccupation with symptoms.

Nursing interventions

These nursing interventions may be appropriate for a person with somatisation disorder.

• Acknowledge the person's symptoms and support her efforts to function and cope despite distress. Don't tell her that her symptoms are imaginary – but do inform her of diagnostic test results and their implications.

• Negotiate a plan of care with input from the person and, if possible, her family. Encourage and help them to understand her need for troublesome symptoms.

Strength in compliments

> Emphasise the person's strengths and point out her accomplishments.

• Emphasise the person's strengths. For example, say, 'It's good that you can still work even though you're in pain. You can be pleased with that accomplishment.'

• Gently point out the link between stressful events and the onset of physical symptoms.

• Keep in mind that your goal is to help the person manage symptoms, not eliminate them. Interpersonal relationships commonly are linked to symptoms, so remedying the symptoms may impair her interactions with others.

Attitude assessment

• Check your own feelings and attitudes periodically. If you think you've developed an attitude that says, 'This person doesn't really want to get better, so why should I waste my time?', acknowledge your feelings honestly. If appropriate, regular clinical supervision will help you develop an effective way to deal with your feelings.

Quick quiz

1. Manifestation of physical symptoms caused by psychological distress is termed:

    A. pain disorder.
    B. somatisation.
    C. conversion disorder.
    D. psychosomatic disorder.

Answer: B. Somatisation occurs when a psychological state causes or contributes to the development of physical symptoms.

2. A person concerned with an imagined or slight defect in physical appearance is most likely to be suffering from:
    A.   BDD.
    B.   conversion disorder.
    C.   hypochondriasis.
    D.   somatisation.

Answer: A. In BDD, the person is preoccupied with an imagined or an actual slight defect in physical appearance.

3. A person who reports paralysis with no specific cause but has a history of a recent stressful event has a probable diagnosis of:
    A.   hypochondriasis.
    B.   somatic illness.
    C.   conversion disorder.
    D.   pain disorder.

Answer: C. In conversion disorder, symptoms suggest a physical disorder, but physical examination and diagnostic tests find no physiological cause.

4. Misinterpretation of bodily sensations or symptoms is a chief feature of:
    A.   body dysmorphic disorder.
    B.   somatisation.
    C.   conversion disorder.
    D.   hypochondriasis.

Answer: D. A person with hypochondriasis misinterprets the severity and significance of bodily sensations or symptoms as indications of illness.

Scoring

☆☆☆   If you answered all four items correctly, kudos! You've obviously converted all the information in this chapter to your brain!

☆☆   If you answered two or three items correctly, nice job! There's nothing factitious about your understanding of psychosomatic disorders.

☆   If you answered fewer than two items correctly, don't convert your disappointment into symptoms. Just flood yourself with the concepts in this chapter, and then give it another shot.

8

Dissociative disorders

Just the facts

In this chapter, you'll learn:

♦ general characteristics of dissociation

♦ diagnostic tools used to evaluate dissociative disorders

♦ proposed causes of dissociative disorders

♦ signs and symptoms of dissociative disorders

♦ assessment and interventions for service users with dissociative disorders.

A look at dissociative disorders

Dissociative disorders are marked by disruption of the fundamental aspects of waking consciousness – memory, identity, consciousness and the general experience and perception of oneself and the surroundings. The person uses dissociation as an unconscious defence mechanism to separate anxiety-provoking feelings and thoughts from the conscious mind.

Actually, dissociation is a common occurrence that ranges from normal to pathological. Normal types of dissociation include daydreams, highway hypnosis (a trancelike feeling that can occur when driving) and getting 'lost' in a book, movie or television programme to the point that you don't notice the time or surroundings. Pathological dissociation occurs in dissociative disorders.

This chapter discusses depersonalisation disorder, dissociative amnesia, dissociative fugue and dissociative identity disorder (DID). Depersonalisation disorder alters the experience and perception of oneself. Dissociative amnesia affects mainly memory, whereas dissociative fugue and DID affect both identity and memory.

One type of dissociation is highway hypnosis, a trancelike feeling that occurs when driving.

Too awful to remember

Usually, dissociative disorders result from overwhelming stress caused by a traumatic event that has been experienced or witnessed, or by intolerable psychological conflict. The disorder occurs as the mind isolates the unacceptable information and feelings.

Dissociative disorders (especially dissociative amnesia) related to 'forgotten' childhood traumas and repressed memories gained significant interest in the last few years. Some experts believe dissociation is a common defence mechanism used by a child who's traumatised, especially by abuse.

Dissociation is a poorly understood phenomenon, and controversy and lawsuits have arisen over the accuracy of 'recovered' childhood memories.

A brief episode or lasting impairment?

Dissociative disorders are rare, and affect more females than males. Symptoms may arise suddenly or gradually.

Many dissociative episodes are transient. But if they persist, such episodes may cause functional impairments.

Causes

Psychological, biological and learning theories have been proposed to explain dissociative disorders.

Psychological theories

According to psychological theories, dissociative disorders are a response to severe trauma or abuse. To cope with the trauma or abuse, the person tries to repress the unpleasant experience from awareness. If repression fails, dissociation occurs as a defence mechanism: the person separates the experience from the conscious mind because it's too traumatic to integrate it. (See *Delving into dissociation*.)

Biological theories

Biological theories are most closely linked with depersonalisation disorder. Researchers point out that this disorder shares a key symptom – a sense of

Please Mummy dearest, spare me the abuse, or a dissociative disorder you might induce.

Myth busters

Delving into dissociation

Dissociation is a mysterious and often misunderstood phenomenon.

Myth: A person who experiences dissociation after a traumatic event can consciously control the dissociation.

Reality: Dissociation occurs because the traumatic event has overwhelmed the person's ability to cope using any other method. It's beyond conscious control.

Myth: People in dissociative fugue states behave in a confused manner.

Reality: Most people in dissociative fugue states behave in a normal manner.

loss of one's own reality – with certain neurological disorders (such as epilepsy and tumours), several mental health disorders and the effects of certain drugs (most notably, barbiturates, benzodiazepines and hallucinogens).

Learning theory

According to learning theory, dissociative disorders represent a learned response of avoiding stress and anxiety. With opportunity and practice, a person can become highly skilled at dissociating. This learned behaviour of forcing the memory from awareness is common in people with a history of abuse.

Evaluation

Because a dissociative disorder can mimic a physical illness or another mental disorder, the person should undergo a complete physical examination.

Treasure trove of trauma

In addition, a mental health professional should obtain a careful personal history from the person and family members. The interview should include questions about childhood and adult trauma, as well as any of these experiences:
* blackouts or 'lost' time
* fugues – travel away from home with no memory of what happened on these trips
* unexplained possessions
* relationship changes
* fluctuations in skills and knowledge
* unclear or spotty recollection of the life history
* spontaneous trances
* spontaneous age regression
* out-of-body experiences
* awareness of other personalities within oneself.

A person with a dissociative disorder may find herself far from home with no memory of how she got there.

Diagnostic toolbox

Service users with dissociative disorders may be evaluated with any of these diagnostic tools.
* Dissociative Experiences Scale. This brief self-report scale measures the frequency of dissociative experiences. The person quantifies her experiences for each item. If she scores high, she should undergo further evaluation using the Dissociative Disorders Interview Schedule or the Structured Clinical Interview for Dissociative Disorders.
* Dissociative Disorders Interview Schedule. This highly structured interview is used to diagnose trauma-related disorders. The person answers questions that the examiner asks in a precisely designated order. The interview takes 30–45 minutes.

- Structured Clinical Interview for Dissociative Disorders (SCID-D). This semi-structured interview assesses the nature and severity of five dissociative symptoms – amnesia, depersonalisation, derealisation, identity confusion and identity alteration. It also enables the clinician to diagnose a dissociative disorder based on the criteria from the *Diagnostic and Statistical Manual of Mental Disorders*, Fourth Edition, Text Revision (*DSM-IV-TR*).
- Diagnostic Drawing Series. This test is used by art therapists to aid diagnosis of dissociative disorders. The person is instructed to draw a tree and a picture of how she's feeling.

> An art therapist may use the Diagnostic Drawing Series to help diagnose a dissociative disorder.

Depersonalisation disorder

Depersonalisation disorder is marked by a persistent or recurrent feeling that one is detached from one's own mental processes or body. The person seldom loses touch with reality completely. However, depersonalisation episodes may cause severe distress and sometimes impair functioning.

Honey, I've shrunk!

During episodes of depersonalisation, self-awareness (or a portion of it) is altered or lost temporarily. The sense of depersonalisation may be restricted to a single body part, such as a limb – or it may encompass the whole self. The person may feel as if a body part or the entire body has shrunk or grown.

Watching the world go by

The person may perceive the change in consciousness as a barrier between herself and the outside world. She may feel as if she's passively watching her mental or physical activity or as if the external world is unreal or distorted.

We're all space cadets

Although depersonalisation disorder is rare, the experience of depersonalisation isn't. It occurs in many 'normal' people for brief periods and shouldn't be confused with a mental health disorder.

For example, many people occasionally feel 'spaced out' or as if they're in a dream or looking at themselves from the outside. When intoxicated, some people feel they're out of control of their actions. Depersonalisation symptoms also can arise from meditation or certain religious practices. (See *Dissociation and cultural considerations*, page 265.)

More of it than you'd think

Actually, depersonalisation is the third most common mental health symptom and often follows life-threatening danger, such as accidents, assaults and serious illnesses and injuries. It can occur as a symptom in many other mental health disorders as well as in seizure disorders.

Dissociation and cultural considerations

If the individual has symptoms of a dissociative disorder, make sure to find out about her cultural and religious practices before drawing conclusions about her mental state.

Possession trances

Meditative and trancelike practices are a part of some religions and cultures. Some of these practices may resemble a dissociative disorder (particularly depersonalisation disorder).

For instance, certain cultural groups in Indonesia, Malaysia, the Arctic, Latin America and India experience 'possession trances'. During the trance, a person's customary identity is replaced with a new identity, which is attributed to the influence of a deity, spirit or power. In many cases, people in these trances make stereotyped 'involuntary' movements, which they experience as being beyond their control.

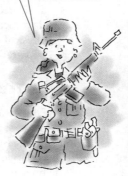

Combat experiences may lead to depersonalisation disorder in some people.

While the symptom of depersonalisation is brief and has no lasting effect, depersonalisation *disorder* is a chronic illness.

Prevalence and onset

The prevalence of depersonalisation disorder isn't known. Onset is sudden, usually in adolescence or early adulthood.

The disorder progresses and often becomes chronic, with exacerbations and remissions. Resolution occurs gradually.

Causes

As a separate disorder, depersonalisation disorder hasn't been studied widely and its exact cause is unknown. It typically occurs in people who have experienced severe stress, such as combat, violent crime, accidents or natural disasters.

Other factors linked to its development include:

* sensory deprivation
* neurophysiological factors, such as epilepsy or a concussion
* history of physical or mental abuse
* history of substance abuse
* history of obsessive–compulsive disorder (OCD).

Signs and symptoms

A person with depersonalisation disorder may report that she feels detached from her entire being and body, as if watching herself from a distance or living in a dream. She may report sensory anaesthesia, loss of self-control, difficulty speaking and feelings of derealisation and losing touch with reality.

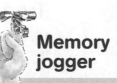

Memory jogger

ABCDES of depersonalisation

A Altered perceptions of self

B Belief that one is observing oneself from outside the body

C Characteristics of the body are perceived as altered

D Detachment from the environment

E Errors in the perceived sense of time

S Sense of unreality

Rumination and disconsolation

Other signs and symptoms may include:
- obsessive rumination
- depression
- anxiety
- fear of going insane
- disturbed sense of time
- slow recall
- physical complaints, such as dizziness
- impaired social and occupational functioning.

Diagnosis

The doctor must rule out physical disorders, substance abuse and other dissociative disorders. Psychological tests and special interviews may aid diagnosis. Standard tests include the Dissociative Experiences Scale and the Dissociative Disorders Interview Schedule, both of which can demonstrate the presence of dissociation.

The diagnosis is confirmed if the person meets the criteria established in the *DSM-IV-TR*. (See *Diagnostic criteria: Depersonalisation disorder*.)

Treatment

Even without treatment, many people recover completely. Treatment is warranted, however, if the disorder is persistent, recurrent or distressing.

Diagnostic criteria: Depersonalisation disorder

The diagnosis of depersonalisation disorder is confirmed when the person meets these criteria from the *Diagnostic and Statistical Manual of Mental Disorders*, Fourth Edition, Text Revision.

- The person has persistent or recurrent experiences of depersonalisation, as indicated by a feeling of being detached from her mind or body (as if observing herself from the outside) or feeling as if she's in a dream.
- During the depersonalisation episode, the person isn't psychotic and is able to perceive or discern the qualities of the surroundings.
- Depersonalisation causes clinically significant distress or impairment in social, occupational or other important areas of functioning.
- The depersonalisation experience doesn't occur only during the course of another mental disorder (such as schizophrenia, panic disorder, acute stress disorder or another dissociative disorder) and doesn't result from the direct physiological effects of a substance or a general medical condition.

Treatment measures include psychotherapy, cognitive-behaviour therapy, hypnosis and pharmacological agents. For the treatment to succeed, all stressors linked to onset of the disorder must be identified and addressed.

Untangling the trauma

If depersonalisation disorder is linked to a traumatic event, psychotherapy focuses on helping the person recognise the event and anxiety it has evoked. Then the therapist teaches the person to use reality-based coping strategies instead of detaching herself from the situation.

Pharmacological therapy

Selective serotonin reuptake inhibitors (SSRIs) and clomipramine, a tricyclic antidepressant, have been moderately successful in treating depersonalisation disorder. The doctor may also prescribe tranquillisers.

Nursing interventions

These nursing interventions may be appropriate for a person with depersonalisation disorder.
- Establish a therapeutic, nonjudgemental relationship with the service user.
- If she experienced a traumatic event, encourage her to recognise that depersonalisation is a defence mechanism she's using to deal with anxiety caused by the trauma.
- Help the person recognise and deal with anxiety-producing experiences by implementing behavioural techniques to cope with stressful situations, if appropriate.
- Assist the person in establishing supportive relationships.

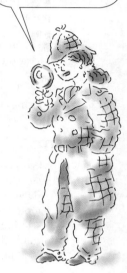

For treatment to succeed, all stressors linked to onset of the disorder must be identified.

Dissociative amnesia

The key feature of dissociative amnesia is an inability to recall important personal information (usually of a stressful nature) that can't be explained by ordinary forgetfulness. Commonly, the person forgets basic autobiographical information, such as her name, people she spoke to recently and what she said, thought, experienced or felt recently.

In most cases, the acute memory loss is triggered by severe psychological stress. Recovery is usually complete and recurrence is rare, although the person may be unable to recall certain life events. (See *Myths about memory lapses*.)

Types of dissociative amnesia

Dissociative amnesia occurs in five main types.

In *localised amnesia*, the person can't remember events that took place during a specific period of time – usually, the first few hours after an extremely stressful or traumatic event.

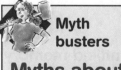

Myth busters

Myths about memory lapses

Myth: Memory lapses are a sign of insanity.

Reality: Occasional, brief memory lapses are common – and normal – experiences. If these lapses recur often and cause impairment, they may reflect an injury or an underlying mental or physical disorder.

In *selective amnesia*, the person can recall some, but not all, of the events during a circumscribed time period. For instance, a soldier may be able to recall only some parts of a violent combat experience.

In *generalised amnesia*, the person suffers prolonged loss of memory – possibly encompassing an entire lifetime.

In *continuous amnesia*, the person forgets all events from a given time forward to the present.

In *systematised amnesia*, the service user's memory loss is limited to a specific type of information. For instance, she may have no memories related to a specific person.

Time warp

Most people with dissociative amnesia are aware that they have 'lost' some time. But a few have 'amnesia for amnesia' – they realise they have lost time only after seeing evidence that they have done things they don't recall. Some people are distressed over their amnesia; others aren't.

Unlike other types of amnesia, dissociative amnesia doesn't result from an organic disorder (such as a stroke or dementia) or physical trauma (such as a closed head injury).

Prevalence and onset

The prevalence of dissociative amnesia is unknown. Most common in adolescents and young women, the disorder is also seen in young men after combat. It may resolve quickly, but sometimes becomes chronic.

Unfilled memory voids

Although most people recover, some never break through the barriers to reconstruct their missing past. The prognosis depends mainly on life circumstances, particular stresses and conflicts associated with the amnesia and the person's overall psychological adjustment. (See *Person safety and family strain*.)

Person safety and family strain

During an episode of dissociative amnesia or fugue, the person may pose a safety risk to herself because of her impaired memory and reduced awareness of surroundings. Not only is she at high risk for falls and other injuries, if she appears obviously confused, she's also an easy prey for con artists and criminals. Her self-care may suffer, too.

Family strain

If the person experiences frequent amnesia or fugue episodes, her family may feel helpless to cope with her behaviour. Concerned for her well-being, they may change their daily routines – a burden that could lead to strained relationships and, possibly, abuse.

Causes

Dissociative amnesia probably results from severe stress associated with a traumatic experience, major life event or severe internal conflict. Some people – such as those who are easily hypnotised – may be predisposed to amnesia.

Factors that may contribute to development of this disorder include:
- altered identity
- low self-esteem
- history of a traumatic event
- history of physical, emotional or sexual abuse.

> During an amnesiac episode, the person may wander aimlessly, seeming disoriented and perplexed.

Signs and symptoms

During an amnesiac episode, the person may seem perplexed and disoriented, wandering aimlessly. She's unable to remember the event that precipitated the episode and usually doesn't even recognise her inability to recall information. She may have mild to severe social impairment.

Once the amnesia episode ends, the person usually isn't aware that she has experienced a memory disturbance.

Diagnosis

Dissociative amnesia can mimic many physical disorders. The person should undergo a thorough physical examination to rule out an organic cause for her symptoms. Blood and urine tests may be done to rule out drug use and other conditions. EEG can exclude a seizure disorder.

Say it in pictures

The person also should undergo a mental health examination. Psychological tests help characterise the nature of her dissociative experiences. These tests include the Diagnostic Drawing Series, Dissociative Experiences Scale and Dissociative Disorders Interview Schedule.

The diagnosis of dissociative amnesia is confirmed if the person meets the criteria in the *DSM-IV-TR*. (See *Diagnostic criteria: Dissociative amnesia*, page 270.) However, when dissociative amnesia occurs as a symptom of another mental health disorder, it isn't diagnosed separately.

Treatment

Psychotherapy aims to help the person recognise the traumatic event that triggered the amnesia and the anxiety it has produced. A supportive, trusting therapeutic relationship is essential to achieving this goal. An accepting environment may in itself enable the person to gradually recover her missing memories. The psychotherapist subsequently attempts to teach her reality-based coping strategies.

Diagnostic criteria: Dissociative amnesia

The diagnosis of dissociative amnesia is confirmed when the person meets these criteria from the *Diagnostic and Statistical Manual of Mental Disorders*, Fourth Edition, Text Revision.

- The main disturbance is an episode marked by the sudden inability to recall important personal information (usually of a stressful or traumatic nature) that's too extensive to attribute to normal forgetfulness.
- The disturbance doesn't occur only during the course of dissociative fugue, dissociative identity disorder, acute stress disorder, post-traumatic stress disorder or somatisation disorder and doesn't result from the direct physiological effects of a substance or a general medical condition.
- Symptoms cause clinically significant distress or impairment of social, occupational or other areas of functioning.

Recovery and clarification

Filling in the memory gaps can be useful in restoring the continuity of the service user's identity and sense of self. Once these gaps have been filled, treatment helps the person clarify the trauma or conflicts and resolve the problems associated with the amnesic episode.

Mission: Memory retrieval

When the need to recover memories is urgent, the person may be questioned under hypnosis or in a drug-induced semi-hypnotic state. However, such memory-retrieval techniques must be used cautiously because the circumstances that triggered the memory loss are likely to be highly distressing to the service user.

Also, the validity of 'recovered' memories is controversial, and external corroboration is required to validate their accuracy. (See *First do no harm*, page 271.)

Pharmacological therapy

Drugs used to treat dissociative amnesia may include benzodiazepines, such as alprazolam and lorazepam, and SSRIs.

Nursing interventions

These nursing interventions may be appropriate for a person with dissociative amnesia.
- Establish a therapeutic, nonjudgemental relationship.
- Encourage the person to verbalise feelings of distress.
- Help her recognise that memory loss is a defence mechanism used to deal with anxiety and trauma.

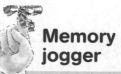

Advice from the experts

First do no harm

Dissociative amnesia usually arises as a reaction to a trauma too overwhelming for the service user to integrate into her waking consciousness. In other words, she has experienced something she wants to forget.

Although you may encourage the person to express her feelings, don't try to elicit forgotten memories. Only a mental health professional with special competence in addressing unconscious memories should attempt to do this. The techniques used to elicit memories, such as hypnosis, guided imagery and free association, carry certain risks and could prove harmful to the person.

- Help the person deal with anxiety-producing experiences.
- Teach and assist the person in using reality-based coping strategies under stress rather than strategies that distort reality.

Dissociative fugue

Dissociative fugue is marked by sudden, unexpected travel away from one's home or workplace, along with an inability to recall one's past and confusion about one's personal identity (or assumption of a new identity). The degree of impairment varies with the duration of the fugue and the nature of the personality state it invokes.

Travel may range from brief trips lasting hours or days to complex wandering for weeks or months. In some cases, the person travels thousands of miles.

Maybe she's in the witness protection programme

Occasionally, a person forms a new identity during a dissociative fugue. She assumes a new name, takes up a new residence and engages in social activities with no hint that she has a mental disorder. Typically, the new identity is more outgoing and less inhibited than the former one.

During the fugue, she may appear normal and attract no attention. However, confusion about her identity – or the return of her original identity – may make her aware of her memory loss or may cause distress.

Who am I? Where am I?

In some cases, the person is brought to the attention of the police or is taken to a hospital – usually because she can't remember recent events or her personal identity. Once she returns to her pre-fugue state, she may have no memory for the events that took place during the fugue.

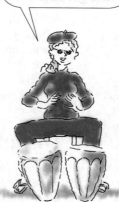

You claim I used to trade options on Wall Street? I don't remember that gig!

Prevalence and onset

Dissociative fugue is rare, with an estimated prevalence of 0.2%. Age of onset varies.

The disorder is most common among people who have experienced wars, accidents, violent crimes and natural disasters. Fugue behaviours also occur in people with DID.

Dissociative fugue usually resolves rapidly. The prognosis for complete recovery is good. Although the disorder can recur, service users with frequent episodes may more appropriately be diagnosed with DID.

Causes

The precise cause of dissociative fugue isn't known. The disorder typically follows an extremely stressful event, such as combat experience, a natural disaster, a violent or abusive confrontation or personal rejection. Heavy alcohol use may be a predisposing factor.

The function of a fugue

Many fugues seem to represent disguised wish fulfillment. Some appear to protect the person from suicidal or homicidal impulses.

A fugue also may be a mechanism that the person uses unconsciously to absolve herself from accountability for her actions or to reduce her exposure to a hazard. For this reason, some people view it as a form of malingering.

Signs and symptoms

A fugue in progress is rarely recognised. Others may suspect it only if the person seems confused about her identity or puzzled about her past – or if she grows confrontational when her new identity (or absence of identity) is challenged.

A rough landing

Although the person may be asymptomatic during a fugue, she may experience various symptoms when it ends – depression, discomfort, grief, shame, intense conflict, even suicidal or aggressive impulses. Failure to remember the events that took place during the fugue may cause confusion, distress or even terror.

The psychosocial history of a person with dissociative fugue may include episodes of violent behaviour.

Diagnosis

Mental health examination may reveal that the person has assumed a new, more uninhibited identity. If the new personality is still evolving, she may avoid social contact.

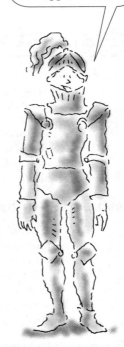

Heads up: when a fugue ends, the person may feel terrified and aggressive.

Diagnostic criteria: Dissociative fugue

The diagnosis of dissociative fugue is confirmed when the person meets these criteria from the *Diagnostic and Statistical Manual of Mental Disorders,* Fourth Edition, Text Revision.

- The predominant disturbance is sudden, unexpected travel away from home or the person's customary place of work, with an inability to recall the past.
- The person assumes a new identity (either partial or complete) or is confused about her personal identity.
- The disturbance doesn't occur only during the course of dissociative identity disorder and doesn't result from the direct physiological effects of a substance or a general medical condition.
- Symptoms cause clinically significant distress or impairment in social, occupational or other important areas of functioning.

On the other hand, the person may have travelled to a distant location, set up a new residence and developed a well-integrated network of social relationships – circumstances that don't suggest a mental alteration.

A thorough physical examination should be done to rule out medical disorders (such as seizure) or medication or substance use as the cause of the person's symptoms.

All too real

However, diagnosis may not be possible until the fugue ends and the person resumes her pre-fugue identity. She may then become distressed at finding herself in unfamiliar circumstances.

The diagnosis of dissociative fugue is confirmed if the person meets the criteria documented in the *DSM-IV-TR.* (See *Diagnostic criteria: Dissociative fugue.*)

Treatment

Psychotherapy aims to help the person recognise the traumatic event that triggered the fugue state and to develop reality-based strategies for coping with anxiety. A trusting, therapeutic relationship is crucial for successful therapy.

Restoration project

Hypnosis may be used to prompt the person to recall events and feelings and, ultimately, to assist her in restoring her memory.

Cognitive therapy may be valuable in helping her to examine maladaptive thought patterns and to link them to irrational behaviours, such as fleeing.

Group therapy may provide ongoing support and can help the person gain self-esteem and increase socialisation. Family therapy can explore the person's traumatic experiences and teach family members about the disorder.

Singing away the sorrows

Creative therapies, such as music or art therapy, are sometimes used, too. These therapies permit the person to explore her emotions within a safe environment.

Nursing interventions

These nursing interventions may be appropriate for a person with dissociative fugue.
- Encourage the person to identify emotions that occur under stress.
- If the person is resolving a dissociative fugue state, monitor her for signs of overt aggression towards herself or others.
- Teach the person effective coping skills.
- Encourage her to use available social support systems.

Dissociative identity disorder

Formerly called *multiple personality disorder*, DID is marked by two or more distinct identities or subpersonalities (or alters) that recurrently take control of the person's consciousness and behaviour. Each identity may exhibit unique behaviour patterns, memories and social relationships.

Made famous by movies and books such as *Sybil* and *The Three Faces of Eve*, DID is the most severe type of dissociative disorder.

Sugar or spice, naughty or nice

In many cases, the primary personality is religious with a strong moral sense, while the subpersonalities are radically different. They may behave aggressively and lack sexual inhibitions. They may have a different gender, sexual orientation, religion or race than the primary personality – and may even differ in hand dominance, vocal qualities, intelligence level and EEG readings.

The primary personality may be unaware of the subpersonalities and may wonder about lost time and unexplained events. Subpersonalities are more likely to be aware of the existence of other personalities and may even interact with one another.

OK, which one of you subpersonalities swiped my stethoscope?

About face!

The transition from one personality to another often is triggered by stress or a meaningful social or environmental cue. Although usually sudden (seconds to minutes), the transition can take hours or days.

Prevalence and onset

Estimates of the prevalence of DID range from 1 in 500 to 1 in 5,000 people. DID is four times as common in women, and tends to be chronic.

It can get very complicated

DID may lead to severe social and occupational impairment, depending on the nature of the subpersonalities and their interrelationships. Often, one or more of the subpersonalities have an overlapping mental disorder, such as generalised anxiety disorder, borderline personality disorder or mood disorder. Suicide attempts, self-mutilation, externally directed violence and psychoactive drug dependence may occur.

Causes

No known single cause for DID exists, but many experts believe the disorder results primarily from trauma or extreme stress – especially when experienced before age 15. Researchers have found a strong connection between DID and a history of severe childhood abuse.

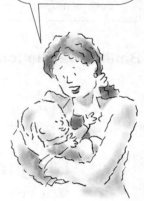

Be kind to your kids. A child who suffers trauma may develop multiple personalities.

Survival through splitting

Some psychiatrists believe victims of severe trauma and abuse develop DID as a survival mechanism. A child exposed to overwhelming trauma may evolve multiple personalities to dissociate herself from the traumatic situation. The dissociated contents then become linked with one of many possible influences that shape personality organisation.

Besides emotional, physical or sexual abuse, factors that may contribute to DID include:
- genetic predisposition
- lack of nurturing experiences to assist in recovering from abuse
- low self-esteem.

Signs and symptoms

Signs and symptoms of DID may include:
- lack of recall beyond ordinary forgetfulness
- hallucinations, particularly auditory and visual
- post-traumatic symptoms, such as flashbacks, nightmares and an exaggerated startle response
- recurrent depression
- sexual dysfunction and difficulty forming intimate relationships
- sleep disorders
- eating disorders
- somatic pain disorders
- substance abuse
- guilt and shame
- suicidal tendencies or other self-harming behaviours, such as excessive risk-taking, unprotected sex with multiple partners, self-neglect or excessive drinking, smoking or eating.

> ## Diagnostic criteria: Dissociative identity disorder
>
> The diagnosis of dissociative identity disorder is confirmed when the person meets these criteria from the *Diagnostic and Statistical Manual of Mental Disorders*, Fourth Edition, Text Revision.
>
> - Two or more distinct identities or personality states (each with its own relatively lasting pattern of perceiving, relating to and thinking about the self and the environment) exist within the person.
> - At least two of these identities or personality states recurrently take control of the person's behaviour.
> - The person's inability to recall important personal information is too extensive to result from ordinary forgetfulness.
> - The disturbance doesn't stem from direct physiological effects of a substance or a general medical condition.

Baffling vacillations

The person's history may include unsuccessful mental health treatment, periods of amnesia and disturbances in time perception. Family members and friends may describe incidents that the person can't recall as well as pronounced changes in her facial presentation, voice and behaviour.

Diagnosis

Many service users with DID spend months or even years in the mental health system before they're diagnosed correctly. Common misdiagnoses are schizophrenia and bipolar disorder with psychotic episodes.

Standard tests for DID include the Diagnostic Drawing Series, Dissociative Experiences Scale, Dissociative Disorders Interview Schedule and the SCID-D. These tests all demonstrate the presence of dissociation.

The diagnosis is confirmed if the person fulfills the criteria in the *DSM-IV-TR*. (See *Diagnostic criteria: Dissociative identity disorder*.)

Treatment

Treatment of DID is a long-term process, taking five or more years. The goal of therapy is to integrate all personalities of the service user and to prevent the personality from splitting again.

Can't they all just get along?

After stabilising the service user, the therapist tries to decrease the degree of dissociation, enhance cooperation and co-consciousness among the subpersonalities, and ultimately merge them into one personality.

Advice from the experts

Promoting recovery from dissociative identity disorder

Integrating the subpersonalities is the goal of therapy for a person with dissociative identity disorder (DID). Certain actions by the therapist and caregivers can promote connectedness among the subpersonalities, but the following actions are counterproductive:

- *Don't* encourage the person to create additional subpersonalities.
- *Don't* suggest that she adopt names for unnamed subpersonalities.
- *Don't* encourage subpersonalities to function more autonomously.
- *Don't* encourage the person to ignore certain subpersonalities.
- *Don't* exclude unlikable subpersonalities from therapy.

Unifying the parts

Although the therapist may address the different personalities separately, an increased connectedness is the measure of success. Treatment success is linked to the strength of the therapist's relationship with each subpersonality.

Whether disagreeable or congenial, all of the service user's personalities must be treated with equal respect and empathetic concern. (See *Promoting recovery from dissociative identity disorder*.)

Respecting boundaries

Clearly delineating boundaries is also important in treating service users with DID. Many grew up in environments without clear boundaries or where personal boundaries weren't always respected.

Family focus

Family and couples therapy also may be indicated. Many service users have difficulty parenting and admit to being abusive towards their children.

Hypnosis

Some therapists may use hypnosis for:
- helping the person revisit the traumatic experience
- managing crises – for instance, reducing spontaneous flashbacks and reorienting the person to reality
- strengthening the service user's ego
- stabilising the person between therapy sessions.

Tiffs over trances

However, the role of hypnosis in ongoing DID treatment is controversial. For one thing, service users and therapists may become overconfident in the accuracy of information arrived at during a hypnotic trance. To reduce the risk that the person will alter details of what she recalls during hypnosis, the therapist must minimise the use of leading questions.

Informed consent should be obtained before the use of hypnosis, and its benefits, risks and limitations should be discussed. Also, the therapist should tell the person that anything she recalls while in a trance isn't likely to be admissible evidence used in legal actions.

Pharmacological interventions

Drugs used to treat DID include benzodiazepines, SSRIs and tricyclic antidepressants.

Nursing interventions

These nursing interventions may be appropriate for a person with DID.
• Establish a trusting relationship with each subpersonality. If the person has a history of abuse, be aware that she may have difficulty trusting others.
• Promote interventions that help the person identify each subpersonality, with the goal of integration.

Memory jogger

ABREACTION refers to the purging of distressing memories or feelings. This term will help you remember key interventions for service users with dissociative identity disorder.

A Abuse is identified

B Blend or integrate all the personalities into one personality

R Recall the trauma in detail and process it

E Encourage the person to maintain a safe environment

A Anxiety is decreased

C Conflict resolution is taught

T Talk about the service user's feelings, especially guilt and shame

I Inform the person about the use of hypnosis to help mobilise memories

O Orient the person to surroundings as necessary

N New coping strategies are developed

- Encourage her to identify emotions that occur under stress.
- Recognise even small gains that the person makes.
- Teach the person effective defence mechanisms and coping skills, including the use of available social support systems.

Preach patience

- Stress the importance of continuing with psychotherapy. Prepare the person to expect the need for prolonged therapy, with alternating successes and failures, and the possibility that one or more of the subpersonalities may resist treatment.
- Monitor the person for violence directed at others.
- Monitor the person for suicidal ideation and behaviour. Implement precautions as needed.

Quick quiz

1. In people with dissociative disorders, the defence mechanism most often used to block traumatic experiences is:
    A.   passive aggression.
    B.   reaction formation.
    C.   denial.
    D.   repression.

Answer: D. Repression is the defence mechanism used most often to block traumatic experiences. Neither reaction formation nor denial is relevant in these disorders.

2. Feelings of a dreamlike state or of being a detached observer typically occur in:
    A.   dissociative fugue.
    B.   dissociative amnesia.
    C.   depersonalisation disorder.
    D.   dissociative identity disorder.

Answer: C. Depersonalisation disorder is characterised by a sense of being in a dreamlike state or being a detached observer.

3. Multiple personality disorder is also known as:
    A.   dissociative fugue.
    B.   depersonalisation disorder.
    C.   dissociative amnesia.
    D.   DID.

Answer: D. DID was formerly known as multiple personality disorder.

4. Factors that may contribute to DID include all of these except:
   A. history of seizures.
   B. emotional, physical or sexual abuse.
   C. genetic predisposition.
   D. extreme stress and trauma.

Answer: A. A history of seizures hasn't been linked to the development of DID.

5. Signs and symptoms of dissociative fugue are most pronounced:
   A. weeks before the fugue episode.
   B. during the fugue episode.
   C. after the fugue episode.
   D. hours before the fugue episode.

Answer: C. After a fugue, the person may experience depression, grief, shame, intense conflict, confusion, terror or suicidal or aggressive impulses. In contrast, a fugue in progress is rarely recognised. There are no warning signs of an impending fugue episode.

Scoring

☆☆☆ If you answered all five items correctly, unreal! You've integrated all aspects of dissociative disorders into your conscious mind.

☆☆ If you answered three or four items correctly, fantastic. It's all coming together for you nicely.

☆ If you answered fewer than three items correctly, don't go to pieces! Just thumb through the chapter again and try to fill in those memory gaps.

9

Personality disorders

Just the facts

In this chapter, you'll learn:

♦ major features of personality disorders

♦ proposed causes of personality disorders

♦ assessment findings and nursing interventions for people with personality disorders

♦ recommended treatments for people with personality disorders.

A look at personality disorders

A personality disorder occurs when personality traits – behaviour patterns that reflect how a person perceives and relates to others and himself – become rigid, maladaptive and fixed. The disorder affects the person's cognition, behaviour and style of interacting with others.

Generally, people with personality disorders have trouble getting along with others. They may be irritable, demanding, hostile, fearful or manipulative. Many sufferers have inadequate coping mechanisms and thus have trouble dealing with everyday stresses.

Severe personality disorders impose a hefty financial and emotional burden.

Stress, symptoms and sequelae

When mild, a personality disorder may have little effect on a person's social, family or work life. However, if symptoms get worse – as they commonly do during times of increased stress – the disorder can seriously interfere with emotional, psychological, social and occupational functioning.

When severe, personality disorders result in hospitalisation, poor work performance and lost productivity. Their emotional toll – unhappiness, domestic violence, child abuse, imprisonment and even suicide – is equally staggering.

Myth busters

The fix is in

Relationship problems may arise if the individual's family and friends don't understand the nature of personality disorders.

Myth: If someone with a personality disorder seems normal, that means he's capable of changing his behaviour.

Reality: With a personality disorder, personality traits are fixed and not conducive to change. Yet with a mild personality disorder, the individual's behaviour seems normal, so friends and family may assume he can easily change his behaviour. When he doesn't change, they may think he isn't willing to – when the problem is that he *can't*.

Relationship woes

People with personality disorders have trouble adjusting to others, so others are forced to adjust to them. This can create a major strain: If others don't or can't adjust, the person with the disorder may become angry, frustrated, depressed or withdrawn. This sets up a vicious cycle of interaction in which the sufferer persists with the maladaptive behaviour until his needs are met – further angering those around him. (See *The fix is in*.)

Common features

To one degree or another, most people with personality disorders share the following features:
- disturbances in self-image
- inappropriate range of emotions
- poor impulse control
- maladaptive ways of perceiving themselves, others and the world
- long-standing problems in personal relationships, ranging from dependency to withdrawal
- reduced occupational functioning, ranging from compulsive perfectionism to intentional self-sabotage.

All in the mix

These features mix together to create a pervasive pattern of behaviour that differs markedly from the norms of the person's cultural or ethnic background. (See *Culture and personality disorders*, page 283.)

Personality disorder clusters

The *Diagnostic and Statistical Manual of Mental Disorders*, Fourth Edition, Text Revision (*DSM-IV-TR*) groups personality disorders into three clusters:

Cluster A – paranoid, schizoid and schizotypal personality disorders. These disorders share odd or eccentric behaviour.

Bridging the gap

Culture and personality disorders

Before concluding that a person has a personality disorder, always consider his cultural, ethnic and religious background. According to the *Diagnostic and Statistical Manual of Mental Disorders*, Fourth Edition, Text Revision, the person's signs and symptoms must deviate markedly from the expectations of his culture to qualify for the diagnosis of a personality disorder.

Stoics vs. expressives

Asian and Northern European cultures place a high value on emotional restraint. Thus, stoic behaviour in a person of Japanese descent may be mistaken for avoidant personality disorder.

On the other hand, people from Hispanic, Middle Eastern and Mediterranean backgrounds tend to be more expressive. Keep that in mind

before concluding that a person with this background has histrionic personality disorder.

Skirting the stereotypes

At the same time, avoid stereotyping people. Individuals within a culture – or even within a particular family – may vary widely in personality traits and emotional expression.

Cluster B – antisocial, borderline, histrionic and narcissistic personality disorders. Dramatic, emotional or erratic behaviour highlights these disorders.

Cluster C – avoidant, dependent and obsessive – compulsive personality disorders. These disorders are marked by anxious or fearful behaviour.

Each disorder produces characteristic signs and symptoms, which may vary among people and even within the same person at different times.

Demographic dynamics

Personality disorders are relatively common, affecting an estimated 10% of the UK population. Gender plays a role in their prevalence. For example, antisocial and obsessive – compulsive personality disorders are more common in men, whereas borderline, dependent and histrionic personality disorders are more prevalent in women.

Age and intensity

Personality disorders are lifelong conditions with an onset in adolescence or early adulthood. Cluster A and B disorders tend to grow less intense in middle age and late life, whereas cluster C disorders tend to become exaggerated. People with cluster B disorders are susceptible to substance abuse, impulse control and suicidal behaviour, which may shorten their lives.

Piling on

Personality disorders commonly overlap with other psychiatric disorders, such as substance abuse disorders, mood disorders and anxiety disorders.

Causes

No one knows the exact cause of personality disorders. Most likely, they represent a combination of genetic, biological, social, psychological, developmental and environmental factors.

> More women have borderline and dependent personality disorders, whereas more men have antisocial personality disorder.

Chain of influence

Genetic factors influence the biological basis of brain function as well as basic personality structure. In turn, personality structure affects how a person responds to and interacts with life experiences and the social environment. Over time, each person develops distinctive ways of perceiving the world and of feeling, thinking and behaving.

Out-of-control emotions

Some researchers suspect that poor regulation of the brain circuits that control emotion increases the risk for a personality disorder – when combined with such factors as abuse, neglect or separation.

For a biologically predisposed person, the major developmental challenges of adolescence and early adulthood (such as separation from the parents, identity and independence) may trigger a personality disorder. Perhaps this explains why personality disorders usually emerge during those years.

Psychodynamic theories

Psychodynamic theories propose that personality disorders stem from deficiencies in ego and superego development. These deficiencies may relate to mother – child relationships highlighted by unresponsiveness, overprotectiveness or early separation.

Social theories

According to social theories, personality disorders reflect the responses that a person learns through the processes of reinforcement, modelling and aversive stimuli. When even low levels of stress occur, chronic trauma or long-term stressors may create new neurochemical pathways. As a result, the person 'acts out' old patterns.

Evaluation

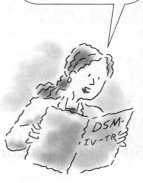

All the diagnostic criteria are right here in black and white. What a handy tome!

A person with a suspected personality disorder should undergo a physical examination to rule out an underlying physical or organic cause for his symptoms. (See *Personality changes and physical illness*.)

A psychological evaluation can exclude other psychiatric disorders – or it may suggest additional ones. Psychological tests may support or guide the diagnosis. The Structured Clinical Interview for *DSM-IV-TR* for Axis II Disorders also aids diagnosis.

For official diagnosis of a personality disorder, the person must meet the criteria established in the *DSM-IV-TR*. Some people meet the criteria for multiple personality disorders, making diagnosis a particular challenge. (See *General diagnostic criteria for personality disorders*.)

Personality changes and physical illness

Be aware that a personality change may be the first sign of a serious neurological, endocrine or medical illness – which may be reversible if detected early.

For example, a person with a frontal lobe tumour may show changes in personality and motivation, even though the results of a neurological assessment are otherwise negative. Such problems should be ruled out before the person is diagnosed with a personality disorder.

General diagnostic criteria for personality disorders

The general criteria below, from the *Diagnostic and Statistical Manual of Mental Disorders*, Fourth Edition, Text Revision, applies to everyone with a personality disorder. However, each particular disorder has additional criteria that the person must meet.

Enduring pattern and areas affected

The person exhibits an enduring pattern of behaviours and inner experiences that deviates significantly from the norms and expectations of his culture. This pattern affects two or more of the following areas:

- cognition (ways of interpreting and perceiving oneself, other people and events)
- affectivity (the degree, range, lability and appropriateness of emotional responses)
- interpersonal functioning
- impulse control.

Features of the pattern

- The pattern of behaviours and inner experiences is inflexible and extends to a broad range of personal and social situations.
- The pattern leads to clinically significant distress or impairment of social, occupational or other important areas of functioning.
- The pattern is stable and enduring, with an onset that can be traced back to early adulthood or adolescence.
- The pattern isn't better explained by another mental disorder.
- The pattern doesn't result directly from the physiological effects of a medication or other substance.

Substance screening

Toxicology screening may be warranted because intoxication with certain substances can mimic the features of a personality disorder.

Approach to treatment

Personality disorders are among the most challenging psychiatric disorders to treat – partly because, by definition, a personality disorder is an integral part of what defines the individual and his self-perceptions. Rather than aiming for a cure, treatment typically focuses on enhancing the person's coping skills, solving short-term problems and building relationship skills through psychotherapy and education.

The road to rapport

Traditionally, long-term psychotherapy has been the treatment of choice. Effective psychotherapy always requires a trusting relationship with the therapist.

Adjunctive medication

Today, many people also receive drugs to relieve associated symptoms, such as acute anxiety or depression. However, drugs should be used only as an adjunct to psychotherapy – not as a cure for the personality disorder.

Prescribing by the cluster

Here are general guidelines for drug use:
• People with cluster A personality disorders may benefit from low-dose antipsychotic drugs.
• People with cluster B disorders who suffer from marked mood reactivity, impulsivity or rejection hypersensitivity may respond well to antidepressant drugs.
• People with cluster C disorders may benefit from antidepressant drugs. Mood stabilisers may also reduce impulsiveness and aggression.

Paranoid personality disorder

Paranoid personality disorder is marked by a distrust of other people and a constant, unwarranted suspicion that others have sinister motives. Sufferers place excessive trust in their own knowledge and abilities. They search for hidden meanings and hostile intentions in everything that others say and do.

Conspiracy theorists

Quick to challenge the loyalties of friends and loved ones, many people with this disorder seem cold and distant. They shift blame to others and carry long grudges. Because they tend to drive people away, they have few friends – which only bolsters their suspicions of a conspiracy against them.

Prevalence
The prevalence of paranoid personality disorder is estimated at 0.5–2.5% of the general population. In clinical samples (and possibly in the general population as well), it's more common in males.

Causes

The specific cause of paranoid personality disorder is unknown. Its higher incidence in families with a schizophrenic member suggests a possible genetic influence.

Some experts believe that the disorder results (at least partly) from negative childhood experiences and a threatening domestic atmosphere – for example, extreme unfounded rage or condescension by the parents, which can produce profound insecurity in the child.

Signs and symptoms

The hallmarks of paranoid personality disorder are suspicion and distrust of others' motives. Other signs and symptoms include:
- refusal to confide in others
- inability to collaborate with others
- hypersensitivity
- inability to relax (hypervigilance)
- need to be in control
- self-righteousness
- detachment and social isolation
- poor self-image
- sullenness, hostility, coldness and detachment
- humourlessness
- anger, jealousy and envy
- bad temper, hyperactivity and irritability
- lack of social support systems.

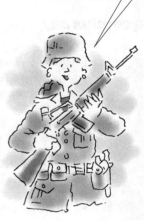

At ease, soldier! Someone with paranoid personality disorder may be unable to relax.

Diagnosis

The diagnosis is confirmed if the person meets the criteria in the *DSM-IV-TR*. (See *Diagnostic criteria: Paranoid personality disorder*, page 288.)

Treatment

Few people with paranoid personality disorder seek treatment on their own. When they do, health care providers may have difficulty establishing a rapport because of these people's suspicious, distrustful nature. The challenge is to engage the person in a collaborative working relationship based on trust.

Diagnostic criteria: Paranoid personality disorder

The diagnosis of paranoid personality disorder is confirmed when the person meets these criteria from the *Diagnostic and Statistical Manual of Mental Disorders*, Fourth Edition, Text Revision.

Misinterpretation of others' actions

Since early adulthood, the person has exhibited a pervasive distrust and suspiciousness of others, interpreting their actions as deliberately malicious or threatening. This pattern is indicated by at least four of the following behaviours:

- suspicion, without sufficient basis, that others are exploiting, deceiving or harming him
- preoccupation with unjustified doubts about the loyalty and trustworthiness of friends and associates
- reluctance to confide in others because of unwarranted fears that the information will be used against him
- reading hidden negative meanings into benign events or remarks
- bearing prolonged grudges
- belief that others are attacking his reputation or character and reacting quickly with anger or a counterattack
- questioning, without justification, the fidelity of a spouse or sexual partner.

Other features

These symptoms don't occur exclusively during the course of schizophrenia or a delusional disorder and don't result from the direct physiological effects of a general medical condition.

Psychotherapy

Individual psychotherapy is preferred over group therapy because of the person's suspicious nature. The most effective psychotherapy for a paranoid person takes a simple, honest, business-like approach rather than an insight-oriented approach. It focuses on the current problem that brought the person to therapy.

As therapy progresses, the person may begin to trust the therapist more and, eventually, start to disclose some of his paranoid ideations.

Pharmacological therapy

Some doctors recommend medication for people with paranoid personality disorder. Prescribed agents may include:
- antipsychotic drugs (such as olanzapine or risperidone) to treat severe agitation or delusional thinking (given in one-tenth to one-fourth the usual dosage used in people who are psychotic)
- selective serotonin reuptake inhibitors (SSRIs) such as fluoxetine to treat irritability, anger and obsessional thinking
- anxiolytic drugs to treat severe anxiety that interferes with normal functioning.

Doubts about drugs

However, a person with paranoid personality disorder may distrust medications and, in particular, may resent the suggestion that he needs an antipsychotic agent. For this reason, some therapists delay considering medication until the person asks about it.

Drug therapy should be limited to the briefest course possible. The person should receive thorough teaching about possible side effects so he doesn't get more suspicious if these occur.

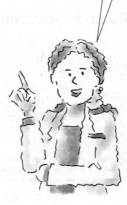

> The paranoid person may distrust medications – especially if they cause side effects.

Nursing interventions

These nursing interventions may be appropriate for a person with paranoid personality disorder:
* Use a straightforward, honest, professional approach rather than a casual or friendly approach.
* Offer persistent, consistent and flexible care.
* Provide a supportive, nonjudgemental environment in which the person can safely explore his feelings.
* Establish a therapeutic relationship by actively listening and responding.

Don't get too personal

* Avoid inquiring too deeply into his life or history unless it's relevant to clinical treatment.
* Don't challenge the person's paranoid beliefs. Such beliefs are delusional and aren't reality based, so it's useless to argue them from a rational point of view.
* Avoid situations that threaten the person's autonomy.
* Be aware that the person may not respond well to interviewing. (See *Guidelines for an effective interview*.)

You call that funny?

* Use humour cautiously. A paranoid person may misinterpret a remark that was meant to be humorous.

Advice from the experts

Guidelines for an effective interview

You may have difficulty establishing a rapport with a person with a personality disorder. These guidelines may be helpful:

* Start the interview with a broad, empathetic statement: 'You look distressed. Tell me what's bothering you today.'
* Explore normal behaviours before discussing abnormal ones: 'What do you think has enabled you to cope with the pressures of your job?'
* Phrase questions sensitively to ease the person's anxiety: 'Things were going well at home and then you became depressed. Tell me about that.'
* Ask the person to clarify vague statements: 'Explain to me what you mean when you say, "They're all after me".'
* If the person rambles, help him focus on his most pressing problem: 'You've talked about several problems. Which one bothers you the most?'
* Interrupt a nonstop talker as tactfully as possible: 'Thank you for your comments. Now let's move on.'
* Express empathy towards a tearful, silent or confused person who has trouble describing a problem: 'I realise it's difficult for you to talk about this.'

- Encourage the person to take part in social interactions to expose him to others' perceptions and realities and to promote social skills development.
- Help the person identify negative behaviours that interfere with his relationships so he can see how his behaviour affects others.
- Encourage the expression of feelings, self-analysis of behaviour and accountability for actions.

Distance yourself

- Recognise the person's need for physical and emotional distance.
- Avoid defensiveness and arguing.
- Assess the person's coping skills. As necessary, teach him effective strategies to alleviate stress and reduce anxiety.
- Teach the person about his prescribed medications.
- Encourage him to continue therapy for optimal results.

> Keep your distance – both physically and emotionally – from a paranoid person.

Schizoid personality disorder

The hallmarks of schizoid personality disorder are detachment, social withdrawal, indifference to others' feelings and a restricted emotional range in interpersonal settings. People with this disorder are commonly described as loners, with solitary interests and occupations and no close friends. Typically, they maintain a social distance even from family members and seem unconcerned about others' praise or criticism.

They want to be left alone

Most people with this disorder function adequately in everyday life but don't develop many meaningful relationships. Although they fare poorly in groups, they may excel in positions where they have minimal contact with others. (See *What's in a name?*)

Myth busters

What's in a name?

Psychiatric disorders with similar names don't necessarily share common traits.

Myth: Schizoid personality disorder is similar to schizophrenia.

Reality: People with schizoid personality disorder don't have schizophrenia. (*Schizotypal* personality disorder, on the other hand, does share certain features with schizophrenia.) Unfortunately, because the names sound alike, people with schizoid personality may be misunderstood or even discriminated against.

Prevalence

Schizoid personality disorder affects only about 0.7% of the general population. More males have this disorder than females; they also suffer more impairment from it.

Some people with schizoid personality disorder also have additional personality disorders – most commonly schizotypal, paranoid or avoidant personality disorder.

Causes

As with the other personality disorders, the exact cause of schizoid personality disorder isn't known. Some researchers think it may be inherited. Other possible causes may include:
* a sustained history of isolation during infancy and childhood
* cold or grossly deficient early parenting
* parental modelling of interpersonal withdrawal, indifference and detachment.

Signs and symptoms

Assessment of a person with schizoid personality disorder may reveal:
* emotional detachment
* inability to experience pleasure
* lack of strong emotions and little observable change in mood
* indifference to others' feelings, praise or criticism
* avoidance of activities that involve significant interpersonal contact
* little desire for or enjoyment of close relationships
* no desire to be part of a family
* strong preference for solitary activities
* little or no interest in sexual experiences with another person
* lack of close friends or confidants other than immediate family members
* shyness, distrust and discomfort with intimacy
* loneliness
* feelings of utter unworthiness coexisting with feelings of superiority
* self-consciousness and feeling ill at ease with people
* oversensitivity to slights.

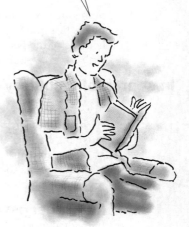

Some people might call me lonely, but I truly prefer solitary activities.

Diagnosis

No specific tests diagnose schizoid personality disorder. Schizoid personality disorder must be distinguished from schizotypal or avoidant personality disorders, which also involve social isolation and withdrawal.

The diagnosis of schizoid personality disorder is confirmed if the person meets the criteria in the *DSM-IV-TR*. (See *Diagnostic criteria: Schizoid personality disorder*, page 292.)

Diagnostic criteria: Schizoid personality disorder

The diagnosis of schizoid personality disorder is confirmed when the person meets these criteria from the *Diagnostic and Statistical Manual of Mental Disorders*, Fourth Edition, Text Revision.

Pattern of social indifference

Since early adulthood, the person has exhibited a pervasive pattern of indifference to social relationships and a restricted range of emotional experience and expression in various contexts. This pattern is indicated by at least four of the following behaviours:

- neither wanting nor enjoying close relationships (such as being part of a family)
- almost always choosing solitary activities
- showing little or no desire for sexual experiences with another person
- taking pleasure in few, if any, activities

- having no close friends or confidants other than first-degree relatives
- seeming indifferent to others' praise or criticism
- displaying constricted affect, emotional coldness or detachment.

Other features

These symptoms don't occur exclusively during the course of schizophrenia or another psychotic disorder, delusional disorder or pervasive developmental disorder. Also, they don't stem from the direct physiological effects of a general medical condition.

Treatment

Someone with schizoid personality disorder isn't likely to seek treatment unless he's under great stress. Additionally, treatment poses a challenge because of the person's initial inability or lack of desire to form a relationship with a therapist or other health care professional.

In search of a solitary niche

Treatment goals include:
- helping the person find the most comfortable solitary niche and cultivate satisfying hobbies that allow him to be on his own
- decreasing his resistance to change
- reducing his social isolation and improving his social interaction
- enhancing his self-esteem.

Individual psychotherapy

Individual psychotherapy should be short term, focusing on solving the person's immediate concerns or problems. Generally, long-term psychotherapy for the schizoid person has a poor outcome and isn't recommended.

Developing a rapport and trusting therapeutic relationship with this person is usually a slow, gradual process. To avoid confrontations, the therapist should make every effort to help him feel secure and acknowledge his boundaries.

Fears and fantasies

When the person opens up, he may reveal fantasies, imaginary friends and fears of unbearable dependency. He may also fear growing dependent on the therapist and prefer to remain in fantasy and withdrawal. The therapist should bring such feelings into proper focus.

Support, not smothering

Stability and support for the person are essential – but the therapist must take care not to smother him and should expect and tolerate some acting-out behaviours.

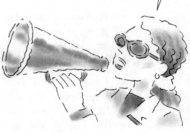

Once more, with some feeling! The therapist should expect some acting-out behaviours in a schizoid person.

Cognitive therapy

Cognitive restructuring may be useful in dealing with illogical thoughts that impede the person's coping ability and functioning. In this technique, the person learns to identify his pattern of thoughts, emotions and behaviour – and then to change his thinking to benefit his mental health.

Group therapy

Initially, group therapy isn't a good treatment choice because most people with schizoid personality disorder can't tolerate being in a social group. However, a person who's graduating from individual to group therapy may have developed adequate social skills to tolerate group therapy. Supportive group members can help the person overcome fears of closeness and feelings of isolation.

People who don't need people

In a group therapy session, the person is usually quiet, seeing little or no reason for social interaction. The group leader should expect this behaviour and not pressure him into participating more fully until he's ready. Also, the leader should protect him from criticism by other group members. Eventually, if the group can tolerate his silence, the person may participate more.

Self-help support groups

Self-help support groups can play an important role in promoting healthier social relationships, enhanced functioning, greater ability to cope with unexpected stressors and reducing fears of closeness and feelings of isolation. Within the group, the person can try out new coping skills and learn that social attachments don't have to be rife with rejection or fear.

Pharmacological therapy

Drug therapy isn't warranted if the person is comfortable with his symptoms. However, medications may be prescribed if he has an overlapping psychiatric disorder such as major depression or needs relief from other acute symptoms. People with psychotic ideations may benefit from low-dose treatment with a novel or atypical antipsychotic, such as olanzapine or risperidone. Generally, long-term drug treatment is avoided.

Nursing interventions

These nursing interventions may be appropriate for a person with schizoid personality disorder:
- Respect the person's need for privacy, and slowly build a trusting therapeutic relationship so that he finds more pleasure than fear in relating to you.
- Offer persistent, consistent, flexible care. Take a direct, involved approach to gain the person's trust.

No crowding allowed

- Recognise the person's need for physical and emotional distance.
- Remember that he needs close human contact but is easily overwhelmed.

Time, space and social skills

- Give the person plenty of time to express his feelings. Keep in mind that pushing him to do so before he's ready may cause him to retreat.
- Teach the person social skills, and reinforce appropriate behaviour.
- Encourage him to express his feelings, analyse his own behaviour and take accountability for his actions.
- Avoid defensiveness and arguing.

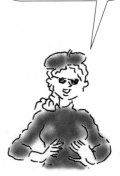

Stay cool, sister. Keep the rhythm slow and steady when trying to build a rapport with a schizoid person.

Schizotypal personality disorder

Schizotypal personality disorder is marked by a pervasive pattern of social and interpersonal deficits, along with acute discomfort with others. People with this disorder have odd thought and behavioural patterns.

During times of extreme stress, some people also have cognitive or perceptual disturbances – although these psychotic symptoms aren't as fully developed as in schizophrenia. Any psychotic episode is short lived, resolving with the use of an appropriate antipsychotic drug.

Figures of speech

The person commonly exhibits eccentric behaviour and has trouble concentrating for long periods. His mannerisms and dress may be peculiar and his speech may be unusual – overly elaborate, vague, metaphorical and hard to follow.

A schizophrenic link?

Some experts think schizotypal personality disorder represents mild schizophrenia. The person may have magical thinking, strange fantasies, odd beliefs (such as thinking he has extrasensory abilities), unusual perceptions and bodily illusions, social isolation and paranoid ideas. However, unlike a person with schizophrenia, a person with schizotypal personality disorder isn't psychotic.

Party of one

Typically, the person has severe social anxiety – usually because he's paranoid about others' motivations. He may relate to others in a stiff or inappropriate way or fail to respond to normal interpersonal cues. Although some people with this disorder marry, most have no more than one person they relate to closely.

Prevalence

Schizotypal personality disorder is found in about 3% of the general population. It's slightly more common in men than in women.

This disorder takes a chronic course and occasionally progresses to schizophrenia. From 30% to 50% of people with schizotypal personality disorder also have major depression. A large number have an additional personality disorder, especially paranoid or avoidant personality disorder.

Causes

Schizotypal personality disorder may have a genetic basis. Family, twin and adoption studies show an increased risk of the condition in people with a family history of schizophrenia. Environmental factors (such as severe stress) may determine whether schizotypal personality disorder or schizophrenia manifests.

Dopamine deviance

Some evidence suggests that people with schizotypal personality disorder have poor regulation of dopamine pathways in the brain.

Psychological and cognitive theories

Psychological and cognitive explanations for schizotypal personality disorder focus on deficits in attention and information processing. These people perform poorly on tests that assess continuous performance tasks, which require the ability to maintain attention on one object and to look at new stimuli selectively.

Neutrality is nicer

They also tend to do poorly on tasks that involve emotionally laden words – suggesting they may have a cognitive bias towards neutral words.

Psychoanalytical theories

Two psychoanalytical theories attempt to explain schizotypal personality disorder. One proposes that people with this disorder have ego boundary problems; the other, that they were raised by parents with inadequate parenting skills, poor communication skills and loose association of words.

It says here that schizotypal personality disorder is similar to schizophrenia, but without the psychotic component.

Signs and symptoms

Assessment findings in a person with schizotypal personality disorder may include:

- odd or eccentric behaviour or appearance
- inaccurate beliefs that others' behaviour or environmental phenomena are meant to have an effect on the person
- odd beliefs or magical thinking (such as thinking that one's thoughts or desires can influence the environment or cause events to occur)
- unusual perceptual experiences, including bodily illusions
- vague, circumstantial, metaphorical, overly elaborate or stereotypical speech or thinking
- unfounded suspicion of being followed, talked about, persecuted or under surveillance
- inappropriate or constricted affect
- lack of close relationships other than immediate family members
- social isolation
- excessive social anxiety that doesn't abate with familiarity
- a sense of feeling different and not fitting in with others easily.

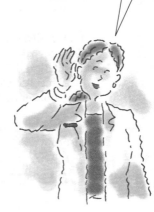

The schizotypal person may speak in a vague, metaphorical or elaborate way.

Diagnosis

The diagnosis is confirmed if the person meets the criteria in the *DSM-IV-TR*. (See *Diagnostic criteria: Schizotypal personality disorder*.)

Diagnostic criteria: Schizotypal personality disorder

The diagnosis of schizotypal personality disorder is confirmed when the person meets these criteria from the *Diagnostic and Statistical Manual of Mental Disorders*, Fourth Edition, Text Revision.

Social and interpersonal deficits

Since early adulthood, the person has exhibited a pervasive pattern of interpersonal and social deficits in various contexts. The pattern is marked by acute discomfort with and reduced capacity for close relationships and by cognitive or perceptual distortions and behavioural eccentricities.

Five or more of the following behaviours are present:

- ideas of reference (excluding delusions of reference)
- odd beliefs or magical thinking that influence the person's behaviour and aren't consistent with subcultural norms (such as superstitiousness, belief in clairvoyance or telepathy)
- unusual perceptual experiences (such as bodily illusions)

- odd speech and thinking (vague, circumstantial, metaphorical, elaborate or stereotypical)
- paranoid ideation or suspiciousness
- inappropriate or narrow range of affect
- odd or eccentric behaviour or appearance
- absence of close friends or confidants (aside from first-degree relatives)
- excessive social anxiety that doesn't abate with familiarity and seems to be associated with paranoid feelings rather than negative judgements about oneself.

Other features

These symptoms don't occur exclusively during the course of schizophrenia or a pervasive developmental disorder.

Treatment

Treatment options for a person with schizotypal personality disorder include individual psychotherapy, family therapy, group therapy, cognitive-behavioural therapy, self-help measures and medications. The person may also benefit from social skills training and other behavioural approaches that emphasise the basics of social interactions.

Psychoanalytical intervention focuses on defining ego boundaries. Cognitive-behavioural therapy attempts to help the person interpret his odd beliefs and teach him valuable coping and interpersonal skills.

Shun challenges

Initially, individual therapy is usually preferred. A warm, supportive, person-centred approach helps establish rapport. The therapist should avoid directly challenging the person's delusional or inappropriate thoughts.

Group prejudice

Group therapy may be considered as the person makes progress. However, a person with this disorder may have trouble tolerating a group because he's mistrustful and suspicious.

Pharmacological therapy

Antipsychotic agents (such as clozapine) may be used to treat psychotic symptoms; they're usually given in low doses. SSRIs have also been effective in some cases.

Nursing interventions

These nursing interventions may be appropriate for a person with schizotypal personality disorder:
- Offer persistent, consistent, flexible care. Take a direct, involved approach to promote the person's trust.
- Know that the person is easily overwhelmed by stress. Give him plenty of time to make difficult decisions.

He likes me, can't stand you

- Be aware that the person may relate unusually well to certain staff members but not at all to others.
- Recognise the person's need for physical and emotional distance.

Social skills and self-analysis

- Teach the person social skills, and reinforce appropriate behaviour.
- Encourage the person's expression of feelings, self-analysis of behaviour and accountability for actions.
- Avoid defensiveness and arguing.

The schizotypal person may relate well to you but not your colleagues – or vice versa.

Antisocial personality disorder

The highlight of antisocial personality disorder is chronic antisocial behaviour that violates others' rights or generally accepted social norms. This disorder predisposes a person towards criminal behaviour.

Other features of this disorder include impulsivity, egocentricity, disregard for the truth and aggression. The antisocial person can't tolerate boredom and frustration. He's reckless, irritable and unable to maintain consistent, responsible functioning at work, at school or as a parent. He lacks remorse and exhibits few, if any, feelings. (See *Insight into antisocial personality disorder*.)

Crime and politics

Although most common among people who get into trouble with the law, antisocial personality disorder also occurs in milder forms. Examples include the politician who's comfortable lying to the public continuously, the husband who continually cheats on his wife and the con artist who scams others out of their money.

Prevalence

In the general population, the prevalence of antisocial personality disorder is about 2–3%. In prison populations, it may be as high as 50%. Roughly one-half of people with this disorder have a history of arrest.

The testosterone effect?

Antisocial personality disorder affects three to four times as many males as females. During adolescence, common coexisting disorders are conduct disorder and oppositional defiant disorder.

Myth busters

Insight into antisocial personality disorder

Do you think you understand the antisocial personality? Think again.

Myth: Most people with antisocial personality disorder are powerful and are always 'out for Number 1'.

Reality: People with antisocial personality disorder see themselves as victims. They seek revenge and don't accept responsibility for their actions.

Causes

Genetic and biological factors may influence the development of antisocial personality disorder. Biological factors include:

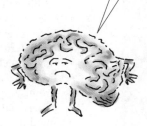

Poor serotonin regulation in certain brain regions may factor into antisocial personality disorder.

poor serotonin regulation in certain brain regions, which may decrease behavioural inhibition

reduced autonomic activity and developmental or acquired abnormalities in the prefrontal brain systems.

Such biological factors may underlie the low arousal, poor fear conditioning and decision-making deficits seen in people with antisocial personality disorder.

Children at risk

Other possible causes or risk factors include attention deficit hyperactivity disorder, large families and childhood exposure to these conditions:
*   substance abuse
*   criminal behaviour
*   physical or sexual abuse
*   neglectful or unstable parenting
*   social isolation
*   transient friendships
*   low socioeconomic status.

Memory jogger

Each letter in ANTISOCIAL stands for a feature of antisocial personality disorder.

A Abuses substances (some people)

N No satisfying interpersonal relationships

T Tends to manipulate others

I Irresponsible and exploitative

S Social norms are disregarded

O Obnoxious towards others (no sense of guilt, shame or remorse)

C Cold and callous

I Intimidates others

A Argumentative

L Legal problems

Signs and symptoms

A person with antisocial personality disorder has a long-standing pattern of disregarding others' rights and society's values. Other assessment findings may include:

- repeatedly performing unlawful acts
- reckless disregard for his own or others' safety
- deceitfulness
- lack of remorse
- consistent irresponsibility
- power-seeking behaviour
- destructive tendencies
- impulsivity and failure to plan ahead
- superficial charm
- manipulative nature
- inflated, arrogant self-appraisal
- irritability and aggressiveness
- inability to maintain close personal or sexual relationships
- disconnection between feelings and behaviours
- substance abuse.

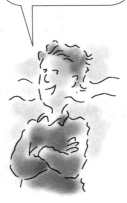

I'm too charming to have antisocial personality disorder. Don't you agree, gorgeous?

Diagnosis

The person with antisocial personality disorder rarely seeks evaluation or treatment on his own. Much more commonly, he's mandated by the court or pressured by family members to seek help.

Not all criminals qualify

Because not all criminals have antisocial personality disorder, the doctor must differentiate this condition from simple criminal activity, adult antisocial behaviour or other behaviours that don't justify the personality disorder as a diagnosis. Formal psychological testing may prove invaluable. (See *Personality and projective tests*, page 301.)

The diagnosis of antisocial personality disorder is confirmed if the person meets the criteria in the *DSM-IV-TR*. (See *Diagnostic criteria: Antisocial personality disorder*, page 302.)

Treatment

Working with an antisocial person can be challenging because he seems to neither show nor feel emotions – especially guilt after doing something wrong. For therapy to be effective, he needs help in drawing the connection between his feelings and behaviours.

Psychotherapy is the usual treatment of choice. Options include individual psychotherapy, group therapy, family therapy and self-help support groups. If needed, the person should also undergo drug or alcohol rehabilitation.

Personality and projective tests

Personality and projective tests elicit person responses that provide insight into mood, personality or psychopathology. These tests include the Beck Depression Inventory (BDI), draw-a-person test, Minnesota Multiphasic Personality Inventory-2 (MMPI-2), sentence completion test and thematic apperception test.

Beck Depression Inventory

A self-administered, self-scored test, the BDI asks people to rate how often they experience symptoms of depression, such as poor concentration, suicidal thoughts, guilt feelings and crying. Questions focus on cognitive symptoms, such as impaired decision-making, and physical symptoms such as appetite loss.

The sum of 21 items gives the total, with a maximum possible score of 63. A score of 11–16 indicates mild depression; a score above 17 indicates moderate depression.

You may help people to complete the BDI by reading the questions – but be careful not to influence their answers. Instruct them to choose the answer that describes them most accurately.

If you suspect depression, a BDI score above 17 may provide objective evidence of the need for treatment. To monitor the person's depression, repeat the BDI during the course of treatment.

Draw-a-person test

In the draw-a-person test, the person draws a human figure of each sex. The psychologist interprets the drawing systematically and correlates the interpretation with diagnosis. The draw-a-person test also provides an estimate of a child's developmental level.

Minnesota Multiphasic Personality Inventory-2

The MMPI-2 is a structured paper-and-pencil test that provides a practical way to assess personality traits and ego function in adolescents and adults. Most people who read English need little assistance in completing it. The MMPI – the original version of this test – was developed at the University of Minnesota and introduced in 1942. The MMPI-2 was released in 1989 and subsequently revised in early 2001.

The MMPI-2 has 567 questions and takes 60–90 minutes to complete. (A short form consists of the first 370 questions of the long-form version.) Questions are designed to evaluate the thoughts, emotions, attitudes and behavioural traits that comprise personality.

A psychologist translates the person's answers into a psychological profile and then combines the profile with data gathered from the interview. Test results shed light on the person's coping strategies, defences, personality strengths and weaknesses, sexual identification and self-esteem. The MMPI-2 may also identify certain personality disturbances or mental deficits caused by neurological problems.

A person's test pattern may strongly suggest a diagnostic category. If the results reveal a risk of suicide or violence, monitor the person's behaviour. If they show frequent somatic complaints indicating possible hypochondria, evaluate the person's physical status. If the complaints lack medical confirmation, help the person explore how these symptoms may signal emotional distress.

Sentence completion test

In the sentence completion test, the person completes a series of partial sentences. A sentence might begin, 'When I get angry, I . . .' The response may reveal the person's fantasies, fears, aspirations or anxieties.

Thematic apperception test

In the thematic apperception test, the person views a series of pictures depicting ambiguous situations and then tells a story describing each picture. The psychologist evaluates these stories systematically to help analyse the person's personality, particularly regarding interpersonal relationships and conflicts.

Diagnostic criteria: Antisocial personality disorder

The diagnosis of antisocial personality disorder is confirmed when the person meets these criteria from the *Diagnostic and Statistical Manual of Mental Disorders*, Fourth Edition, Text Revision.

Disregard for others' rights

Since age 15, the person has displayed a pervasive pattern of disregard for and violation of others' rights, as shown by a history of three or more of the following behaviours:

- failure to conform to social norms with respect to lawful behaviours, as shown by repeatedly performing acts that are grounds for arrest
- deceitfulness, as shown by repeatedly lying, using aliases or conning others for personal profit or pleasure
- impulsivity or failure to plan ahead
- irritability and aggressiveness, as shown by repeated physical fights or assaults
- reckless disregard for his own or others' safety
- consistent irresponsibility, as shown by repeated failure to sustain consistent work or honour financial obligations

- lack of remorse, manifested by indifference to or rationalisation of hurting, mistreating or stealing from another person.

Other features

- None of these symptoms occurred exclusively during the course of schizophrenia or a manic episode.
- The person is at least 18 years old.

Previous evidence of conduct disorder

The person displayed some signs of conduct disorder before age 15. Manifestations of conduct disorder fall into four major categories:

- aggression towards people and animals
- property destruction
- deceitfulness or theft
- serious violations of rules.

Individual psychotherapy

Many people with antisocial personality disorder are mandated to have therapy, sometimes in a forensic or prison setting.

Prison talk

In a confined setting, therapy should focus on alternative life issues, such as:
- goals the person can pursue after his release from custody
- improvement in social or family relationships
- learning new coping skills.

In an outpatient setting, therapy should focus on discussing the person's antisocial behaviour and lack of feelings.

Ultimatums are unwise

Threats are never an appropriate motivating factor for any type of treatment and are least effective in people who are antisocial and have been mandated by the courts to have therapy. Instead of threatening to report the person's lack of motivation to the courts or the prison warden, the therapist should try to help the person find good reasons to want to work on his problem – for example, avoiding more jail time or further trouble with the law.

Advice from the experts

Confidentiality in criminal cases

If you're caring for a person who has been mandated by the courts to have treatment, you may be required by law to disclose confidential person information to the authorities. Some laws create an exemption to the privilege doctrine in criminal cases, which gives the courts access to all essential information.

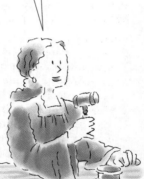

Judges see the consequences of antisocial personality disorder all too often.

Emotional breakthrough

Intensive psychoanalytical approaches aren't indicated for a person with this disorder. Instead, therapy should focus on reinforcing appropriate behaviours, helping him gain greater access to his feelings and helping him make connections between his actions and feelings.

The person may be unfamiliar with the feelings associated with various emotional states, such as depression. Getting him to experience these feelings is crucial. In fact, experiencing intense affect usually is a sign of progress.

Keeping confidences

A therapeutic relationship can occur only when the person and therapist establish a solid rapport and the person can trust the therapist implicitly. However, fears about confidentiality may pose an obstacle to the person's trust. (See *Confidentiality in criminal cases*.)

For example, if he was mandated to have therapy, the therapist must report on his progress occasionally. Although this can be done in a way that doesn't reveal specific details about the content of therapy, the person may be suspicious and distrustful of the therapist – especially at first.

To ease the person's fears, caregivers should honestly disclose what they'll reveal to the courts. In time, the person can learn that what he says in therapy won't necessarily become common knowledge.

Consequences, not conscience

If the person is morally and ethically deficient, dwelling on this problem may bring little progress. A better approach is to try to have the person face up to the consequences of his behaviour. Eventually, this may motivate him to continue with therapy.

Group therapy

After the person overcomes his initial fears over joining a group, he may find group therapy beneficial. Ideally, the group should consist exclusively of people with antisocial personality disorder. In such a group, the person has a greater reason to contribute and share.

Brag sessions

However, the group leader must make sure that the group doesn't become a how-to course in criminal behaviour or a forum to brag about criminal exploits.

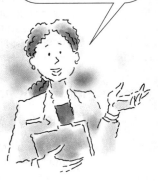

The group leader must make sure that the group doesn't become a forum for people to brag about their criminal exploits.

Family therapy

Family therapy can help the family understand the person's antisocial behaviour. Open discussion should be encouraged – especially regarding confusion, guilt, temptation to make restitution for the person's criminal acts and the frustrations of being with someone who's ill but resists treatment.

Inpatient care

Although people with antisocial personality disorder rarely require inpatient hospital care, they may be hospitalised for treatment of a crisis or major depression. Inpatient care may be intensive and expensive, and is rarely sought out by individuals themselves.

To maintain treatment gains, the person needs community follow-up and support by the hospital staff or professionals or possibly, a self-help support group, after discharge.

Pharmacological therapy

Although research doesn't support using medications to treat antisocial personality disorder directly, drugs may be given to treat disorganised thinking, stabilise mood swings or ease the acute symptoms of concurrent psychiatric disorders. Lithium or a beta-adrenergic blocker (such as propranolol) may be useful in controlling aggressive outbursts.

Nursing interventions

These nursing interventions may be appropriate for a person with antisocial personality disorder:
• Keep in mind that the person may seem charming and convincing.
• Using a straightforward, matter-of-fact approach, set limits on acceptable behaviour. Encourage and reinforce positive behaviour. (See *Setting limits effectively*, page 305.)
• Clearly convey your expectations of the person, as well as the consequences if he fails to meet them.

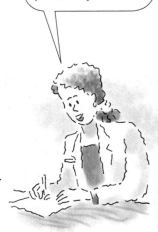

You may have to draw up a behavioural 'contract' with a person who has antisocial personality disorder.

Managing manipulative behaviour

• Anticipate manipulative efforts. Help the person identify such behaviours so that he can learn that other people aren't just extensions of himself.
• Expect the person to refuse to cooperate in an effort to gain control.
• Establish a behavioural 'contract' to communicate to the person that other behaviour options are available.
• Hold the person responsible for his behaviour to promote the development of a collaborative relationship.

Advice from the experts

Setting limits effectively

In a therapeutic setting, placing limits on behaviour gives the person a sense of security and self-control. It also communicates caring on the part of the staff. Limit-setting establishes boundaries, for example that the person may not hurt others or destroy property. It also helps you avoid getting angry and frustrated with the person and increases the effectiveness of the therapeutic relationship. The person benefits from developing a sense of responsibility for his actions.

To set effective limits, follow these guidelines.

Choosing battles wisely

- Choose your battles wisely by setting limits only as needed.
- Set limits when you first sense that the person is violating others' rights. Don't tolerate his behaviour for several days and then launch an angry tirade.
- Avoid using limits as punishment or retaliation. Don't set limits only when you're angry or under stress, because this will hurt your efforts to build a therapeutic relationship.
- Let the person express his feelings about what the limits mean to him. He may perceive them as a message that you no longer like him or may feel increased anxiety because he isn't used to external controls.

Focusing on behaviour

- Establish limits strictly for the person's *behaviour*, not his feelings. If he oversteps the limits, convey that although you don't accept his behaviour, you accept him as a person. If instead you focus on such feelings as anger, the person may sense that his emotions are unacceptable.
- Make sure that the person knows exactly what behaviour you expect.
- Apply the rules consistently and, when possible, offer alternatives to unacceptable behaviour.

Ensuring consistency

- Inform other staff members of the limits you've set. Otherwise, a manipulative person may try split the staff into factions that he can pit against one another.
- Apply the same principles when working with the person's family. Many people come from families that have had little success in establishing discipline. Explain to them that rules may be enforced in a way that communicates love, caring and acceptance.

No-struggle zone

- Avoid power struggles and confrontations so as to maintain the opportunity for therapeutic communication.
- Avoid defensiveness and arguing.

Anger alert

- Observe for physical and verbal signs of agitation.
- Help the person manage anger.
- Teach the person social skills and reinforce appropriate behaviour.
- Encourage the person to express his feelings, analyse his own behaviour and be accountable for his actions.

Borderline personality disorder

A disorder of poor regulation of emotions, borderline personality disorder is marked by a pattern of instability in interpersonal relationships, mood, behaviour and self-image. Although people with this disorder may experience it in various ways, most find it hard to distinguish reality from their own misperceptions of the world. Their emotions overwhelm their cognitive functioning, creating many conflicts with others.

Alternating extremes of anger, anxiety, depression and emptiness are common in people who are borderline. However, intense bouts of these emotions typically last only hours, or at most a day.

Fluctuations and flip-flops

Distortions in cognition and sense of self can lead to frequent changes in long-term goals, jobs and career plans, friendships, values and even gender identity.

The person may see herself as fundamentally bad or unworthy. She may feel misunderstood, mistreated, bored and empty, with little idea of who she really is.

Shopping 'til they drop

People with borderline personality disorder tend to act impulsively without considering the consequences. Impulsive behaviours may include promiscuity, substance abuse and eating or spending binges.

Outbursts of intense anger may lead to violence, which are easily triggered when others criticise or thwart their impulsive acts. Some even have brief psychotic-like experiences.

All or nothing at all

A person with borderline personality disorder tends to have intense and stormy relationships, alternating between a black and white view of others. Her perceptions of family members and friends may shift suddenly from great admiration and love to intense anger and dislike.

For example, she may adore and idealise another person – but when a slight separation or conflict occurs, she may switch unexpectedly to the other extreme and angrily accuse that person of not caring for her.

Called *splitting*, this tendency to view others as either heroes or villains is a defence mechanism meant to protect her from the perception of dangerous anxiety and intense affects. However, instead of offering real protection, splitting leads to destructive behaviour and turmoil.

Rejection blues

With borderline personality comes extreme sensitivity to rejection. The person may react with anger and distress to even mild separations from loved ones, such as vacations, business trips or a sudden change in plans.

Self-mutilation

To escape from her inner turmoil, the person may resort to self-destructive behaviours, such as self-mutilation (cutting or burning herself), substance abuse, eating disorders and suicide attempts. These symptoms commonly are triggered by fear of abandonment.

Prevalence

Borderline personality disorder affects 2–3% of the general population, about 11% of psychiatric outpatients and nearly 20% of psychiatric inpatients. It's three times more common in females than in males.

Age and stability

The disorder usually begins in early childhood and peaks in adolescence and early adulthood. It can take a tumultuous course, resulting in the high use of health care resources by people in their late teens and 20s. However, by their 30s and 40s, up to 60% of people achieve some stability in their work and personal life (although significant areas of dysfunction remain).

Borderline personality disorder commonly overlaps with other personality disorders as well as bipolar disorder, depression, anxiety disorders and substance abuse.

Causes

The precise cause of borderline personality disorder is unknown, but several theories are being investigated. Because it's five times more common in first-degree relatives of people who have it, researchers suspect genetics may play a role.

Biological factors may involve:
- dysfunction in the brain's limbic system or frontal lobe
- decreased serotonin activity
- increased activity in alpha-2-noradrenergic receptors.

Early losses and abuse

Prolonged separation from their parents, other major losses early in life and physical, sexual or emotional abuse or neglect seem to be more common in people with this disorder than in the general population.

Signs and symptoms

Major signs and symptoms of borderline personality disorder fall into four main categories – unstable relationships, unstable self-image, unstable emotions and impulsivity. Symptoms are most acute when the person feels isolated and without social support, causing her to make frantic efforts to avoid being alone.

Assessment findings may include:
- a pattern of unstable and intense interpersonal relationships
- splitting (viewing others as either extremely good or extremely bad)
- intense fear of abandonment, as displayed in clinging and distancing manoeuvres
- rapidly shifting attitudes about friends and loved ones
- desperate attempts to maintain relationships
- unstable perceptions of relationships, with estrangement over ordinary disagreements
- manipulation, as in pitting people against one another
- limited coping skills
- dissociation (separating objects from their emotional significance)
- transient, stress-related paranoid ideation or severe dissociative symptoms
- inability to develop a healthy sense of oneself
- uncertainty about major issues, such as self-image, identity, life goals, sexual orientation, values, career choices or types of friends
- imitative behaviour
- rapid, dramatic mood swings, from euphoria to intense anxiety to rage, within hours or days
- acting out of feelings instead of expressing them appropriately or verbally
- inappropriate, intense anger or difficulty controlling anger
- chronic feelings of emptiness
- unpredictable self-damaging behaviour, such as driving dangerously, gambling, sexual promiscuity, overeating, spending and abusing substances
- self-destructive behaviour, such as physical fights, recurrent accidents, self-mutilation and suicidal gestures.

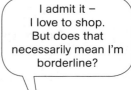

I admit it – I love to shop. But does that necessarily mean I'm borderline?

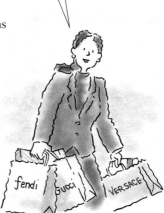

Diagnosis

Standard psychological tests may reveal a high degree of dissociation in a person with borderline personality disorder. The diagnosis is confirmed if the person meets the criteria in the *DSM-IV-TR*. (See *Diagnostic criteria: Borderline personality disorder*, page 309.)

Treatment

Treatment of borderline personality disorder may involve:
- individual psychotherapy
- group therapy
- family therapy
- milieu therapy
- alcohol and drug rehabilitation as indicated.

Psychotherapy

Psychotherapy is usually the treatment of choice for this disorder. Although borderline personality disorder can be hard to treat, individual and group therapies are at least partially effective for many people.

Diagnostic criteria: Borderline personality disorder

The diagnosis of borderline personality disorder is confirmed when the person meets these criteria from the *Diagnostic and Statistical Manual of Mental Disorders*, Fourth Edition, Text Revision.

Pattern of instability

Since early adulthood, the person has exhibited a pervasive pattern of instability of mood, interpersonal relationships and self-image in a variety of contexts. This pattern is indicated by at least five of the following behaviours:

- frantic efforts to avoid real or imagined abandonment
- unstable and intense interpersonal relationships, alternating between extremes of idealising and devaluating others
- markedly and persistently unstable self-image or sense of self
- impulsivity in at least two areas that are potentially self-damaging (such as substance abuse, sex, spending, binge eating or reckless driving)
- recurrent suicidal threats, gestures or behaviour or self-mutilating behaviour
- unstable affect (such as intense irritability or anxiety), usually lasting only a few hours and seldom more than a few days
- chronic feelings of emptiness or boredom
- inappropriate, intense anger or lack of control over anger (such as frequent displays of temper or recurrent physical fights)
- transient and stress-related severe dissociative symptoms or paranoid ideation.

The person's unstable relationships and intense anger can cause difficulty in establishing a therapeutic relationship with health care professionals. She may fail to respond to therapeutic efforts and may make considerable demands on her caregiver's emotional resources, especially when suicidal behaviours are prominent.

Sign on the dotted line

Initially, the therapist should contract with the person to ensure that she doesn't commit suicide or perform self-destructive behaviour. Suicidal potential should be carefully assessed and monitored throughout the entire course of treatment. A person at high risk for suicide may require medication and hospitalisation.

Borderlines with boundaries

A structured therapeutic setting is important. The borderline person may try to test the therapist's limits, so the therapist must set boundaries for the relationship when therapy begins. Everyone involved in her care should maintain these boundaries consistently.

Dialectical behaviour therapy

Within the past 15 years, a psychosocial treatment called dialectical behaviour therapy (DBT) – developed specifically to treat borderline personality disorder – has proven effective in helping people cope with the disorder.

In this comprehensive approach, the person is taught to better control her life and emotions through self-knowledge, emotion regulation and cognitive restructuring.

Treatment modes

DBT involves four primary modes of treatment:

- individual therapy
- group skills training
- telephone contact with the therapist
- therapist consultation.

Individual therapy sessions

The main work of therapy occurs in individual therapy sessions. (The therapist may add group therapy and other treatment modes as appropriate.) Between sessions, the person is offered telephone contact with the therapist to give her help and support in applying the skills she's learning to real life situations – and to help her avoid self-injury.

Therapeutic hierarchy

In individual therapy sessions, goals are dealt with according to the following hierarchy:

- decreasing suicidal behaviours

- decreasing behaviours that interfere with therapy
- decreasing behaviours that interfere with the quality of life
- increasing behavioural skills
- decreasing behaviours related to post-traumatic stress
- improving self-esteem
- individual goals negotiated with the person.

Skills training

Skills training usually is carried out in a group. In the group, people learn:

- core mindfulness skills (meditation-like techniques)
- interpersonal effectiveness skills (which focus on effective ways to achieve one's objectives with others)
- emotion modulation skills (ways of changing distressing emotional states)
- distress tolerance skills (techniques for coping with the emotional states that can't be changed for the time being).

Some people have had success with a psychosocial treatment called *dialectical behaviour therapy*. (See *Dialectical behaviour therapy*.)

Other types of psychotherapy

Therapies that focus on social learning theory and conflict resolution may also be used to treat borderline personality disorder. However, these solution-focused therapies may neglect the person's core problems, such as difficulty expressing appropriate emotions and problems forming emotional attachments to others because of faulty cognitions.

Hospitalisation

Long-term care in a hospital setting is rarely appropriate. However, during an episode of acute depression or another crisis, the person may be seen in an Accident & Emergency department, an inpatient unit or a local community health centre.

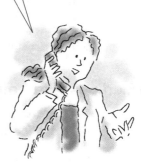

Crisis hotlines, Internet chat rooms and self-help groups are good alternatives to hospitalisation for a borderline person.

Milieu therapy

Whether it takes place in the hospital or in a community setting, milieu therapy uses the person's setting or environment to help her overcome psychiatric disorders. If the person is undergoing this type of therapy, follow these guidelines.

Person preparation

Explain the purpose of milieu therapy to the person. Tell her what you expect of her, and explain how she can participate in the therapeutic community. Orient her to the community's routines, such as the schedule for various activities. Introduce her to other people and staff.

Monitoring and aftercare

Regularly evaluate the person's symptoms and therapeutic needs.

Oversee her activities, encouraging her to keep a schedule typical of life outside the hospital. Also encourage her to interact with others so that she doesn't become withdrawn or feel secluded. Point out the importance of respecting others and her environment.

Home care instructions

If the person eventually returns to the outside community, encourage her to keep follow-up appointments with her therapist.

Because hospital visits are costly, the person should be encouraged instead to find additional social support within the community from such sources as:
- telephone or personal contact with the therapist or doctor
- self-help support groups (including those available through the Internet)
- crisis hotlines.

Pharmacological therapy

The person may receive drugs to relieve specific symptoms, especially during a crisis. These drugs may include:
- antidepressants, such as SSRIs (for example, fluoxetine) or monoamine oxidase inhibitors (MAOIs), to treat depression
- anxiolytic drugs, such as buspirone, to ease anxiety
- antipsychotic drugs, such as risperidone or olanzapine, to ease dissociative symptoms or self-destructive impulses
- mood stabilising drugs, such as valproate or lithium, to treat mood swings

Overdose alert

Dosages should be kept low, prescriptions must be closely monitored because the person may overdose impulsively if she has an adequate drug supply.

Self-help support groups

Many communities have self-help support groups for people with borderline personality disorder. In these groups, people can try out new coping skills, learn to regulate emotions, develop new and healthier social relationships and learn how to reduce stress and anxiety. These techniques help them cope better on their own and avoid situational crises.

Nursing interventions

These nursing interventions may be appropriate for a person with borderline personality disorder:

- Encourage the person to take responsibility for herself. Don't try to rescue her from the consequences of her actions (except suicidal and self-mutilating behaviours).
- Convey empathy and support, but don't try to solve problems she can solve herself.
- Maintain a consistent approach in all interactions with the person, and ensure that other team members use the same approach.
- Avoid sympathetic, nurturing responses.

Manipulation and expectation

- Recognise behaviours that the person uses to manipulate people so that you can avoid unconsciously reinforcing them.
- Set appropriate expectations for social interactions, and praise the person when she meets these expectations.
- To promote trust, respect the person's personal space.

Staff subjects

- Be aware that the person may idealise some staff members and devalue others.
- Don't take sides in the person's disputes with staff members.
- Avoid defensiveness and arguing.
- Try to limit her interactions to assigned staff, to decrease splitting behaviours. Know that using only a few consistent staff members helps maintain consistent treatment.

Cheek checks

- If the person is taking medications, monitor her for 'cheeking' (holding medications in the cheek) or hoarding of medications for overdose at a later time.
- Encourage the person to express her feelings, analyse her behaviour and be accountable for her actions.

Skills expansion

- Help the person develop problem-solving skills.
- Review and encourage relaxation techniques.
- Suggest that the person start an exercise regimen. Exercise promotes stability by decreasing mood swings and aiding the release of anger.

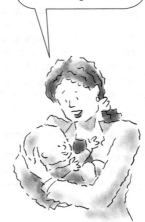

Mothering a baby is appropriate. But mothering a person with borderline personality disorder does more harm than good.

Histrionic personality disorder

Histrionic personality disorder is characterised by a pervasive pattern of excessive emotionality and attention seeking. People with this disorder are drawn to momentary excitements and fleeting adventures.

Charming, dramatic and expressive, they can be easily hurt, vain, demanding, capricious, excitable, self-indulgent and inconsiderate. The words and feelings they express seem shallow and simulated, not real or deep. As a result, they often come across as manipulative and phony. Despite their emotional responsiveness, their emotions may shift instantly from rage to friendliness.

Tone it down, please! You're chewing up the scenery.

Sarah Bernhardt syndrome

Their style of speech is excessively impressionistic, if not downright theatrical, and their gestures are exaggerated. They use grandiose language to describe everyday events and value words more for their emotional content than their factual accuracy.

'Look at me!'

People with histrionic personality disorder need to be the centre of attention at all times. They place great emphasis on physical appearance, often dressing provocatively and behaving seductively. Consumed with superficialities, they devote little time or attention to their internal lives.

Chameleon effect

With limited self-knowledge, they may have no sense of who they are, aside from their identification with others. They may change their attitudes and values depending on the views of significant others. (See *Watching the watchers*.)

Watching the watchers

People with histrionic personality disorder rarely gain an understanding of others. Instead, they devote their intense observation skills to determining which behaviours, attitudes or feelings are most likely to win others' admiration and approval. Essentially, they watch other people watch them.

Because of their limited understanding of how others feel, they tend to see their relationships as closer or more significant than they really are. They don't realise when they're being humoured or placated by someone who has lost patience with their constant need for attention and their inability to relate in an honest way.

Exaggerations and embroidery

People with histrionic personality disorder may exaggerate their illnesses to gain attention, interrupt others so that they can dominate the conversation and seek constant praise. They exaggerate friendships and relationships, believing that everyone loves them. They consider friendships and relationships to be far more intimate than they are.

From fairytale to nightmare

Because they don't view others realistically, people with histrionic personality disorder have trouble developing and sustaining satisfactory relationships. Typically, their relationships start out as ideal and end up as disasters. They idealise the significant other early in the relationship and may see the connection as more intimate than it really is.

If others start to pull back from the incessant demands, the histrionic person becomes dramatic and demonstrative in an attempt to bind the other person to the relationship. To avoid rejection, she may resort to crying, coercion, temper tantrums, assault and suicidal gestures.

Do as I say, not as I do

Despite her attempts to bind others to her, the person with histrionic personality disorder often lacks fidelity and loyalty.

Prevalence

Histrionic personality disorder affects an estimated 2–3% of the general population. Although more commonly diagnosed in women, it may be just as common in men.

Without treatment, the disorder can lead to social, occupational and functional impairments. However, many people function at a high level and succeed at work (although frequent disruption of intimate relationships is common).

Histrionic personality disorder commonly coexists with psychosomatic and mood disorders.

Causes

The cause of histrionic personality disorder isn't known. A genetic component may be involved, as hysterical traits are more common in relatives of those with this disorder. However, little research has been done on the biological origins of this disorder.

Childhood events may come into play as well. Psychoanalytical theories focus on seductive and authoritarian attitudes by fathers of these people.

Signs and symptoms

Assessment of a person with histrionic personality disorder may reveal:
• constant craving for attention, stimulation and excitement
• intense affect

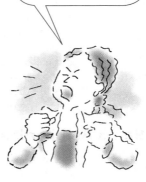

I know I'm being histrionic, but yikes – this chapter is long!!

- shallow, rapidly shifting expression of emotions
- vanity
- flirting and seductive behaviour
- overinvestment in appearance
- exaggerated, vague speech
- self-dramatisation
- impulsivity
- exhibitionism
- suggestibility and impressionability
- egocentricity, self-indulgence and lack of consideration for others
- intolerance of frustration, disappointment and delayed gratification; impatience
- somatic (physical) preoccupations and symptoms
- angry outbursts and tantrums
- sudden enraged, despairing or fearful states
- intense anger towards people viewed as withholding
- divisive, manipulative behaviour
- intolerance of being alone
- suppression or denial of internal distress, weakness, depression or hostility
- dread of growing old
- demanding and manipulative nature
- use of alcohol or drugs to quickly alter negative feelings
- depression
- suicidal gestures and threats.

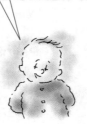

Would you believe I'm the same age as Bob Dylan? Thanks to facelifts and Botox, I plan to stay forever young.

Cultural histrionics

When assessing a person for histrionic personality disorder, keep in mind that to some extent, attention seeking and emotionalism may be culturally determined.

Diagnosis

No specific tests can diagnose histrionic personality disorder; however, personality and projective tests can be helpful. If the person has somatic complaints, physiological disorders must be ruled out.

The diagnosis of histrionic personality disorder is confirmed if the person meets the criteria in the *DSM-IV-TR*. (See *Diagnostic criteria: Histrionic personality disorder*, page 316.)

Treatment

A person with histrionic personality disorder rarely seeks treatment unless a crisis occurs or a situational factor causes functional impairments and ineffective coping. The goal of treatment isn't to cure the person but to relieve the worst elements of her behaviour. Psychotherapy is the treatment of choice.

Diagnostic criteria: Histrionic personality disorder

The diagnosis of histrionic personality disorder is confirmed when the person meets these criteria from the *Diagnostic and Statistical Manual of Mental Disorders*, Fourth Edition, Text Revision.

Pattern of excessive emotionality and attention seeking

Since early adulthood, the person has exhibited a pervasive pattern of excessive emotionality and attention seeking in various contexts. This pattern is indicated by at least five of the following behaviours:

- discomfort when not the centre of attention
- inappropriate sexually seductive or provocative behaviour

- shallow and rapidly shifting expression of emotions
- consistent use of physical appearance to gain attention
- excessively impressionistic and vague style of speech
- self-dramatisation, theatricality and exaggerated expression of emotion
- suggestibility (easily influenced by others)
- perception that relationships are more intimate than they actually are.

Psychotherapy

Psychotherapy focuses on solving problems in the person's life rather than producing long-term personality changes. Individual therapy is preferred over group or family therapy because a group environment may trigger the person's dramatic, attention-seeking behaviour. Likewise, self-help support groups aren't recommended, either.

While establishing a rapport and trust with the person, the therapist must avoid a dependent situation with a needy person who sees the therapist as her rescuer.

Insight, shminsight

Insight-oriented and cognitive approaches aren't especially effective because histrionic people have little capacity or inclination to examine their unconscious motives and thoughts. Instead, the therapist should try to help the person view her interactions objectively and explore and clarify her emotions.

Let's get real

A person with histrionic personality disorder may use such mechanisms as suppression, disavowal, denial and avoidance to block information that could cause emotional distress. If so, the therapist should focus on the issues that the person usually avoids to help her live with reality on its terms.

Serious about suicide

The person should be assessed regularly for suicidal potential, and suicidal thoughts and plans should be taken seriously. Some therapists draw up a 'suicide contract' that specifies under what conditions the person may contact the therapist when she feels like hurting herself.

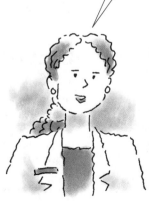

A histrionic person may try to block out distressing information.

Pharmacological therapy

Medications usually aren't indicated for histrionic personality disorder; however, they may relieve associated symptoms, such as anxiety or depression.

In a crisis, the person may seek drugs for self-destructive or harmful purposes. Also, she may respond to the side effects of medications with intense, dramatic overreactions.

Nursing interventions

These nursing interventions may be appropriate for a person with histrionic personality disorder:
• Give the person choices in care options, and incorporate her wishes into the treatment plan as much as possible. Increasing her sense of self-control may lower her anxiety.
• Be aware that the person will want to 'win over' caregivers and – at least initially – is responsive and cooperative.

Role modelling

• Teach the person appropriate social skills and reinforce appropriate behaviour.
• Help the person learn to think more clearly.
• Promote the person's expression of her feelings, self-analysis of her behaviour and accountability for her actions.
• Encourage warmth, genuineness and empathy.

Crisis management

• Teach the person stress-reducing techniques, such as deep breathing and an exercise regimen.
• Help her manage crisis situations and feelings.
• Monitor her for suicidal thoughts and behaviour.

Narcissistic personality disorder

The hallmarks of narcissistic personality disorder are self-centredness, self-absorption and an inability to empathise with the effects of one's behaviour on others. A person with this disorder takes advantage of people to achieve his own ends, using them without regard to their feelings. He has an inflated sense of himself and an intense need for admiration.

Image control

The narcissist tries to maintain an image of perfection and invincibility to prevent others from discovering his weaknesses and imperfections. However, beneath the image is an insecure person with low self-esteem.

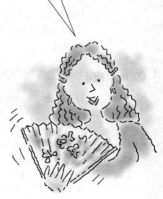

Sure, I'm a tad self-centred. But with my looks, who wouldn't be?

Superior species?

The narcissist expects to be recognised as superior. Preoccupied with fantasies of brilliance and unlimited success or power, he believes he's special and entitled to favoured treatment. He expects others to comply with his wishes automatically and believes he should associate only with other special or high-status people.

Cream of the narcissistic crop

Many narcissists are driven and achievement oriented. In fact, this personality disorder is common among politicians, business tycoons, movie producers, surgeons and criminal lawyers.

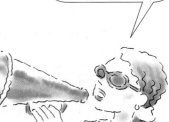

Many narcissists are achievement oriented. The disorder is common among movie producers.

Shattered illusions

The narcissist's illusion of greatness may be shattered by a threat to his ego, as from:
• physical illness
• loss of a job
• loss of a relationship
• feelings of emptiness and depression despite material wealth and success.
    Such threats trigger panic. He feels his world is falling apart and his life is unravelling.

Prevalence

Narcissistic personality disorder is found in less than 1% of the general population. It affects about three times as many males as females.

    Although it develops by early adulthood, this disorder may not be identified until middle age, when the person experiences the sense of a loss of opportunity or faces personal limitations. Many people with narcissistic personality disorder also have histrionic or borderline personality disorder.

Causes

The exact cause of narcissistic personality disorder is unknown. A psychodynamic theory proposes that it arises when a child's basic needs go unmet.

Love thyself, hate thyself

Another theory holds that people with this disorder have an ambivalent self-perception: An idealised (or overidealised) view of the self coexists with deep feelings of inferiority and low self-esteem. Thus, the grandiose image is an effort to cover feelings of inferiority.

    According to this theory, the person received little encouragement and support from his parents during childhood and tends to internalise the process by looking for these feelings within himself.

Signs and symptoms

In a person with narcissistic personality disorder, assessment findings may include:
- arrogance or haughtiness
- self-centredness
- unreasonable expectations of favourable treatment
- grandiose sense of self-importance
- exaggeration of achievements and talents
- preoccupation with fantasies of success, power, beauty, brilliance or ideal love
- manipulative behaviour
- constant desire for attention and admiration
- lack of empathy
- lack of concern over whom he offends
- taking advantage of others to achieve his own goals
- rage, shame or humiliation in response to criticism.

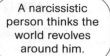

A narcissistic person thinks the world revolves around him.

Diagnosis

The people should undergo psychological evaluation and personality and projective testing. However, no specific tests diagnose narcissistic personality disorder.

The diagnosis is confirmed if the person meets the criteria in the *DSM-IV-TR*. (See *Diagnostic criteria: Narcissistic personality disorder*.)

Diagnostic criteria: Narcissistic personality disorder

The diagnosis of narcissistic personality disorder is confirmed when the person meets these criteria from the *Diagnostic and Statistical Manual of Mental Disorders*, Fourth Edition, Text Revision.

Pattern of grandiosity

Since early adulthood, the person has exhibited a pervasive pattern of grandiosity (in behaviour or fantasy), lack of empathy and the need for admiration in various contexts. This pattern is indicated by at least five of the following behaviours:

- grandiose sense of self-importance (as shown by exaggerating achievements and talents or expecting to be viewed as superior)
- preoccupation with fantasies of unlimited power, success, beauty, brilliance or ideal love

- belief that he's special and unique and can be understood only by other 'special' people
- need for excessive admiration
- sense of entitlement (unreasonable expectations of favourable treatment or automatic compliance with his wishes)
- exploitation of interpersonal relationships (takes advantage of others to achieve his own ends)
- lack of empathy
- envy of others or a belief that others envy him
- arrogant, haughty behaviours or attitudes.

Treatment

Most people with narcissistic personality disorder seek treatment only in a crisis and terminate it as soon as their symptoms ease. Those who don't terminate treatment may be seeking help for depression or interpersonal difficulties.

Long-term psychotherapy is the treatment of choice because it helps establish a strong alliance between the person and the therapist. Therapy should focus on making small, not large, changes in personality traits.

Pulling away the pedestal

The goals of therapy include placing the person's exaggerated self-importance in perspective, helping him develop empathy and teaching him how to handle slights and rejections without feeling extremely threatened.

Group therapy tends to be ineffective because the person typically dominates the group. Others may tire of hearing about his accomplishments and talents; if they criticise him, he's likely to drop out of group therapy.

Inpatient treatment

Hospitalisation may be necessary for a person with severe symptoms, such as self-destructive behaviour and poor reality testing. However, hospitalisation should be brief, with treatment specific to the particular symptoms.

Milieus for weak egos

People with little motivation for outpatient treatment, chronic destructive acting out and chaotic lifestyles may need longer therapy. Inpatient care can offer intensive milieu therapy, individual psychotherapy, family involvement or a specialised residential environment. Such treatment may be appropriate for people with severe ego weakness, helping them to improve their self-concept.

Nursing interventions

These nursing interventions may be appropriate for a person with narcissistic personality disorder:
- Convey respect and acknowledge the person's sense of self-importance so that he can reestablish a coherent sense of self. However, don't reinforce either pathological grandiosity or weakness.
- Focus on the person's positive traits or on his feelings of pain, loss or rejection.

Don't play Judge Judy

- If the person makes unreasonable demands or has unreasonable expectations, tell him in a matter-of-fact way that he's being unreasonable. However, remain nonjudgemental because a critical attitude may make him even more demanding and difficult. Don't avoid him as this could increase his maladaptive attention-seeking behaviour.

You may have put yourself on a pedestal, but I'm not going to reinforce your grandiosity.

- Avoid defensiveness and arguing.
- Offer persistent, consistent and flexible care. Take a direct, involved approach to ensure the person's trust.
- Teach the person social skills and reinforce appropriate behaviour.

Avoidant personality disorder

Avoidant personality disorder is marked by feelings of inadequacy, extreme social anxiety, social withdrawal and hypersensitivity to others' opinions. People with this disorder have low self-esteem and poor self-confidence. They dwell on the negative and have difficulty viewing situations and interactions objectively.

To rationalise their avoidance of new situations, they exaggerate the potential difficulties involved. They may create fantasy worlds to substitute for the real one.

Wallflower syndrome

The avoidant person yearns for social relations but fears being rejected or embarrassed in front of others. In fact, he isn't willing to enter into social relationships without the assurance of uncritical acceptance. He even seeks out jobs that require little contact with others.

Prevalence

In the adult general population, the prevalence of avoidant personality disorder is estimated at 0.5–1.0%. It affects males and females equally and develops by early adulthood.

Many people with avoidant personality disorder also have other psychiatric disorders, including social phobia, schizoid or dependent personality disorder, agoraphobia, obsessive–compulsive disorder, generalised anxiety disorder, dysthymia, major depressive disorder, psychosomatic disorders, dissociative disorder and schizophrenia.

Causes

Avoidant personality disorder most likely results from a combination of genetic, biological, environmental and other factors – although the evidence for genetic and biological causes is weak. From a psychodynamic view, the disorder has been attributed to an overly critical parental style.

Genetic and biological theories

Avoidant personality disorder is closely linked to temperament. Studies of children under age 2 found that some have an apparently inborn tendency to withdraw from new situations or people. In fact, roughly 10% of toddlers are habitually fearful and withdrawn when exposed to new people and situations. Some evidence suggests that a timid temperament in infancy may predispose a person to developing avoidant personality disorder later in life.

> About 10% of toddlers are fearful and withdrawn when exposed to new people and situations.

Information overload

The inherited tendency to be shy may result from overstimulation or an excess of incoming information. The person can't cope with the excess information and withdraws in defence. Inability to cope with the information overload may stem from a low autonomic arousal threshold.

Low threshold, greater response

Research suggests that in people with this disorder, certain structures in the brain's limbic system may have a lower threshold of arousal and a more pronounced response when activated.

Environmental factors

Some experts believe that significant environmental influences during childhood, such as rejection by the parents or peers, leads to the full development of avoidant personality disorder. (See *The rejected child*.)

Signs and symptoms

A person with avoidant personality disorder may exhibit or report:
- shyness, timidity and social withdrawal
- behaviour or appearance that's meant to drive others away (which gives him a sense of control)

The rejected child

Some authorities suspect that avoidant personality disorder results from childhood rejection by the parents or peers.

Parental rejection

Normal, healthy infants may encounter varying degrees of parental rejection. In those who subsequently develop avoidant personality disorder, the amount of rejection seems to be particularly intense or frequent.

Particular types of parental rejection can alter a child's attitude and behaviour in a way that predisposes him to developing avoidant personality disorder later in life. For example, if a parent is aloof or critical when the child expresses positive emotions, the child might learn to spare himself the anguish by keeping positive feelings to himself.

Likewise, if he's repeatedly told that it's bad to feel angry, he might swear off relationships to avoid the intermittent feelings of dissatisfaction or anger that occur in nearly all close relationships.

Peer rejection

Repeated social interactions expose a person to potential rejection over a sustained period. Such rejection can wear down one's self-esteem. After humiliation and rejection by peers, a person may begin to criticise himself.

Feelings of loneliness and isolation worsen with these harsh self-judgements. Deepening feelings of personal inferiority and self-worthlessness contribute to social withdrawal.

Rejection by peers seems to validate rejection by the parents. When a child can't turn to parents, peers or even himself for gratification or validation, he retreats – and avoidant personality disorder may result.

- reluctance to speak or, conversely, overtalkativeness
- constant mistrust or wariness of others
- testing of others' sincerity
- difficulty starting and maintaining relationships
- perfectionism
- rejection of people who don't live up to his impossibly high standards
- limited emotional expression
- tenseness and anxiety
- low self-esteem
- feelings of being unworthy of successful relationships
- self-consciousness
- loneliness
- reluctance to take personal risks or engage in new activities
- frequent escapes into fantasy, such as by excessive reading, watching TV or daydreaming.

Diagnosis

No specific tests can diagnose avoidant personality disorder. The person should undergo a psychological evaluation, along with personality and projective tests.

The diagnosis is confirmed if he meets the criteria in the *DSM-IV-TR*. (See *Diagnostic criteria: Avoidant personality disorder*.)

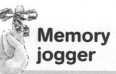

Memory jogger

For an easy way to remember the signs and symptoms of avoidant personality disorder, think of AVOIDANT.

A Anxious and angry with oneself because of the lack of meaningful relationships

V Very socially withdrawn

O Often feels lonely and unwanted

I Intensely shy

D Desires close relationships but has difficulty developing and sustaining them

A Awkward and uncomfortable in others' company

N No natural optimism or positive regard for oneself

T Terrified by the fear of rejection

Diagnostic criteria: Avoidant personality disorder

The diagnosis of avoidant personality disorder is confirmed when the person meets these criteria from the *Diagnostic and Statistical Manual of Mental Disorders*, Fourth Edition, Text Revision.

Pattern of social inhibition

Since early adulthood, the person has displayed a pervasive pattern of social inhibition, feelings of inadequacy and hypersensitivity to criticism in various contexts. This pattern is indicated by at least four of the following behaviours:

- avoidance of work activities that involve significant interpersonal contact because of the fear of disapproval, criticism or rejection
- unwillingness to get involved with people unless he's sure they'll like him
- restraint in intimate relationships for fear of being ridiculed or shamed
- preoccupation with being criticised or rejected in social situations
- inhibition in new interpersonal situations due to feelings of inadequacy
- self-perception as socially inept, inferior or personally unappealing
- marked reluctance to take personal risks or engage in new activities for fear that these will cause embarrassment.

Treatment

People with avoidant personality disorder rarely seek treatment unless something goes wrong in their lives to indicate that they aren't coping adequately. High-functioning people may need psychotherapy only, while others benefit from a combination of medication and psychotherapy.

The goals of treatment are to:
- enhance self-esteem
- improve social interaction and increase confidence in interpersonal relationships
- desensitise the reaction to criticism
- decrease resistance to change
- improve coping
- achieve cognitive restructuring
- develop appropriate affect and expression of emotions.

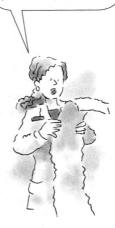

Personality and projective tests can help determine if a person has avoidant personality disorder.

Psychotherapy

Individual psychotherapy, the preferred treatment, is most effective when it's short term and focused on solving specific life problems. As the person progresses through individual therapy, group therapy may be considered.

All's well that ends well

Establishing a solid therapist – person relationship may be difficult, and the person may terminate therapy early. However, a successful ending to the relationship is important because it reinforces for the person the possibility of new relationships.

Pharmacological therapy

If the person has moderate to severe functional impairments, medications may be prescribed as an adjunct to psychotherapy; and may be used to treat such symptoms as anxiety and depression. However, if the person feels disconnected from his emotions, medications may interfere with effective psychotherapeutic management.

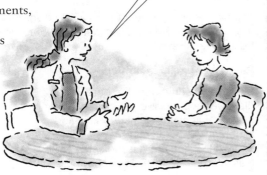

I'm glad you trust me to care for you, but you need to be involved in your care, too.

Nursing interventions

These nursing interventions may be appropriate for a person with avoidant personality disorder:
- Offer persistent, consistent and flexible care. Take a direct, involved approach to gain the person's trust.
- Be aware that the person may become dependent on the few staff members that he feels he can trust. Monitor for signs of dependency, and encourage self-care.
- Assess the person for signs of depression because social impairment increases the risk of mood disorders.

Advice from the experts

Basic requirements for relaxation

According to Dr Herbert Benson, the Harvard professor who first described the relaxation response, four basic elements are needed to elicit this response:

- a quiet environment that's free from distraction
- a sound, process or image to dwell on, such as breathing or a mantra (like that used in transcendental meditation)
- a passive attitude in which the mind is cleared of thoughts and images
- a comfortable position that can be kept easily for at least 20 minutes.

Advance warning

- Make sure that the people knows about upcoming procedures in plenty of time to adjust because he doesn't handle surprises well.
- Inform the person when you will and won't be available if he needs assistance.

Directives and decisions

- Initially, give the person explicit directives rather than ask him to make decisions. Then gradually encourage him to make easy decisions. Continue to provide support and reassurance as his decision-making ability improves.
- Avoid actions that foster dependency.
- Encourage the person's expression of his feelings, self-analysis of his behaviour and accountability for his actions.
- Teach the person relaxation and stress-management techniques to help him cope in times of stress and manage his anxiety level. (See *Basic requirements for relaxation*.)

A basic requirement for relaxation? I'm thinking a week in the Caribbean

Dependent personality disorder

Dependent personality disorder is characterised by an extreme need to be taken care of, which leads to submissive, clinging behaviour and fear of separation or rejection. People with this disorder let others make important decisions for them and have a strong need for constant reassurance and support. To elicit caregiving, they engage in dependent behaviour.

Feeling helpless and incompetent, they comply passively and transfer responsibility to others. In fact, they seek others to dominate and protect them. Some stay in abusive relationships and are willing to tolerate mistreatment.

Replacement therapy

When the break-up of a romantic relationship is imminent, a person with dependent personality disorder may become suicidal. After a close relationship ends, she urgently seeks another relationship as a source of care and support.

People who need people

These behaviours arise from the perception that she can't function adequately without others. She craves attention and validation and may repeatedly request attention to her complaints over such issues as her lifestyle, social relationships, lack of meaning in life or medical problems.

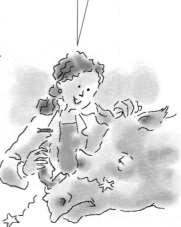

I think this critter has grown overly dependent on me!

That worthless feeling

Overly sensitive to disapproval, she often feels helpless and depressed. She belittles her own abilities and is racked with self-doubt. She takes criticism and disapproval of her as proof that she's worthless.

She's likely to avoid positions of responsibility. If her job requires independent initiative, she may suffer occupational impairments.

Gender patterns

In females, dependent personality disorder is likely to consist of a pattern of submissiveness. In males, it may involve a pattern of autocratic behaviour.

Prevalence

In mental health clinics, dependent personality disorder is among the most frequently reported personality disorders. In the general population, its prevalence is about 1.5%. It affects slightly more females than males.

Abundance of overlap

An estimated 80% of people with dependent personality disorder have an additional personality disorder – most commonly borderline or avoidant. Many also have coexisting mood disorders (especially depression), anxiety disorders, somatoform disorders and dissociative disorders.

Causes

The exact cause of dependent personality disorder isn't known. Because it tends to run in families, it may involve a genetic component.

Dictators and coddlers

According to some experts, authoritarian or overprotective parenting may lead to high levels of dependency. These parenting styles may cause the child to believe that she can't function without others' guidance and protection and that the way to maintain relationships is to give in to others' demands.

Possible contributing factors may include:
- childhood trauma
- closed family system that discourages outside relationships
- childhood physical or sexual abuse
- social isolation.

Signs and symptoms

Assessment findings in a person with dependent personality disorder may include:
- submissiveness
- self-effacing, apologetic manner
- low self-esteem
- lack of self-confidence
- lack of initiative
- incompetence and a need for constant assistance
- intense, unremitting need to be loved in a stable long-term relationship that goes through minimal change
- anxiety and insecurity, especially when deprived of a significant relationship
- feelings of pessimism, inferiority and unworthiness
- hypersensitivity to criticism
- in females, little need to overtly control or compete with others
- clinging, demanding behaviour
- use of cajolery, bribery, promises to change and even threats to maintain key relationships
- fear and anxiety over losing a relationship or being alone
- dependence on a number of people, any one of whom could substitute for the other
- difficulty making everyday decisions without advice and reassurance
- avoidance of change and new situations
- exaggerated fear of losing support and approval.

Don't be so self-effacing. You're a hot, handsome hunk!

Somatically speaking . . .

A person with dependent personality disorder may also present with somatic complaints, such as fatigue and lethargy, as well as tension, anxiety or depression.

Diagnosis

The person should undergo a psychological evaluation and psychological and projective tests, as indicated. If she has somatic complaints, she should be evaluated medically and, as needed, undergo diagnostic tests to rule out underlying medical conditions.

The diagnosis of dependent personality disorder is confirmed if the person meets the criteria in the *DSM-IV-TR*. (See *Diagnostic criteria: Dependent personality disorder*.)

Treatment

Although people with this disorder frequently attend outpatient mental health clinics, they rarely seek treatment for dependency or help in making decisions. Instead, they typically complain of anxiety, tension or depression.

Psychotherapy

Psychotherapy is the treatment of choice. Promoting autonomy and self-efficacy are the overriding treatment goals.

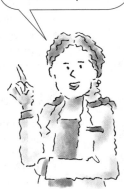

For a dependent person, long-term therapy only reinforces a dependent relationship with the therapist.

Diagnostic criteria: Dependent personality disorder

The diagnosis of dependent personality disorder is confirmed when the person meets these criteria from the *Diagnostic and Statistical Manual of Mental Disorders*, Fourth Edition, Text Revision.

Pattern of submissive behaviour

Since early adulthood, the person has demonstrated a pervasive and excessive need to be taken care of that leads to submissive, clinging behaviour and fear of separation in various contexts. This pattern is indicated by at least five of the following behaviours:

- difficulty making everyday decisions without an excessive amount of advice or reassurance from others
- need for others to take responsibility for most major areas of her life
- difficulty expressing disagreement with others because of unwarranted fears that she'll lose their support or approval
- going to excessive lengths to gain support and nurturance from others, even to the point of volunteering to do unpleasant things
- discomfort or helplessness when alone because of exaggerated fears that she won't be able to care for herself
- urgent seeking of another relationship when a close relationship ends
- unrealistic preoccupation with fears of being left to take care of herself.

Clinging vine

The most effective approach is short term and focuses on helping the person solve specific life problems. Long-term therapy is contraindicated because it only reinforces a dependent relationship with the therapist. (However, some degree of dependency is bound to develop no matter the length of therapy.)

Individual and group therapy may be helpful, although the person may use a group setting to find new dependent relationships.

After-hours attention

The person may be very needy with the therapist and seek tremendous reassurance and attention – especially between therapy sessions. At the start of therapy, the therapist should set boundaries as to how the treatment will be conducted, including such issues as appropriate times to contact the therapist between sessions.

Final endings

Termination of therapy is an important issue because it's a test of how effective the therapy has been. The therapist should set goals for therapy and make it clear to the person that when she attains these goals, therapy will end.

Behavioural approaches

A person with dependent personality disorder can benefit from such behavioural approaches as assertiveness training.

Pharmacological therapy

The doctor may prescribe medications to treat associated symptoms, such as low energy, fatigue and depression. Some people respond well to antidepressants, including SSRIs, tricyclics and MAOIs.

In a crisis, anxiolytic drugs (such as alprazolam or lorazepam) may be prescribed. However, because the person may abuse these drugs, their use should be limited and monitored.

Nursing interventions

These nursing interventions may be appropriate for a person with dependent personality disorder:
- Offer persistent, consistent and flexible care. Take a direct, involved approach to ensure the person's trust.
- Give the person as much opportunity to control her treatment as possible. Offer options and allow her to choose, even if she chooses all of them.
- Verify the person's approval before initiating specific treatment.
- Try to limit caregivers to a few consistent staff members to increase the person's sense of security.

Deter dependency

- Deter actions that promote dependency on caregivers.
- Encourage activities that require decision-making (such as managing a budget, planning meals and paying bills) to promote autonomy.
- Help the person establish and work towards goals to foster a sense of autonomy.
- If the person has physical complaints, don't minimise or dismiss them – but don't encourage them either. Use a simple, matter-of-fact approach.

Aim for assertiveness

- Help the person express her ideas and feelings assertively.
- Be aware that outwardly, the person may seem compliant – perhaps overly compliant – with suggestions for treatment. Despite her passivity, though, she may fail to make real gains in therapy because her compliance is usually superficial.

Monitor medications

- Teach the person about prescribed medications, including exactly what each medication is prescribed for.
- Emphasise that there are no magical drug effects.
- Monitor the person to make sure that she isn't abusing medication. If she's receiving benzodiazepines, check for signs and symptoms of psychological dependence.

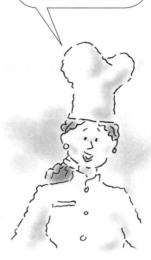

Encourage a dependent person to plan her own meals, manage her own budget and pay bills on her own.

Obsessive–compulsive personality disorder

Obsessive–compulsive personality disorder is marked by a desire for perfection and order at the expense of openness, flexibility and efficiency. The person with this disorder sees the world as black and white.

Along with perfectionism comes relentless anxiety about not getting things perfect. The person with obsessive–compulsive personality disorder places a great deal of pressure on himself and others not to make mistakes. He may have a constant sense of righteous indignation and feel anger and contempt for anyone who disagrees with him.

My way or the highway

His way of doing something is the only right way; all other ways are wrong. His inflexibility extends to interpersonal relationships as well as daily routines. A lifelong pattern of rigid thinking may lead to poor social skills.

Control freak

Someone with obsessive–compulsive personality disorder has an overwhelming need to control the environment. He may force himself and others to follow rigid moral principles and conform to extremely high standards of performance. Conscientious, scrupulous and inflexible about morality, ethics and value, he insists on literal compliance with authority and rules.

Indecisive impasse

In his effort to avoid being wrong, he may suffer severe procrastination and indecisiveness because he can't determine with certainty which choice is correct. He may have trouble even starting a task because of his need to sort out the priorities correctly. His symptoms may cause extreme distress and interfere with occupational and social functioning. (See *A confusing similarity*.)

Prevalence

Obsessive–compulsive personality disorder affects about 1.5% of the general population – about twice as many males as females. In psychiatric settings, its prevalence is estimated at 5–10%.

Incidence may be higher among the oldest children in a family and among people whose occupations require attention to detail and methodical perseverance.

Cluster C confluence

Many people with obsessive–compulsive personality disorder have one or both of the other cluster C personality disorders (avoidant and dependent personality disorders). Some also have paranoid personality disorder as well as various types of anxiety, psychosomatic and depressive disorders.

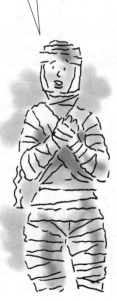

The person with obsessive – compulsive personality disorder is all bound up in self-imposed rules and regulations.

Causes

Genetic and developmental factors may play a role in the development of this disorder. Twin and adoption studies suggest that it runs in families.

Psychodynamic theories view the person as needing control as a defence against feelings of powerlessness or shame.

Signs and symptoms

A person with obsessive–compulsive personality disorder may describe his symptoms in a logical way, attaching little emotion to any physical discomfort. Assessment findings commonly include:
- behavioural, emotional and cognitive rigidity
- perfectionism
- severe self-criticism
- indecisiveness
- controlling manner
- difficulty expressing tender feelings
- poor sense of humour
- cool, distant, formal manner
- solemn, tense demeanour
- emotional constriction
- excessive discipline
- aggression, competitiveness and impatience
- bouts of intense anger when things stray from the person's idea of how things 'should be'
- difficulty incorporating new information into his life
- psychosomatic complaints
- hypochondriasis
- sexual dysfunction
- chronic sense of time pressure and inability to relax
- indirect expression of anger despite an apparent undercurrent of hostility
- miserliness and hoarding of money and other possessions
- preoccupation with orderliness, neatness and cleanliness
- scrupulousness about morality, ethics or values
- signs and symptoms of depression
- physical complaints (commonly stemming from overwork).

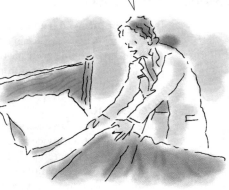

A perfectionistic person simply won't tolerate a poorly made bed.

Diagnosis

The person should undergo a psychological evaluation, including personality and projective tests. The diagnosis of obsessive–compulsive personality disorder is confirmed if he meets the criteria in the *DSM-IV-TR*. (See *Diagnostic criteria: Obsessive–compulsive personality disorder*, page 333.)

Diagnostic criteria: Obsessive–compulsive personality disorder

The diagnosis of obsessive–compulsive personality disorder is confirmed when the person meets these criteria from the *Diagnostic and Statistical Manual of Mental Disorders*, Fourth Edition, Text Revision.

Pattern of perfectionism and control

Since early adulthood, the person has displayed a pervasive pattern of perfectionism, orderliness and mental and interpersonal control at the expense of flexibility, openness and efficiency. Present in various contexts, this pattern is indicated by at least four of the following behaviours:

- preoccupation with details, rules, lists, order, organisation or schedules so that the major point of the activity is lost
- perfectionism that interferes with task completion
- excessive devotion to work and productivity to the exclusion of leisure activities and friendships (not explained by obvious economic need)
- overconscientiousness, scrupulousness and inflexibility regarding matters of morality, values or ethics (not explained by cultural or religious identification)
- inability to discard worn-out or worthless objects even when they lack sentimental value
- reluctance to delegate tasks or work with others unless they exactly follow his way of doing things
- miserliness towards himself and others and a view of money as something to be hoarded for future catastrophes
- rigidity and stubbornness.

Treatment

Typically, a person with obsessive–compulsive personality disorder seeks treatment only if he's depressed, unproductive or under extreme stress – circumstances that tax his limited coping skills. Treatment usually involves individual psychotherapy, possibly in conjunction with medication.

Psychotherapy

Effective psychotherapeutic treatment centres on short-term symptom relief and support for existing coping mechanisms (with new ones taught as therapy progresses). Long-term work on changing the personality is unrealistic because the inherent nature of obsessive–compulsive personality disorder makes it especially resistant to change.

Down to business

The therapist should discuss the nature of the disease process and explain typical treatments in a businesslike, factual manner, rather than give vague impressions. When the person accepts the treatment regimen, he's likely to adhere to it rigorously and strive to be a good person. He's conscientious, honest, motivated and hard-working.

Ideally, therapy should replace skills that aren't working with new skill sets, examine social relationships and identify feeling states. Proper identification and realisation of feelings can help produce changes in the person's life.

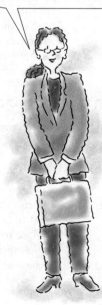

A business-like approach is best if your person has obsessive–compulsive personality disorder.

Focus on feelings

Because the person with obsessive – compulsive personality disorder is likely to be out of touch with his emotions, the therapist should lead him away from describing situations, events and daily happenings. A better approach is to have him express how these events make him feel. Having him keep a daily journal of feelings can help him remember how he felt at any given time.

Cognitive quicksand

Cognitive approaches rarely work with this person, because he's likely to use this type of therapy as a means for verbally attacking the therapist or otherwise taking the focus off himself.

Group therapy

The person may find group therapy intolerable because of the social contact necessary to healthy group dynamics. In fact, group members may ostracise him if he points out their deficits and incorrect ways of doing things.

Pharmacological therapy

Generally, obsessive–compulsive personality disorder doesn't respond to medication. However, if the person suffers from depression, SSRIs or other antidepressants may be helpful.

Nursing interventions

These nursing interventions may be appropriate for a person with obsessive–compulsive personality disorder:
- Offer persistent, consistent and flexible care. Take a direct, involved approach to gain the person's trust.
- Let the person control his own treatment plan by giving him choices whenever possible.
- Maintain a professional attitude. Avoid informality; this person wants strict attention to detail.

Don't get too close

- Recognise the person's need for physical and emotional distance.

Pay attention!

- Be prepared for long monologues centring on the person's goals and ambitions and reasons why family members, friends and work subordinates need to be rigidly controlled. Try to remain attentive.
- Use tolerance and ordinary kindness when dealing with the person. Remember that he's used to causing exasperation in others but doesn't fully understand why.
- Avoid defensiveness and arguing.

No-pressure tactics

- Don't brush aside issues that the person thinks are important in an effort to get on with affective issues. Pressuring him to focus prematurely on emotions will alienate him.
- If appropriate, encourage the person to record his feelings in a journal.
- Remember that the person's defensive structure (which makes him seem arrogant and argumentative) is a cover for his vulnerability to shame, humiliation and dread.

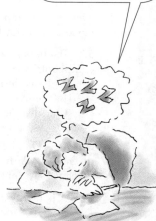

Try to be attentive even if the person rambles on about others' faults.

Teaching topics

- Teach the person social skills, and reinforce appropriate behaviour.
- Teach him about prescribed medication.
- Encourage him to continue therapy for optimal results.

Quick quiz

1. The personality disorder that's characterised primarily by mistrust is:
    A. paranoid personality disorder.
    B. antisocial personality disorder.
    C. dependent personality disorder.
    D. schizotypical personality disorder.

Answer: A. Paranoid personality disorder is characterised by an extreme distrust of others. People with this disorder avoid relationships in which they aren't in control or have the potential of losing control.

2. For people with most personality disorders, the treatment of choice is:
    A. group therapy.
    B. individual psychotherapy.
    C. self-help support groups.
    D. inpatient care.

Answer: B. Individual psychotherapy is usually the treatment of choice for people with personality disorders.

3. Ideas of reference and magical thinking may occur in:
    A. borderline personality disorder.
    B. schizotypal personality disorder.
    C. schizoid personality disorder.
    D. histrionic personality disorder.

Answer: B. Schizotypal personality disorder is marked by ideas of reference, odd beliefs or magical thinking, among other features.

4. The hallmark of borderline personality disorder is:
   A. irresponsibility.
   B. reckless disregard for others.
   C. impulsivity.
   D. unlawful behaviour.

Answer: C. Impulsivity is the most prominent characteristic of borderline personality disorder.

5. If a person with dependent personality disorder reports physical complaints, the nurse should:
   A. overlook the symptoms.
   B. encourage her to talk about her symptoms.
   C. disregard symptoms until emotional issues have been explored.
   D. explore symptoms in a matter-of-fact way.

Answer: D. The nurse should explore the person's symptoms in a matter-of-fact way. Although physical complaints should be evaluated promptly, caregivers shouldn't encourage the person to talk about them.

6. A person who's preoccupied with details and lists is most likely to have:
   A. histrionic personality disorder.
   B. obsessive–compulsive personality disorder.
   C. schizotypal personality disorder.
   D. narcissistic personality disorder.

Answer: B. Obsessive–compulsive personality disorder is marked by a preoccupation with details, lists, rules and schedules.

Scoring

✰✰✰ If you answered all six items correctly, take a bow! We won't hold it against you if you're feeling a bit narcissistic right now.

✰✰ If you answered four or five items correctly, you certainly don't need to be rescued. You're right on the borderline between good and excellent.

✰✰ If you answered fewer than four items correctly, don't get histrionic. Just cling to this chapter a little longer.

10 Eating disorders

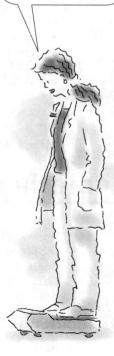

Just the facts

In this chapter, you'll learn:

♦ major features of eating disorders

♦ proposed causes of eating disorders

♦ assessment findings and nursing interventions for people with eating disorders

♦ recommended treatments for people with eating disorders.

> People with eating disorders are preoccupied with their weight and shape.

A look at eating disorders

Eating disorders are severe disturbances in eating behaviour accompanied by distortions in body image and self-perception. The two main eating disorders, anorexia nervosa and bulimia nervosa, share such features as dieting and preoccupation with weight and shape. Additionally, anorexia nervosa and bulimia nervosa can occur simultaneously.

The typical sufferer is a white, middle-class female in her teens or twenties. However, eating disorders can occur in people of all ages and of all economic, ethnic and educational backgrounds.

An eating disorder can be physically and psychologically debilitating. Extreme cases can lead to death from physical complications or suicide. The risk of mortality is especially high if the disorder is long-standing or the person has an overlapping psychiatric problem, such as substance abuse or depression.

Isolation cycle

People with eating disorders face social obstacles, too. Young girls may be ostracised because their peers don't know how to approach them and most boys aren't comfortable dating them. This can establish a vicious cycle that leads to further isolation.

Causes

Theories explaining the cause of eating disorders encompass such factors as genetics, biology, psychodynamics and social and family influences. In all likelihood, a combination of components is involved.

Genetic and biological theories

Eating disorders tend to run in families, with female relatives most often affected. A girl whose sibling has anorexia nervosa runs a 10- to 20-fold higher risk of developing the disorder herself. This finding suggests that genetic factors may predispose some people to eating disorders (or to accepting society's bias towards thinness).

Neurochemical factors have also been linked to eating disorders – although it isn't clear if these factors cause, accompany or follow the development of the eating disorder.

Psychological factors

Psychological factors that may play a role in the development of eating disorders include:
- low self-esteem
- conflicts over identity, role development and body image
- fears concerning sexuality
- chaotic families with few rules or boundaries
- parental overemphasis on, or excessive worry over, the child's weight
- an overly close mother–daughter relationship (in bulimia nervosa)
- sexual abuse.

Social influences

Society sets unrealistic expectations for appearance, equating being thin with being successful, powerful and popular. These expectations are conveyed through omnipresent images of thin, beautiful people on television and in films, magazines and other media.

Anorexia nervosa

Anorexia nervosa is a self-starvation syndrome in which the person relentlessly pursues thinness – sometimes to the point of fatal emaciation – as she becomes preoccupied with food and body image. Despite her extreme thinness, she thinks that she's fat because she has a distorted body image. Generally, a person is deemed to have anorexia nervosa when her weight drops to less than 85% of ideal body weight. (See *Name games*, page 339.)

Disorder forms

Anorexia nervosa occurs in two main forms:
- restricting type, in which food intake is limited

Myth busters

Name games

Many people confuse anorexia nervosa with anorexia.

Myth: Anorexia nervosa is the clinical term for anorexia.

Reality: The two conditions aren't the same thing. *Anorexia* refers to loss of appetite. A common symptom of GI and endocrine disorders, anorexia may also accompany anxiety, chronic pain, poor oral hygiene, increased blood temperature caused by fever or hot weather and aging-related changes in taste or smell. Some drugs may also cause anorexia.

Anorexia nervosa, on the other hand, is an eating disorder marked by a distorted body image, an extreme fear of obesity and refusal to maintain a minimally normal body weight. People with anorexia nervosa think they're overweight even when they're extremely underweight.

- binge-eating or purging type, in which the person also engages in regular binge-eating or purging behaviours, including self-induced vomiting or abuse of laxatives, diuretics or enemas.

Complications

Serious medical complications can result from the malnutrition, dehydration and electrolyte imbalances caused by prolonged starvation, vomiting and laxative abuse. Anorexia nervosa also increases the susceptibility to infection.

Malnutrition may cause hypoalbuminaemia and subsequent oedema or hypokalaemia – possibly leading to ventricular arrhythmias and renal failure. Coupled with laxative abuse, poor nutrition and dehydration produce bowel changes similar to those of chronic inflammatory bowel disease.

Frequent vomiting may cause oesophageal erosion, ulcers, tears and bleeding as well as tooth and gum erosion and dental caries.

Menstrual suspension

Amenorrhoea (cessation of menstrual periods) may occur when the person loses about 25% of her normal body weight. Complications of prolonged amenorrhoea include oestrogen deficiency (which raises the risk of calcium deficiency and osteoporosis) and infertility.

Dis-heartening complications

Cardiovascular complications of anorexia nervosa can be life-threatening. They include:
- heart failure
- decreased left ventricular muscle mass and chamber size
- reduced cardiac output

> If malnutrition leads to oedema or hypokalaemia, ventricular arrhythmias may occur.

> **Myth busters**
>
> # Getting past stereotypes
>
> If you have preconceived notions about who gets anorexia nervosa, you may mistake this disorder for another condition.
>
> **Myth:** Only young women get anorexia nervosa.
>
> **Reality:** Although the typical anorexic is a young female, the disorder is increasingly showing up in males and older women.

- hypotension
- bradycardia
- electrocardiograph (ECG) changes, such as nonspecific ST intervals, T-wave changes and prolonged PR intervals
- sudden death, possibly from ventricular arrhythmias.

Prevalence and onset

Precise statistics on the prevalence of anorexia nervosa aren't available. However, by conservative estimates, 0.5–1% of females in late adolescence and early adulthood meet the diagnostic criteria. Over their entire lifetime, an estimated 0.5–3.7% of females will suffer from it. Only 4% are males.

Person profile

Although more than 90% of those with anorexia nervosa are adolescent and young women, the condition has been diagnosed in males, children as young as age 7 and women up to age 80. (See *Getting past stereotypes*.) Up to 50% of people with anorexia nervosa have additional psychiatric disorders.

Volunteering for help

The prognosis varies, but improves if the person is diagnosed early or seeks help voluntarily. Mortality ranges from 5% to 15%; suicide accounts for about one-third of the deaths.

Causes

No one knows exactly what causes anorexia nervosa. Most likely, the causes are varied.

Genetic causes

Identical twins have a higher risk for anorexia nervosa than fraternal twins, and sisters of anorexics are more likely to suffer from the disorder.

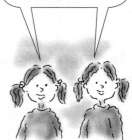

We're identical twins, so if one of us gets anorexia nervosa, the other has an increased risk.

Biological causes

In people with anorexia nervosa, studies have found below-normal levels of the neurotransmitters serotonin and norepinephrine and above-normal levels of cortisol (a 'stress' hormone) and vasopressin. These findings suggest that the disorder is linked to inadequate production of norepinephrine and serotonin.

Behavioural and environmental factors

Because anorexia nervosa occurs mainly in Western and industrialised countries, some experts blame the disorder on societal standards of ideal body shape and the constant pressure to be thin. Additionally, many people first learn about eating disorders from friends and the media. Thus, eating disorders may represent learned behaviours in response to strong social pressures, which are bolstered by society's expectation that women stay thin.

Stress may also play a role. As with other psychiatric disorders, stressful events probably raise the risk of anorexia nervosa.

Psychological factors

Most experts believe low self-esteem, perfectionism and a sense of powerlessness underlie anorexia nervosa. Thus, the disorder is both a symptom of and a defence against feelings of inadequacy.

To compensate for her low self-esteem, the person becomes a perfectionist. In response to failure or rejection, she becomes extremely self-critical, which further weakens her fragile self-esteem.

Power and perfection

Because she doesn't know how to deal with these painful feelings directly, she expresses them through her eating disorder. Feeling powerless and unable to control her life or environment, she strives for a sense of power and control through caloric restriction. She believes that if she can control her eating, she'll be in control of her world, and that if she achieves the 'perfect' body, she'll lead the 'perfect' life.

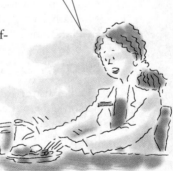

Restricting calories gives the person with anorexia nervosa a sense of power and control.

A shield against sexuality

Some psychiatrists see a refusal to eat as a subconscious effort to protect oneself from dealing with issues surrounding sexuality.

Family dynamics

According to some authorities, families of people with anorexia nervosa tend to demonstrate an interactional pattern that demonstrates enmeshment, rigidity and over-involvement. Some of these behaviour patterns may result from having a chronically ill child. The family may place a high value on achievement. Family members may also have trouble resolving conflict and expressing anger directly.

Memory jogger

The word HUNGER is your signpost to the major features of anorexia nervosa.

H Has an obsession with food and weight

U Underweight or emaciated

N Needs go unmet because of controlling parents or family conflict

G Gross distortion of body image

E Exercises, vomits or uses laxatives and diuretics to lose weight

R Refuses to eat

Families under stress

Other family factors that may play a role in the disorder include:
* sexual, physical or emotional abuse
* one parent who's aggressive and another who's passive
* a mother who's superficially powerful in the family but, in reality, weak
* a father who's distant and withholds his feelings as the daughter becomes an adolescent.

Signs and symptoms

The key feature of anorexia nervosa is self-imposed starvation, despite the person's obvious emaciation. The person's history usually reveals a 15% or greater weight loss with no organic reason, coupled with a morbid dread of being fat and a compulsion to be thin.

Physical findings

Physical findings that suggest anorexia nervosa include:
* emaciated appearance
* skeletal muscle atrophy
* loss of fatty tissue
* breast tissue atrophy
* blotchy or sallow skin
* lanugo (a covering of soft, fine hair) on the face and the body
* dryness or loss of scalp hair
* hypotension
* bradycardia
* painless salivary gland enlargement
* fatigue
* sleep difficulties
* cold intolerance
* constipation

- bowel distention
- slow reflexes
- loss of libido
- amenorrhoea.

Psychosocial findings

Common psychosocial findings of anorexia nervosa include:
- preoccupation with body size
- distorted body image
- descriptions of herself as 'fat'
- dissatisfaction with a particular aspect of the appearance
- low self-esteem
- social isolation
- perfectionism
- ritualism
- paradoxical obsession with food, such as preparing elaborate meals for others
- social regression, including poor sexual adjustment and fear of failure
- feelings of despair, hopelessness and worthlessness
- suicidal thoughts.

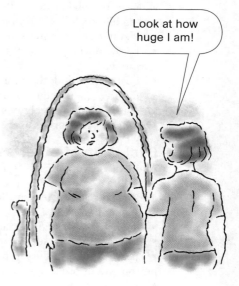

Look at how huge I am!

Behavioural findings

Behavioural signs of anorexia nervosa include:
- wearing of oversized clothing in an effort to disguise body size
- layering of clothing or wearing of unseasonably warm clothing to compensate for cold intolerance and loss of adipose tissue
- restless activity and vigour (despite undernourishment)
- avid exercising with no apparent fatigue
- outstanding academic or athletic performance.

Diagnosis

Although anorexia nervosa should be suspected in any young woman with weight loss, health care providers often miss the diagnosis because the person is secretive about her symptoms. She should undergo a complete physical examination; as indicated, certain laboratory tests should be done.

Laboratory findings

Laboratory tests help rule out endocrine, metabolic and central nervous system abnormalities; cancer; malabsorption syndrome; and other disorders that cause physical wasting (such as acquired immunodeficiency syndrome).

Deviations from the norm

In a person who has lost more than 30% of her normal weight, findings may include:
- below-normal haemoglobin level, platelet count and white blood cell count
- prolonged bleeding time (from thrombocytopenia)

- decreased erythrocyte sedimentation rate
- below-normal levels of serum creatinine, blood urea nitrogen, uric acid, cholesterol, total protein, albumin, sodium, potassium, chloride, calcium and fasting blood glucose (from malnutrition)
- elevated serum amylase levels (unless pancreatitis is present)
- below-normal levels of serum luteinising hormone and follicle-stimulating hormone
- decreased triiodothyronine level (from a lower basal metabolic rate)
- dilute urine (from the kidney's impaired ability to concentrate urine).

An ECG may reveal nonspecific changes in ST intervals and T-waves, prolonged PR intervals and ventricular arrhythmias.

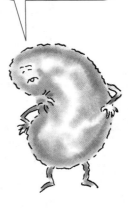

Anorexia nervosa may impair the kidney's ability to concentrate urine.

Exclusion of other psychiatric disorders

Anorexia nervosa must be differentiated from other psychiatric disorders, including:
- substance abuse (especially with stimulants, such as cocaine and amphetamines)
- anxiety disorders (especially obsessive–compulsive disorder)
- mood disorders (such as major depression and bipolar disorder)
- personality disorders (especially histrionic, borderline and narcissistic personality disorders)
- schizophrenia.

The diagnosis of anorexia nervosa is confirmed if the person meets the criteria in the *Diagnostic and Statistical Manual of Mental Disorders*, Fourth Edition, Text Revision (*DSM-IV-TR*). (See *Diagnostic criteria: Anorexia nervosa.*)

Diagnostic criteria: Anorexia nervosa

The diagnosis of anorexia nervosa is confirmed when the person meets these criteria from the *Diagnostic and Statistical Manual of Mental Disorders*, Fourth Edition, Text Revision.

Abnormally low weight and body image distortion

- The person refuses to maintain her weight at or above a minimally normal weight for her age and height (for instance, weight loss leading to maintenance of body weight that's less than 85% of the expected weight) or fails to achieve expected weight gain during a growth period, resulting in a weight less than 85% below that expected.
- Even though she's underweight, the person has an intense fear of gaining weight or becoming fat.
- The person has a distorted perception of her body weight, size or shape; her weight or shape has an undue influence on her self-evaluation; or she denies the seriousness of her underweight condition.

- If the person is of menstruating age, she has missed at least three consecutive menstrual cycles (excluding menses induced by hormone administration).

Subtypes of anorexia nervosa

- The person has the *restricting* type if she hasn't regularly engaged in binge eating or purging (self-induced vomiting or misuse of laxatives, diuretics or enemas) during the current episode of anorexia nervosa.
- The person has the *binge-eating/purging* type if she has regularly engaged in binge eating or purging during the current episode.

Treatment (see National Institute for Clinical Excellence [NICE] guidelines)

Treatment for anorexia nervosa aims to promote weight gain, correct malnutrition and resolve the underlying psychological dysfunction. The most effective strategy has been psychotherapy coupled with weight restoration within 10% of normal.

As appropriate, treatment measures may include:
- a reasonable diet, with or without liquid supplements
- vitamin and mineral supplements
- activity curtailment as needed (such as for arrhythmias or other physical reasons)
- group, family or individual psychotherapy.

Family members, including siblings, should be included in the treatment of children and adolescents with eating disorders. Family interventions may include the sharing of information, advice on behavioural management and facilitating communication.

Hospitalisation

Most people with anorexia nervosa should be managed on an outpatient basis with psychological treatment (with physical monitoring). However, the person who exhibits any of the following signs or symptoms requires inpatient care in a setting that can provide the skilled implementation of feeding with careful physical monitoring in combination with psychosocial interventions:
- rapid weight loss equal to 15% or more of normal body mass
- persistent bradycardia (heart rate of 50 beats/minute or less)
- systolic blood pressure of 90 mmHg or lower
- hypothermia (a core body temperature of 97°F [36.1°C] or less)
- medical complications
- no improvement with appropriate outpatient treatment
- denial of the disorder and the need for treatment
- significant risk of severe self-harm
- significant risk of suicide.

> Hospitalisation is warranted if the person's systolic blood pressure drops to 90 mmHg or lower.

Two years??

Hospitalisation may be as brief as 2 weeks or as long as 2 years or more. Specialist clinical centres have inpatient and outpatient programmes specifically for managing eating disorders. All too often, however, treatment proves difficult and the results can be discouraging.

Psychological treatment

Therapies to be considered for the psychological treatment of anorexia nervosa include cognitive analytical therapy (CAT), cognitive behavioural therapy (CBT), interpersonal psychotherapy (IPT), focal psychodynamic therapy and family interventions focused explicitly on eating disorders. Individual and, where appropriate, carer preference should be taken into account in deciding which psychological treatment is to be offered. The aims of psychological treatment should be to reduce risk, to encourage weight gain and healthy eating, to reduce other symptoms relating to an eating disorder and to facilitate psychological and physical recovery.

Nursing interventions

These nursing interventions may be appropriate for a person with anorexia nervosa:
- During hospitalisation, regularly monitor the person's vital signs, nutritional status and fluid intake and output.
- Help her establish a target weight, and support her efforts to achieve this goal.
- Negotiate an adequate food intake with the person.
- Frequently offer small portions of food or drinks.
- Monitor the person for suicidal potential.

Person to person

- Maintain one-on-one supervision of the person during meals and for 1 hour afterwards to ensure that she's complying with the dietary treatment programme. Remember that for a hospitalised person with anorexia nervosa, food is considered a medication.
- Allow the person to maintain control over the types and amounts of food she eats.
- Teach her how to keep a food journal, including the types of food she eats, eating frequency and feelings associated with eating and exercise.

Liquidation strategy

- Be aware that during an acute anorexic episode, nutritionally complete liquids are more acceptable because they don't require the person to select foods (something people with anorexia nervosa commonly find difficult).

Pound by pound

- Weigh the person daily (before breakfast if possible) on the same scale, at the same time and in the same clothing. Before weighing her, observe her to detect added objects in her pockets or elsewhere or the intake of large amounts of fluids meant to falsely increase her weight.
- Keep in mind that her weight should increase from morning to night.
- Anticipate a weight gain of about 1 lb per week.

Defusing fat fears

- If oedema or bloating occurs after the person resumes normal eating behaviour, reassure her that this is temporary. Otherwise, she may fear that she's getting fat and may stop complying with the treatment plan.
- Encourage the person to recognise and assert her feelings freely. If she understands that she can be assertive, she gradually may learn that expressing her true feelings won't result in her losing control or love.

- Explain to the person how improved nutrition can reverse the effects of starvation and prevent complications.
- Advise family members to avoid discussing food with the person.

Preservation tactics

- Remember that the person with anorexia nervosa may use exercise, preoccupation with food, ritualism and secretive behaviour as mechanisms to preserve the only control she thinks she has in her life.
- If an outpatient requires hospitalisation, maintain contact with her treatment team to promote a smooth return to the outpatient setting.

Post-hospitalisation psychological treatment

Following a period in hospital where weight has been restored, people with anorexia nervosa should be offered outpatient treatment that focuses on both eating behaviour and attitudes to weight and shape, and on wider psychosocial issues, with regular monitoring of both physical and psychological risk. The duration of outpatient psychological treatment and physical monitoring following inpatient weight restoration should typically be at least 12 months.

Bulimia nervosa

Bulimia nervosa has only recently been recognised (1980) as a separate eating disorder from anorexia nervosa with which it shares certain characteristics.

Bulimia nervosa is marked by episodes of binge eating followed by feelings of guilt, humiliation, depression and self-condemnation. Eating binges may occur up to several times a day.

Many sufferers also use measures to prevent weight gain, such as self-induced vomiting, diuretic or laxative use, dieting or fasting. (See *Erroneous beliefs about eating disorders*.)

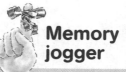

Memory jogger

Give the person and family CUES to eating disorders by covering these topics during teaching:

C Causes of eating disorders

U Understanding how to overcome power struggles and issues of separation and autonomy

E Effects of the eating disorder on physical and mental health

S Symptoms of eating disorders and signs of relapse

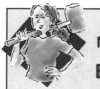

Myth busters

Erroneous beliefs about eating disorders

What you don't know about eating disorders could prevent you from assessing the condition accurately.

Myth: A person who binges but doesn't purge doesn't have bulimia nervosa.

Reality: A person with bulimia nervosa may engage in either the purging or the nonpurging form of this disorder.

Myth: Open conflict and verbal fighting are common among families of adolescents with eating disorders.

Reality: Conflict *avoidance*, not open conflict, is typical in these families.

Common features

- A family history of obesity
- Childhood events resulting in low self-esteem and poor self-identity
- Family concern about weight or diet
- Life events usually involving relationship difficulties triggering the onset of the illness
- Dieting preceding the illness
- Impulsive self-harm

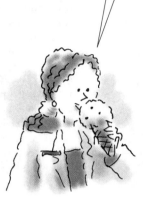

Lucky me! I never feel guilty about a little Chocolate Chip ice cream!

Eating to excess

The typical bulimic is a young woman of normal or nearly normal weight who develops the condition after a history of extended dieting. As dieting continues, she may experience a growing impulse to eat restricted foods. Eventually (usually after an anxiety-producing situation), she eats to excess, temporarily relieving this impulse. She then panics, fearing the food will turn to fat, and induces vomiting or uses diuretics or laxatives (or both) to prevent weight gain.

Catalogue of complications

Unless the person devotes an excessive amount of time to bingeing and purging, bulimia nervosa seldom is incapacitating.

However, during periods of bingeing, gastric rupture may occur. Repetitive vomiting may lead to such physical problems as dental caries, erosion of tooth enamel, parotitis and gum infections. Rarely, frequent vomiting leads to oesophageal inflammation and rupture. If the person uses ipecac syrup to induce vomiting, she may suffer heart failure.

Deadly imbalances

Dehydration or electrolyte imbalances (including metabolic alkalosis, hypochloraemia and hypokalaemia) also may occur, increasing the risk of such serious complications as arrhythmias and sudden death. Laxative abuse may cause chronic irregular bowel movements and constipation.

In addition, bulimics are at higher risk for suicide and psychoactive substance abuse.

Prevalence and onset

Sufferers tend to be women and tend to be slightly older than those with anorexia nervosa. Women from all social classes and between the ages of 19 and 39 are the most common group to present for treatment.

Approximately 3% of females meet the diagnostic criteria for bulimia nervosa – but 5 to 15% of females have some symptoms of the disorder. These numbers may be a gross underestimation because many sufferers are able to hide their symptoms.

Bulimia affects eight or nine females for every male. The condition usually begins in adolescence or early adulthood and may coexist with anorexia nervosa.

Causes

The exact cause of bulimia nervosa is unknown. As with anorexia nervosa, experts suspect it results from an interplay of genetic, biological, behavioural, environmental, family and psychosocial factors.

Genetic and biological factors

Studies show that eating disorders are more common in relatives of people with bulimia. Although this frequency seems to be related to genetics, family influences may also be important.

Also, researchers have linked a specific area of chromosome 10p to families with a history of bulimia nervosa. This provides strong evidence that genes play a determining role in susceptibility to the disorder.

Some studies suggest that altered serotonin levels in the brain also play a role in the development of the disorder.

Other factors

Modern society's overemphasis on appearance and thinness is integral in the development of bulimia nervosa. Other factors that may contribute to the disorder include:
- family disturbances or conflict
- sexual abuse
- maladaptive learned behaviour
- struggle for control or self-identity.

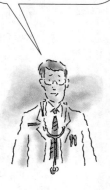

Researchers have linked an area of chromosome 10p to families with a history of bulimia nervosa.

Signs and symptoms

The history of a person with bulimia nervosa typically includes episodic binge eating, occurring up to several times a day. During bingeing episodes, she continues to eat until she's interrupted by abdominal pain, sleep or another person's presence. Most bulimics prefer foods that are sweet, soft and high in calories and carbohydrates.

Physical findings

Physical findings that suggest bulimia nervosa include:
- thin, normal or slightly overweight appearance, with frequent weight fluctuations
- weight within the normal range (through the use of diuretics, laxatives, vomiting and exercise)
- persistent sore throat and heartburn (from vomited stomach acids)
- calluses or scarring on the back of the hands and knuckles (from forcing the hand down the throat to induce vomiting)
- salivary gland swelling, hoarseness, throat lacerations and dental erosion (from repetitive vomiting)
- tooth staining or discolouration
- abdominal and epigastric pain (from acute gastric dilation)
- amenorrhoea.

Memory jogger

Although not all bulimics engage in purging, the term RIDS BODY can help you remember the clinical features of bulimia.

R Recurrent binge-eating episodes

I Intense exercise

D Diuretic, laxative and enema use

S Self-induced vomiting

B Body image distortion

O Ordinary eating alternating with episodes of bingeing and purging

D Depression and anxiety disorders may be present

Y Yo-yo effect of tension relief and pleasure experienced with bingeing, guilt and depression following purging

Psychosocial findings

Stay alert for these psychosocial features:
- perfectionism
- distorted body image
- exaggerated sense of guilt
- feelings of alienation
- recurrent anxiety
- signs and symptoms of depression
- an image as the 'perfect' student, mother or career woman (a child may be distinguished for participating in competitive activities, such as ballet or gymnastics)
- poor impulse control
- chronic depression
- low tolerance for frustration
- self-consciousness
- difficulty expressing such feelings as anger
- impaired social or occupational adjustment
- history of childhood trauma (especially sexual abuse)
- history of unsatisfactory sexual relationships
- parental obesity.

Behavioural findings

Behavioural signs of bulimia nervosa include:
- evidence of binge eating, such as the disappearance of large amounts of food over short periods or the presence of containers and wrappers (indicating consumption of large amounts of food)

- evidence of purging, including frequent trips to the bathroom after meals, sounds and smells of vomiting and the presence of packages of diuretics and laxatives
- peculiar eating habits or rituals
- excessive, rigid exercise regimen despite poor weather, fatigue, illness or injury
- a complex schedule (to make time for binge-and-purge sessions)
- withdrawal from friends and usual activities
- hyperactivity
- frequent weighing
- other behaviours suggesting that weight loss, dieting and control of food are becoming primary concerns.

Diagnosis

The person should undergo a medical evaluation to rule out an upper GI disorder that can cause repeated vomiting. A psychological evaluation and the Beck Depression Inventory can identify depression and other psychiatric disorders. If the person is honest about the length and extent of her behaviour, her history may suggest the seriousness of bulimia nervosa.

Eccentric electrolytes

Laboratory tests can determine the presence and severity of complications. For example:
- serum electrolyte studies may reveal above-normal bicarbonate levels and decreased potassium and sodium levels
- blood glucose testing may detect hypoglycaemia
- baseline ECG may show cardiac arrhythmias, if the person has severe electrolyte disturbances.

The diagnosis of bulimia nervosa is confirmed if the person meets the *DSM-IV-TR* criteria for this disorder. (See *Diagnostic criteria: Bulimia nervosa*, page 352.)

Treatment (see NICE guidelines)

As a possible first step, people with bulimia nervosa should be encouraged to follow an evidence-based self-help programme.

Early treatment of bulimia nervosa is crucial because over time, the person's behaviour pattern becomes more deeply ingrained and more resistant to change. People treated early in the disease course are more likely to recover fully than those who delay treatment for years.

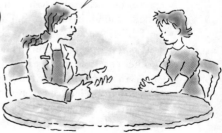

The sooner a person gets treatment for bulimia, the greater the chance of a full recovery.

A focus on the cause, not the symptoms

Treatment is most effective when it centres on the issues that cause the behaviour, not the behaviour itself. Usually, treatment involves individual, group and family therapy; nutrition counselling; and, in many cases, medications.

Diagnostic criteria: Bulimia nervosa

The diagnosis of bulimia nervosa is confirmed when the person meets these criteria from the *Diagnostic and Statistical Manual of Mental Disorders*, Fourth Edition, Text Revision.

Binge eating and behaviours to prevent weight gain

- The person experiences recurrent episodes of binge eating, defined as both of the following criteria:
  - within any 2-hour period, eating an amount of food that's larger than most people would eat during a similar period and under similar circumstances
  - a sense of a lack of control over eating.
- The person recurrently engages in inappropriate compensatory behaviour to prevent weight gain, such as self-induced vomiting; misuse of laxatives, diuretics, enemas or other medications; fasting; or excessive exercise.
- The binge eating and compensatory behaviours occur, on average, at least twice a week for 3 months.

- Body shape and weight unduly influence the person's self-evaluation.
- The disturbance doesn't occur exclusively during episodes of anorexia nervosa.

Subtypes of bulimia nervosa

- The person has the *purging* type of bulimia nervosa if, during the current episode, she has regularly induced vomiting or misused laxatives, diuretics or enemas.
- She has the *nonpurging* type if, during the current episode, she has used other inappropriate compensatory behaviours, such as fasting or excessive exercise, but hasn't regularly induced vomiting or misused laxatives, diuretics or enemas.

Spotlight on structure

At all levels of care, treatment requires a high degree of structure and a behavioural treatment plan based on the person's weight and eating behaviours. Treatment may continue for several years; long-term psychotherapy and medical follow-up are essential.

Psychological treatment

Psychological treatment focuses on breaking the binge–purge cycle and helping the person regain control over her eating behaviour. For the majority of people, treatment can take place in an outpatient setting. It usually includes cognitive behavioural therapy for bulimia nervosa (CBT-BN), a specially adapted form of CBT. A course of treatment should be for 16–20 sessions over 4–5 months. When people with bulimia nervosa have not responded to or do not want CBT, other psychological treatments should be considered, such as IPT.

To supplement psychological treatment, she may receive an antidepressant treatment; selective serotonin reuptake inhibitors (SSRIs) such as fluoxetine are the drugs of first choice for the treatment of bulimia nervosa where the effective dose is 60 mg daily (higher dose than for depression). No drugs other than antidepressants are recommended for the treatment of bulimia nervosa.

Hospitalisation

For people with bulimia nervosa who are at risk of suicide or severe self-harm, psychiatric admission to a setting with experience in managing this disorder may be considered.

Nursing interventions

These nursing interventions may be appropriate for a person with bulimia nervosa:

• Promote an accepting, nonjudgemental atmosphere. Control your reactions to the person's behaviour and feelings.
• Establish a contract with the person that specifies the amount and types of food she must eat at each meal.
• Supervise the person during mealtimes and for a specified period afterwards (usually 1 hour).
• Set a time limit for each meal. Provide a pleasant, relaxed eating environment.
• Teach the person to keep a food journal to monitor her treatment progress.
• Encourage her to recognise and verbalise her feelings about her eating behaviour.
• Identify the person's elimination patterns.
• Encourage the person to talk about stressful issues, such as achievement, independence, socialisation, sexuality, family problems and control.

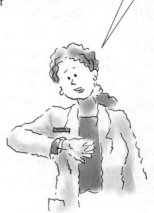

When supervising a bulimic at mealtimes, set a time limit for the meal.

Abuse aversion

• Explain to the person the risks of laxative, emetic and diuretic abuse.
• Provide assertiveness training to help the person gain control over her behaviour and achieve a realistic and positive self-image.
• Assess the person's suicide potential.

Medication minders

• If the person is taking an SSRI, teach her how to recognise signs of central serotonin syndrome – abdominal pain, diarrhoea, sweating, fever, myoclonus, irritability and, in severe cases, hyperpyrexia and cardiovascular shock.

The long haul

• Offer support and encouragement to help the person stay in treatment.

Quick quiz

1. The most serious complication of anorexia nervosa is:
   A. high risk of mortality.
   B. coexisting depression.
   C. poor family relationships.
   D. social isolation.

Answer: A. Anorexia nervosa has a mortality rate of 5–15%.

2. To qualify for the diagnosis of anorexia nervosa, the person's weight must drop below:
    A.   75% of ideal body weight.
    B.   80% of ideal body weight.
    C.   85% of ideal body weight.
    D.   90% of ideal body weight.

Answer: C. The person's weight must drop below 85% of ideal body weight to meet the diagnostic criteria for anorexia nervosa.

3. Purging behaviour is usually triggered by:
    A.   sensations of fullness or bloating.
    B.   guilt, humiliation and self-condemnation.
    C.   fear of being discovered as a binge eater.
    D.   feelings of nausea.

Answer: B. Guilt, humiliation and self-condemnation usually trigger the desire to purge. Physical sensations, such as fullness, bloating or nausea, aren't related to this behaviour, nor is the fear of being discovered.

4. Which of the following medications may be used to treat bulimia nervosa?
    A.   fluoxetine
    B.   amitriptyline
    C.   diazepam
    D.   imipramine

Answer: A. SSRIs such as fluoxetine are commonly used to treat bulimia nervosa. Other antidepressants may be used to treat an underlying depressive illness. A mild tranquilliser such as diazepam is rarely indicated.

Scoring

✰✰✰ If you answered all four items correctly, savour the moment! You've satiated yourself on this chapter and fully deserve the success you're now tasting.

✰✰ If you answered two or three items correctly, swell! You've just gained several pounds of knowledge.

✰ If you answered just one item correctly, don't go off on a binge. Just review the chapter again to bulk up on the information.

11 Substance abuse disorders

Just the facts

In this chapter, you'll learn:

♦ types of substance abuse disorders

♦ street names for commonly abused substances

♦ proposed causes of substance abuse and dependence

♦ how to assess for substance abuse and dependence

♦ nursing interventions for service users experiencing substance withdrawal.

A look at substance abuse disorders

Substance abuse affects males and females of all ages, cultures and socioeconomic groups. People have used alcohol and other psychoactive substances – those that affect the central nervous system (CNS) – for centuries to induce changes in perception, mood, cognition or behaviour. These substances produce a state of consciousness that the user deems pleasant, positive or euphoric.

Substance abuse commonly coexists with – and complicates the treatment of – other mental health disorders. Likewise, many people with emotional disorders or mental illness turn to drugs and alcohol to self-medicate and help them tolerate their feelings.

Suspicious substances

A substance of abuse may be any chemical substance or preparation used therapeutically or recreationally. Commonly abused substances include:
* alcohol
* amphetamines and amphetamine-like drugs
* barbiturates

> Substance abuse has been around for centuries. I wonder if King Tut ever got a little tipsy.

- cocaine – a stimulant derived from the cocoa plant
- crack – cocaine hydrochloride mixed with baking soda
- hallucinogens
- inhalants
- marijuana
- nonbarbiturate sedatives, hypnotics and anxiolytics (primarily benzodiazepines)
- opioids – heroin and morphine.

Many people abuse a combination of substances. Drug mixing is the most dangerous form of substance abuse.

Consequences of substance abuse

Substance abuse commonly leads to physical dependence or psychological dependence or both. It's also associated with illegal activities and may cause unhealthy lifestyles and behaviours, such as a poor diet. Chronic substance abuse impairs social and occupational functioning, creating personal, professional and financial problems.

Teenage wasteland

When drug use begins in early adolescence, it may lead to emotional and behavioural problems resulting in the failure to complete school. In pregnant women, substance abuse jeopardises foetal well-being.

I.V. drug abuse may lead to life-threatening complications (See *Complications of I.V. drug abuse*.)

> Abusing a single drug is bad enough. Mixing several drugs together is especially dangerous.

Complications of I.V. drug abuse

I.V. drug abuse can lead to numerous complications – even beyond those caused by the drugs themselves.

Using contaminated needles, for example, raises the risk of such infections as human immunodeficiency virus, viral hepatitis (especially hepatitis B and C) and bacterial infections. Heroin can cause a nephropathy similar to focal segmental glomerulosclerosis. A condition called *talc granulomatosis* may occur if the drug was adulterated with an inert substance (such as talcum powder).

With chronic I.V. drug abuse, potential complications include:

- skin lesions and abscesses
- thrombophlebitis
- vasculitis
- gangrene
- cardiac and respiratory arrest
- intracranial haemorrhage
- subacute bacterial endocarditis
- septicaemia
- pulmonary emboli
- respiratory infections
- malnutrition
- GI disturbances
- musculoskeletal dysfunction
- depression
- psychosis
- increased suicide risk.

Terrible trips

Few people would voluntarily take a drug they expect to cause an unpleasant experience. However, psychoactive substances often produce negative outcomes – among them, maladaptive behaviour, 'bad trips' and even long-term psychosis.

Not so street-smart

Illicit street drugs pose added dangers. Materials used to dilute street drugs can cause toxic or allergic reactions. Specific effects of street drugs vary with the substance.

Defining the terms

According to the *Diagnostic and Statistical Manual of Mental Disorders*, Fourth Edition, Text Revision (*DSM-IV-TR*), substance use disorders encompass both substance abuse and substance dependence.

• *Substance abuse* is the repeated use of alcohol or other psychoactive drugs that leads to problems but *not* to compulsive use or addiction. Also, reducing or completely stopping the drug use doesn't cause significant withdrawal symptoms.

• *Substance dependence* refers to the persistent use of alcohol or other psychoactive drugs despite problems caused by such use. Compulsive and repetitive use may lead to tolerance of the drug's effects and withdrawal symptoms when the drug use is decreased or stopped. (For other key definitions, see *The language of substance abuse*.)

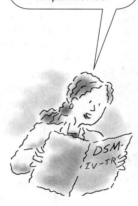

In the *DSM-IV-TR*, the term 'substance use disorders' encompasses both substance abuse and substance dependence.

The language of substance abuse

Here are some important definitions you need to know to fully understand this chapter.

• *Substance abuse:* repeated use of a psychoactive drug that doesn't result in compulsive use or addiction and doesn't lead to withdrawal symptoms when the drug use is terminated.

• *Substance dependence:* compulsive, repetitive use of a psychoactive substance resulting in tolerance to the drug's effects and withdrawal symptoms when the drug use is decreased or stopped.

• *Tolerance:* decreased response to a drug that comes with repeated use. A user who develops a tolerance to the rewarding properties of the abused drug must take increasingly higher amounts to get the desired effect.

• *Physical dependence:* an adaptive state that occurs as a normal physiological response to repeated drug exposure. Physical dependence doesn't necessarily indicate drug abuse or addiction.

• *Withdrawal:* an uncomfortable syndrome that occurs when tissue and blood levels of the abused substance decrease in a person who has used that substance heavily over a prolonged period. Withdrawal symptoms may cause the person to resume taking the substance to relieve the symptoms, thereby contributing to repeated drug use.

• *Intoxication:* a reversible substance-specific syndrome caused by ingestion of or exposure to that substance.

Defining the problem

Substance abuse is a major public health problem. It is increasing in prevalence and young and old alike either abuse or are dependent on alcohol or illicit drugs. Of all 16- to 59-year-olds, 12% had taken an illicit drug and 3% had used a Class A drug in the last year. This equates to around four million illicit drug users and around one million Class A drug users.

Prevalence data in the UK today indicates that:
- drug dependence is experienced by 2.2% of the general population
- drug services are attended by 25,000 people
- alcohol dependence is found in 4.7% of the general population
- approximately 25% of the population drink above safe limits (30% of men and 14% of women)
- an alcohol-related problem is found in 20% of medical inpatients
- Health of the Nation targets are not being met for alcohol consumption
- approximately 25% of the population are addicted to nicotine
- there is increased smoking in the young
- there is a trend towards polydrug use
- increasing use of substances in the young is associated with earlier age of initiation and greater likelihood of dependence
- about one-third of substance misusers have a psychiatric disorder
- about one-third of service users have a substance use disorder.

Teens who toke

Experimentation with drugs commonly begins during adolescence – although recent statistics show a trend towards drug use among preadolescents.

Causes of substance abuse

The exact causes of substance abuse and addiction aren't known but are under intensive investigation. Probable influences include genetic make-up, pharmacological properties of the particular drug, peer pressure, emotional distress and environmental factors.

Genetic theories

Genetic theories propose that inherited mechanisms cause or predispose a person to drug abuse. Genetic factors have been explored most extensively in alcoholism. For example, studies show that many Asians carry a gene that confers a reduced risk for alcoholism.

Other genetic factors may confer an increased risk for alcoholism. Chromosomes 1 and 7 have been linked to susceptibility to alcohol dependence.

Heredity or environment?

Most likely, both heredity and environment influence whether a person becomes a substance abuser. Researchers continue to debate which of the two factors is more important, although results of their studies have been confusing.

For example, on the one hand, many alcoholics have no known alcoholic relatives, and many children of alcoholics don't become alcoholic themselves. On the other hand, children of alcoholics who are adopted into nonalcoholic homes at an early age are more likely to become alcoholics than children of nonalcoholics who are adopted into alcoholic homes.

Neurobiological theories

According to neurobiological theories, chronic exposure to drugs leads to biological and cellular adaptation. Some scientists suspect drug addicts have an inborn deficiency of endorphins – peptide hormones that bind to opiate receptors, reducing the pain sensations and exerting a calming effect. This endorphin deficiency may heighten the sensitivity to pain and confer a greater susceptibility to narcotics abuse.

Endorphins and enzymes

Alternatively, some endorphin scientists suspect regular narcotics use reduces the body's natural endorphin production, causing a reliance on the narcotic for ordinary pain relief.

According to another neurobiological theory, enzymes produced by a given gene might influence hormones and neurotransmitters, contributing to the development of a personality that's more sensitive to peer pressure – including the pressure to use illicit drugs.

Psychobiological theories

Introducing a narcotic into the body may cause metabolic adjustments that require continued and increasing dosages to prevent withdrawal. However, studies haven't yet found cell metabolism changes that are linked to addiction.

Behavioural theories

Behavioural scientists view drug abuse as the result of conditioning, or cumulative reinforcement from drug use. Drug use causes a euphoric experience that the user perceives as rewarding, which motivates him to keep taking the drug. The drug, then, serves as a biological reward.

Right on cue

The stimuli and settings associated with drug use may become reinforcing in themselves – or may trigger drug craving that can lead to a relapse. Many recovering addicts change their environment in an effort to eliminate cues that could promote drug use.

Profile of a drug abuser

A person who's predisposed to psychoactive drug abuse tends to have low self-esteem, an excessive dependence on others and a susceptibility to peer pressure. He may have inadequate coping skills, few mental or emotional resources against stress and a low tolerance for frustration.

Tense, lonely or bored

The typical drug abuser is anxious, angry or depressed. He demands immediate relief from tension or distress, which he gets from taking the drug. The drug gives him pleasure by relieving tension, abolishing loneliness, inducing a temporarily peaceful or euphoric state or simply relieving boredom.

Some people take drugs because of peer pressure or as part of a social ritual.

Social and psychological theories

According to some social and psychological theories, adolescents and young adults take drugs to preserve childhood and avoid having to deal with adult conflicts and responsibilities. Many users see drugs as a way to cope – however dysfunctionally – with their personal and social needs and changing situational demands. (See *Profile of a drug abuser*.)

Following the crowd

In some cultures, drugs may be more available, or social pressures for drug use may be stronger. Social ritual may also play a role by affecting the meaning and style of drug use adopted by a person in a given setting.

Alcohol dependence

Alcohol (ethanol) is a CNS depressant that reduces the activity of neurons in the brain. Chronic uncontrolled alcohol intake is the largest substance abuse problem.

Alcohol dependence is characterised by three main symptom clusters – biological adaptation, loss of control and maladaptive consequences.

Biological adaptation

Some authorities view alcohol dependence simply as a biological adaptation to alcohol, or physical dependence – which manifests as tolerance or withdrawal.

Loss of control

An alcohol-dependent person lacks control over his alcohol use. Lack of control manifests as:
• inability to limit alcohol intake to a moderate amount

- repeated but unsuccessful attempts to cut down on or stop drinking
- compulsive thoughts and actions, with much of the day spent thinking about drinking or recovering from an alcohol binge.

Maladaptive consequences

An alcoholic continues to use alcohol despite reduced occupational functioning and negative psychological, social and health consequences.

Prevalence
Numbers of heavy drinkers

A recent survey conducted by the Office for National Statistics found 27% of men and 14% of women to be exceeding the old 'sensible limits' of regular consumption. The proportions of men exceeding the limits have remained stable over recent years; however, the proportions of women exceeding the limits have increased steadily. Proportions of over-the-limit drinkers are higher in the younger age groups.

Health hazards of alcohol abuse

Alcohol abuse decreases the life span by roughly 15 years. It accounts for nearly 25% of premature deaths in men and 15% in women. (See *Can alcohol kill?*, page 362.)

> Heavy alcohol intake is rough on my buddies the kidney and the brain and . . . Ooohh . . . it's especially rough on yours truly, the liver!

Health-related behaviour in England: Prevalence of alcohol consumption above 21/14 units a week for men/women aged 18 and over.						
	Percentages					
England	1988	1990	1992	1994	1996	1998
Males (above 21 units)						
18–24	35	37	38	36	42	42
25–44	34	33	30	30	31	28
45–64	24	26	24	27	27	30
65 & over	13	14	15	17	18	16
Total	27	28	26	27	28	27
Females (above 14 units)						
18–24	18	18	19	20	22	26
25–44	14	13	14	16	16	16
45–64	9	10	12	13	14	15
65 & over	4	5	5	8	7	6
Total	11	11	12	13	14	14

Myth busters

Can alcohol kill?

Don't assume that alcohol is relatively safe just because it's legal.

Myth: Alcohol intoxication doesn't directly cause death, although it can severely impair a person's functioning level.

Reality: Alcohol intoxication can be fatal if the blood alcohol level exceeds 400 mg/dl.

Way beyond blotto

Heavy alcohol intake adversely affects most body tissues, especially the liver, kidney and brain. Eventually, alcohol abuse can lead to death. (See *Complications of alcohol abuse*, page 363.)

Causes

A definite cause of alcoholism hasn't been identified. Most experts believe genetic, biological, psychological and sociocultural influences are involved.

Genetic factors

These research findings (among others) support a genetic influence in alcoholism:
• Identical twins have a higher risk of alcoholism than fraternal twins do.
• Children of alcoholics have a fourfold increased risk of alcoholism – even if adopted at birth.

Alcoholic markers?

Some researchers believe a genetic marker for vulnerability to alcoholism exists. A follow-up of men originally studied at age 20 found that those with alcoholic fathers had lower response levels to alcohol (including less alcohol-related cognitive and psychomotor impairment and less intense subjective feelings of intoxication). This lower response level was a strong predictor of later alcoholism.

Other genetic influences that may contribute to the risk of alcoholism include such personality traits as higher levels of impulsivity and sensation seeking.

Other factors

Biochemical abnormalities, nutritional deficiencies, endocrine imbalances and allergic responses may contribute to alcoholism.

Psychological factors include the urge to drink alcohol to reduce anxiety or symptoms of mental illness; the desire to avoid responsibility in family, social and work relationships; and low self-esteem.

Complications of alcohol abuse

Alcohol damages body tissues through its direct irritating effects, through changes that occur during its metabolism, by interacting with other drugs, by aggravating existing disease or through accidents brought on by intoxication. Tissue damage can lead to a host of complications.

Cardiopulmonary complications

- Arrhythmias
- Cardiomyopathy
- Essential hypertension
- Chronic obstructive pulmonary disease
- Pneumonia
- Increased risk of tuberculosis

GI complications

- Chronic diarrhoea
- Oesophagitis
- Oesophageal cancer
- Oesophageal varices
- Gastric ulcers
- Gastritis
- GI bleeding
- Malabsorption
- Pancreatitis

Hepatic complications

- Alcoholic hepatitis
- Cirrhosis
- Fatty liver

Neurological complications

- Alcoholic dementia
- Alcoholic hallucinosis
- Alcohol withdrawal delirium
- Korsakoff's syndrome
- Peripheral neuropathy
- Seizure disorders
- Subdural haematoma
- Wernicke's encephalopathy

Mental health complications

- Amotivational syndrome
- Depression
- Foetal alcohol syndrome
- Impaired social and occupational functioning
- Multiple substance abuse
- Suicide

Other complications

- Beriberi
- Hypoglycaemia
- Leg and foot ulcers
- Prostatitis

Sedative, anticholinergic and extrapyramidal effects

High-potency conventional antipsychotics (such as haloperidol) cause minimal sedation and anticholinergic effects, such as rapid pulse, dry mouth, inability to urinate and constipation.

However, these drugs carry a high incidence of extrapyramidal (motor) effects. The most common motor effects are dystonia, Parkinsonism and akathisia.

- *Dystonia* refers to prolonged, repetitive muscle contractions that may cause twisting or jerking movements – especially of the neck, mouth and tongue. It's most common in young males, usually appearing within the first few days of drug treatment.
- Drug-induced *Parkinsonism* results in bradykinesia (abnormally slow movements), muscle rigidity, shuffling gait, stooped posture, flat facial affect, tremors and drooling. It may emerge 1 week to several months after drug treatment begins.

- *Akathisia* causes restlessness, pacing and an inability to rest or sit still.

Intermediate-potency conventional antipsychotics (such as molindone) have a moderate incidence of extrapyramidal effects. Low-potency agents (such as chlorpromazine) are highly sedative and anticholinergic but cause few extrapyramidal effects.

Orthostatic hypotension

Low-potency antipsychotics may cause orthostatic hypotension (low blood pressure when standing).

Tardive dyskinesia

With prolonged use, antipsychotics may cause tardive dyskinesia – a disorder characterised by repetitive, involuntary, purposeless movements. Signs and symptoms include grimacing, rapid eye blinking, tongue protrusion and smacking, lip puckering or pursing and rapid movements of the hands, arms, legs and trunk.

Symptoms may persist long after the service user stops taking the antipsychotic drug. With careful management, however, some symptoms eventually lessen or even disappear.

Neuroleptic malignant syndrome

In up to 1% of service users, antipsychotic drugs cause neuroleptic malignant syndrome. This life-threatening condition leads to fever, extremely rigid muscles and altered consciousness. It may occur hours to months after drug therapy starts or the dosage is increased.

Stress and social attitudes

Sociocultural factors include easy access to alcohol, group or peer pressure to drink, an excessively stressful lifestyle and social attitudes that approve of frequent alcohol consumption.

Signs and symptoms

Many alcoholics hide or deny their addiction and temporarily manage to maintain a functional life – which can make assessment a challenge. Nonetheless, certain physical and psychosocial symptoms suggest alcoholism.

For example, the service user may have many minor complaints that are alcohol-related – malaise, dyspepsia, mood swings or depression, and an increased incidence of infection. Also check for poor personal hygiene and untreated injuries, such as cigarette burns, fractures and bruises, that he can't fully explain. Note an unusually high tolerance for sedatives and narcotics. Assess for signs of nutritional deficiency, including vitamin and mineral deficiencies.

Watch for secretive behaviour, which may be an attempt to hide the disorder or the alcohol supply.

An alcoholic with no other alcohol source may drink mouthwash.

Desperation tactics

When deprived of his usual supply of alcohol, an alcoholic may consume it in any form he can find – mouthwash, aftershave lotion, hair spray and even lighter fluid. Suspect alcoholism in a service user who buys inordinate amounts of aftershave lotion or mouthwash and doesn't use it in the expected way.

Denial, blame and projection

Characteristically, the alcoholic denies he has a problem – or rationalizes the problem. He also tends to blame others and to rationalize problem areas in his life. He may project his anger or feelings of guilt or inadequacy onto others to avoid confronting his illness.

Overt signs and symptoms

Overt indications of excessive alcohol use include:
- episodes of anaesthesia or amnesia during intoxication (blackouts)
- violent behaviour when intoxicated
- the need for daily or episodic alcohol use to function adequately
- inability to stop or reduce alcohol intake.

Withdrawal symptoms

A heavy drinker who stops drinking or abruptly reduces his alcohol intake is likely to go through withdrawal. Symptoms begin shortly after the drinking stops and last for up to 10 days.

Initially, the service user experiences anorexia, nausea, anxiety, fever, insomnia, diaphoresis, agitation, tremor progressing to severe tremulousness and, possibly, hallucinations and violent behaviour. Major motor seizures (sometimes called 'rum fits') may occur.

Deadly delirium

About 5–10% of alcoholics experience alcohol withdrawal delirium, formerly called *delirium tremens* (DTs). A life-threatening complication, this syndrome manifests as delirium accompanied by tremor, severe agitation and autonomic overactivity – dramatic increases in pulse, respirations and blood pressure. (See *Assessing for alcohol withdrawal.*)

Advice from the experts

Assessing for alcohol withdrawal

Alcohol withdrawal symptoms may vary from mild (morning hangover) to severe (alcohol withdrawal delirium). Formerly known as delirium tremens or DTs, alcohol withdrawal delirium is marked by acute distress brought on by drinking cessation in a person who's physically dependent on alcohol.

Signs and symptoms	Mild withdrawal	Moderate withdrawal	Severe withdrawal
Motor impairment	Inner tremulousness with hand tremor	Visible tremors, obvious motor restlessness and painful anxiety	Gross, uncontrollable shaking, extreme restlessness and agitation with intense fearfulness
Sleep disturbance	Restless sleep or insomnia	Marked insomnia and nightmares	Total wakefulness
Appetite	Impaired appetite	Marked anorexia	Rejection of all food and fluid except alcohol
GI symptoms	Nausea	Nausea and vomiting	Dry heaves and vomiting
Confusion	None	Variable	Marked confusion and disorientation
Hallucinations	None	Vague, transient visual and auditory hallucinations and illusions (commonly nocturnal)	Visual and, occasionally, auditory hallucinations, usually with fearful or threatening content; misidentification of people and frightening delusions related to hallucinatory experiences
Pulse rate	Tachycardia	Pulse 100–120 beats/minute	Pulse 120–140 beats/minute
Blood pressure	Normal or slightly elevated systolic	Usually elevated systolic	Elevated systolic and diastolic
Sweating	Slight	Obvious	Marked hyperhidrosis
Seizures	None	Possible	Common

Diagnosis

Various laboratory tests may suggest alcoholism and help evaluate for complications such as cirrhosis of the liver.
- A blood alcohol level of 0.10% weight/volume (200 mg/dl) indicates alcohol intoxication. Although this test can't confirm alcoholism, it can reveal how recently the service user has been drinking – and thus when to expect withdrawal symptoms if he's a heavy drinker.
- Urine toxicology may uncover the use of other drugs.
- Serum electrolyte analysis may identify electrolyte abnormalities associated with alcohol use.
- Blood urea nitrogen level rises and serum glucose level drops in a service user with severe liver disease.
- Increased plasma ammonia level indicates severe liver disease, as in cirrhosis.
- Liver function studies may point to alcohol-related liver damage.
- Haematological screening may identify anaemia, thrombocytopenia and increased prothrombin and partial thromboplastin times.
- Echocardiography and electrocardiography (ECG) may reveal cardiac problems related to alcoholism such as an enlarged heart (cardiomegaly).

> Alcoholism can cause an enlarged heart.

Think patterns, not pints

However, the diagnosis of alcohol abuse or dependence centres on a pattern of difficulties associated with alcohol use – *not* on the amount and frequency of alcohol consumption. The diagnosis of alcohol dependence or alcohol abuse is confirmed when the service user meets the criteria listed in the *DSM-IV-TR*. (See *Diagnostic criteria: Substance dependence*, page 367 and *Diagnostic criteria: Substance abuse*, page 367.)

Treatment

Acute alcohol intoxication calls for symptomatic treatment, which may involve respiratory support, fluid replacement, I.V. glucose to prevent hypoglycaemia, correction of hypothermia or acidosis and emergency measures for trauma, infection or GI bleeding, as needed.

Managing acute withdrawal

Because abrupt alcohol withdrawal can cause death, withdrawal should take place in a monitored therapeutic setting. The service user may require I.V. glucose administration and administration of fluids containing thiamin and other B-complex vitamins to correct nutritional deficiencies and aid glucose metabolism.

Other treatment measures may include:
- furosemide, to ease overhydration
- magnesium sulphate, to reduce CNS irritability
- anticonvulsants, antiemetics or antidiarrhoeals, as needed, to ease withdrawal symptoms
- antipsychotics, to control hyperactivity and psychosis
- sedatives.

Diagnostic criteria: Substance dependence

The diagnosis of substance dependence is confirmed when the service user meets these criteria from the *Diagnostic and Statistical Manual of Mental Disorders*, Fourth Edition, Text Revision.

Maladaptive pattern

The service user exhibits a maladaptive pattern of substance use resulting in clinically significant impairment or distress, as indicated by three or more of the following criteria during the same 12-month period:

- tolerance, as defined by either:
  - a need for markedly increased amounts of the substance to reach intoxication or the desired effect
  - markedly decreased effect with continued use of the same amount of the substance
- withdrawal, as manifested by either:
  - a characteristic withdrawal syndrome
  - use of the substance (or a closely related one) to relieve or avoid withdrawal symptoms
- taking the substance in larger amounts or over a longer period than intended
- persistent desire or unsuccessful efforts to cut down or control substance use
- significant time spent trying to obtain the substance (for example, driving long distances or visiting multiple doctors), to use the substance or to recover from its effects
- giving up or cutting back on important social, occupational or recreational activities because of substance use
- continued use of the substance despite knowledge of having a persistent or recurrent physical or psychological problem that's likely to have been caused or worsened by the substance.

Other features

- Physiological dependence is *present* if the service user exhibits evidence of tolerance or withdrawal (as defined above).
- Physiological dependence is *absent* if the service user doesn't exhibit evidence of tolerance or withdrawal.

Diagnostic criteria: Substance abuse

The diagnosis of substance abuse is confirmed if the service user meets these criteria from the *Diagnostic and Statistical Manual of Mental Disorders*, Fourth Edition, Text Revision.

Maladaptive pattern

The service user exhibits a maladaptive pattern of substance use resulting in clinically significant impairment or distress, as indicated by one or more of the following criteria within a 12-month period:

- recurrent substance use causing failure to fulfil major obligations at home, work or school – for example, neglect of children or household or repeated absences or poor work performance related to substance use, substance-related absences, suspensions or expulsions from school
- recurrent substance use in situations in which such use poses physical hazards – such as driving a vehicle or operating a machine when impaired by substance use
- recurrent legal problems related to substance use – for example, arrests for substance-related disorderly conduct
- continued substance use despite persistent or recurrent social or interpersonal problems caused or worsened by the effects of the substance – such as physical fights or arguments with family members over the effects of intoxication.

Absence of substance dependence

The service user has never met the criteria for substance dependence for the particular class of substance he uses.

Home detoxification

Popular in the UK: Home detoxification (detox) involves the systematic withdrawal from an alcohol in the comfort and security of the service user's home, typically under the care of an appropriately trained drug worker and with support of a local primary health care team (general practitioner [GP] and nurse). Home detoxification provides a safe, efficient and cost-effective intervention. Given the relative paucity of residential detoxification places, it is essential that communities provide a home detoxification programme linked into other drug services. Available literature suggests that most people can be detoxified at home.

There are several key factors that determine suitability.

• Service users must be well motivated to reduce their levels of drug taking and/or alcohol consumption. They must express a clear desire to detoxify and agree to comply with the instructions of the detox worker and GP.

• Service users must have a supportive environment for the home detoxification. Home supervision is essential and this must be provided by a sensible and reliable person, preferably a relative or friend, who does not misuse drugs or alcohol. The carer must be available 24 hours a day during the first week of the detoxification. This may be reduced in the later stage of the detoxification.

• Service users must have no concurrent mental or physical health problems that may be exacerbated by the withdrawal process. Exclusion factors include recent overdose, a history of seizures, delirium tremens, major heart, liver or respiratory problems or pregnancy. Service users who may experience severe withdrawal are also not suitable for home detoxification.

• Service users must have a GP who is willing to prescribe for them. If a person wants to enter the programme but does not have a GP who is willing to support his request and provide a prescription, then he has to consider other options.

• Service users can try to detoxify by using acupuncture provided by one of the detox workers, or they can receive full support from a drugs worker whilst going 'cold turkey'.

Treatment of chronic alcoholism

Alcohol dependence has no known cure, and total abstinence is the only effective treatment. Management commonly involves:

• medications that deter alcohol use (as in aversion, emetic or antagonist therapy) and treat withdrawal symptoms

• measures to relieve associated physical problems

• psychotherapy, usually involving behaviour modification, group therapy and family therapy

• counselling and ongoing support groups to help the service user overcome alcohol dependence.

Aversion therapy

In aversion therapy, the service user receives a daily oral dose of disulfiram (Antabuse) to prevent compulsive drinking. Disulfiram impedes alcohol metabolism and increases blood acetaldehyde levels. Consuming alcohol within 2 weeks of disulfiram intake causes an immediate unpleasant reaction that resembles a bad hangover.

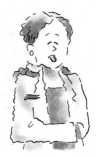

You think I look sick? This is nothing compared to what happens when someone takes alcohol and disulfiram together.

The agonies of Antabuse

Signs and symptoms of a disulfiram reaction include:

- flushing
- throbbing of the neck and head
- nausea and vomiting
- headache
- shortness of breath or other respiratory difficulties
- sweating
- thirst
- chest pain
- palpitations
- tachycardia
- hyperventilation
- hypotension
- syncope
- weakness
- vertigo
- blurred vision
- confusion.

Even small quantities of alcohol, such as the amount in food sauces and cough medicines, or inhaled traces from shaving lotion or furniture varnish may induce these symptoms.

> Good thing I never went through aversion therapy. A disulfiram reaction can cause vertigo!

Aversion through emesis

Another form of aversion therapy attempts to induce aversion by administering alcohol along with an emetic agent.

Antagonist therapy

Naltrexone, a narcotic antagonist, may reduce alcohol craving and help prevent an alcoholic from relapsing to heavy drinking, when it's combined with counselling. Naltrexone blocks the brain's so-called pleasure centres, reducing the urge to drink.

If the service user is also addicted to narcotics or admits using them, they must stop taking all narcotics 7–10 days before starting naltrexone therapy. Usually, naltrexone therapy lasts at least 12 weeks.

Counselling and psychotherapy

For long-term abstinence, supportive programmes that offer detoxification, rehabilitation and aftercare – including continued involvement in Alcoholics Anonymous (AA) – provide the best results. Along with individual, group or family psychotherapy, these programmes improve the service user's ability to cope with stress, anxiety and frustration and help him gain insight into the problems that may have led him to abuse alcohol.

Other types of support

For alcoholics who have lost contact with family and friends and have a long history of unemployment, trouble with the law or other problems related to alcohol abuse, rehabilitation may involve job training, sheltered workshops, halfway houses or other supervised facilities.

Nursing interventions

For general nursing interventions during and after an episode of acute alcohol intoxication, see *General interventions for acute drug intoxication*. These interventions may also be appropriate for an alcoholic service user:

- If the service user is taking disulfiram, warn him that even a small amount of alcohol (such as the amount in cough medicines, mouthwashes and liquid

---

Advice from the experts

General interventions for acute drug intoxication

Care for a substance-abusing service user starts with an assessment to determine which substance he's abusing. Signs and symptoms vary with the substance and dosage.

During the acute phase of drug intoxication and detoxification, care focuses on maintaining the service user's vital functions, ensuring his safety and easing discomfort.

During rehabilitation, caregivers help the service user acknowledge his substance abuse problem and find alternative ways to cope with stress. Health care professionals can play an important role in helping service users achieve recovery and stay drug-free.

These general nursing interventions are appropriate for service users during and after acute intoxication with most types of psychoactive drugs.

During an acute episode

- Continuously monitor the service user's vital signs and urine output. Watch for complications of overdose and withdrawal, such as cardiopulmonary arrest, seizures and aspiration.
- Maintain a quiet, safe environment. Remove harmful objects from the room. Institute appropriate measures to prevent suicide attempts and assaults, according to facility policy. Use restraints only if you suspect the service user might harm himself or others.
- Approach the service user in a nonthreatening way. Limit sustained eye contact, which he may perceive as threatening.

- Institute seizure precautions.
- Administer I.V. fluids to increase circulatory volume.
- Give medications, as prescribed; monitor and record their effectiveness.

During drug withdrawal

- Administer medications, as prescribed, to decrease withdrawal symptoms. Monitor and record their effectiveness.
- Maintain a quiet, safe environment because excessive noise may agitate the service user.

When the acute episode has resolved

- Carefully monitor and promote adequate nutrition.
- Administer drugs carefully to prevent hoarding. Check the service user's mouth to ensure that he has swallowed oral medication. Closely monitor visitors who might supply him with drugs.
- Refer the service user to rehabilitation as appropriate. Give him a list of available resources.
- Encourage family members to seek help regardless of whether the abuser seeks it. Suggest private therapy or community mental health clinics.
- Develop self-awareness and an understanding and positive attitude towards the service user. Control your reactions to his undesirable behaviours – commonly, psychological dependency, manipulation, anger, frustration and alienation.
- Set limits when dealing with demanding, manipulative behaviour.

vitamins) will induce an adverse reaction. Tell him that the longer he takes the drug, the greater his alcohol sensitivity will be. Also inform him that paraldehyde, a sedative, is chemically similar to alcohol and may provoke a disulfiram reaction.

• As appropriate, offer to arrange a visit from a concerned religious advisor who can help provide the motivation for a commitment to sobriety.

The A's have it

• Tell the service user about AA, a self-help group with more than a million members worldwide that offers emotional support from others with similar problems. Stress how this organisation can provide the support he'll need to abstain from alcohol. Offer to arrange a visit from an AA member.

• Inform a female service user that she may prefer a women's AA group, rather than a mixed group where she might hesitate to explore her feelings fully.

• Teach the service user's family about Al-Anon and Alateen, two other self-help groups. By joining these groups, family members learn to relinquish responsibility for the alcoholic's drinking so that they can live meaningful and productive lives. Point out that family involvement in rehabilitation also reduces family tensions.

• Refer adult children of alcoholics to the National Association for Children of Alcoholics. This organisation may provide support in understanding and coping with the past.

Amphetamine abuse

Amphetamines increase arousal, reduce fatigue and can make a person feel stronger, more alert and more decisive. Although they have a few medical uses (mainly in treating obesity and narcolepsy), most abusers take them for their stimulant or euphoric effects or to counteract the 'down' feeling of alcohol or tranquillisers.

The amphetamine group includes amphetamine sulphate, methamphetamine and dextroamphetamine. On the street, amphetamine sulphate tablets are called *bennies, grannies* or *cartwheels*. Methamphetamine is known as *speed, meth, crank* or *crystal*. Made in illegal laboratories, it has a high potential for abuse and dependence. Dextroamphetamine sulphate may be referred to as *dexies, hearts* or *oranges*.

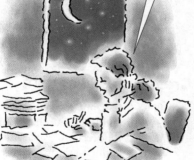

Some people take amphetamines when they have to stay up all night to cram for a test. Not very smart!

Pleasure rush

Amphetamines may be taken orally or by injection, snorting or smoking. Immediately after methamphetamine is injected or smoked, the user experiences an intensely pleasurable sensation (a 'rush') that lasts a few minutes. Snorting produces a long-lasting high rather than a rush, which may last up to half a day.

Users can become addicted quickly, with rapid dose escalation. Higher doses may lead to increasing toxicity and complications.

Prevalence

Use of the drug, which is a form of crystallised methamphetamine, has reached epidemic levels in parts of America and Australia.

How amphetamines produce their effects

Amphetamines increase the release of the neurotransmitters dopamine, norepinephrine and serotonin into brain synapses. The 'rush' or 'high' experienced with these drugs probably results from high levels of dopamine in the brain areas that regulate feelings of pleasure.

Detrimental to dopamine

Amphetamines may also have a neurotoxic effect, damaging brain cells that contain dopamine and serotonin. Studies suggest that over time, methamphetamine reduces dopamine levels, possibly leading to Parkinsonian-like symptoms.

Health hazards of amphetamine abuse

Adverse physiological effects of methamphetamine abuse include headache, poor concentration, poor appetite, abdominal pain, vomiting or diarrhoea, sleep difficulties, paranoid or aggressive behaviour and psychosis.

Besides leading to addiction, chronic methamphetamine abuse can inflame the heart lining. Injection may damage blood vessels and cause skin abscesses. Some methamphetamine abusers have episodes of violent behaviour, paranoia, anxiety, confusion and insomnia. With heavy use, progressive social and occupational deterioration may occur.

Running on meth

Users who become drug tolerant must take higher or more frequent doses or change their method of drug intake. In some cases, they forgo food and sleep while indulging in a form of bingeing known as a 'run', injecting as much as 1 g of methamphetamine every 2–3 hours over several days until the drug supply runs out or the user becomes too disorganized to continue.

Creepy crawly critters

Chronic methamphetamine abuse may damage the brain's frontal areas and basal ganglia. Some chronic abusers experience a toxic psychosis that resembles paranoid schizophrenia – intense paranoia, rages, auditory hallucinations, mood disturbances and delusions. For example, some abusers experience formication – the sensation of insects creeping on the skin. Psychotic symptoms may last months or years after drug use ceases.

Causes

As with all types of substance abuse, the exact causes of amphetamine abuse are hard to identify. Some people abuse amphetamines in an effort to relieve fatigue, induce euphoria or ease depression or other uncomfortable feelings.

> During an amphetamine binge, the user may not eat or sleep for days. Not my style at all!

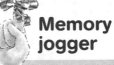

Memory jogger

SPEED helps when assessing a service user for amphetamine use.

S Sweating (diaphoresis)

P Psychotic behaviour

E Exhaustion

E Everything up (hyperactive tendon reflexes, hypertension, hyperthermia, tachycardia)

D Dilated pupils

Signs and symptoms

In a service user under the influence of amphetamines, assessment findings may include:
- euphoria
- hyperactivity and increased alertness
- diaphoresis (sweating)
- shallow respirations
- dilated pupils
- dry mouth
- exhaustion
- anorexia and weight loss
- nausea or vomiting
- tachycardia
- hypertension
- hyperthermia
- tremors
- seizures
- altered mental status, such as confusion, agitation or paranoia
- psychotic behaviour (with prolonged use).

Findings in amphetamine intoxication

Severe methamphetamine intoxication may cause the signs and symptoms listed above, plus:
- arrhythmias
- heart failure
- subarachnoid haemorrhage
- stroke
- cerebral haemorrhage
- coma
- death.

Amphetamine withdrawal symptoms

Abrupt amphetamine withdrawal may trigger CNS depression, ranging from lethargy to coma. Some service users experience hallucinations, while others show signs of overstimulation, including euphoria and violent behaviour. (For additional withdrawal symptoms, see *Assessing for amphetamine withdrawal*, page 374.)

Diagnosis

Urine drug screening may be performed if amphetamine abuse is suspected. Other diagnostic tests depend on the service user's symptoms. For example, an electrocardiogram (ECG) may be done if he reports chest pain.

The diagnosis of amphetamine abuse or dependence is confirmed if the service user meets the criteria documented in the *DSM-IV-TR*. (See *Diagnostic criteria: Substance abuse*, page 367 and *Diagnostic criteria: Substance dependence*, page 367.)

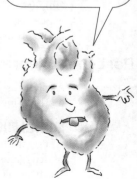

An amphetamine user who reports chest pain may undergo an ECG.

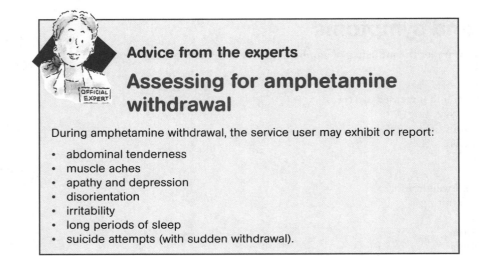

Advice from the experts

Assessing for amphetamine withdrawal

During amphetamine withdrawal, the service user may exhibit or report:

- abdominal tenderness
- muscle aches
- apathy and depression
- disorientation
- irritability
- long periods of sleep
- suicide attempts (with sudden withdrawal).

Treatment

A service user with acute amphetamine intoxication may require airway management, fluid resuscitation or vigorous cooling measures. Arrhythmias may warrant cardioversion, defibrillation and antiarrhythmic drugs. Vital signs must be monitored closely. If the drug was ingested, vomiting is induced or gastric lavage is performed; activated charcoal and a saline or magnesium sulphate cathartic may be given.

Other treatments are symptomatic. For example, the service user may require fluid replacement and nutritional and vitamin supplements. Ammonium chloride or ascorbic acid may be added to the I.V. solution to acidify urine to a pH of 5. Mannitol may be given to induce diuresis.

Sedatives may be given to induce sleep, anticholinergics and antidiarrhoeal agents to relieve GI distress and anxiolytic drugs for severe agitation and symptomatic treatment of complications.

Managing drug dependence

Cognitive-behavioural therapy is commonly used to treat methamphetamine dependence. The goal of this approach is to modify the service user's thinking, expectations and behaviours and increase his ability to cope with stress.

Post-meth depression

Antidepressants may help combat the depression commonly seen in methamphetamine users who have recently become abstinent.

Rehabilitation

After withdrawal, the service user needs rehabilitation to prevent a relapse of drug abuse. Both inpatient user and outpatient rehabilitation programmes are available. They usually last a month or longer and may include individual, group and family psychotherapy.

During and after rehabilitation, participation in a drug-oriented self-help group may be recommended as an adjunct to behavioural interventions and to promote long-term drug-free recovery.

Life after speed

Aftercare means a lifetime of abstinence, usually aided by participation in Narcotics Anonymous (NA) or a similar self-help group.

Nursing interventions

For appropriate nursing interventions during and after an episode of acute amphetamine intoxication, see *General interventions for acute drug intoxication*, page 370.

Caffeine intoxication

A mild CNS stimulant, caffeine may be used to restore mental alertness when a person feels tired, weak or drowsy. However, when used in excess, caffeine causes uncomfortable symptoms of stimulation. Caffeine intoxication can occur with consumption of more than 250 mg of caffeine (equivalent to about 2½ cups of coffee).

Age and body size influence caffeine effects. A child or a small adult may feel the effects more strongly than a large adult. Also, some people are more sensitive to caffeine, feeling the effects at smaller doses.

Caffeine habit

Caffeine can be habit forming – most experts agree that some heavy caffeine users may develop caffeine tolerance or dependence. Someone who abruptly stops using caffeine may experience headache, fatigue or drowsiness.

Cupboards full of caffeine

Dietary sources of caffeine include coffee, tea, chocolate and cola drinks. Caffeine also comes in some prescription and over-the-counter (OTC) drugs. (See *Where's the caffeine?*)

How caffeine produces its effects

Scientists aren't exactly sure how caffeine exerts its effects. A leading theory suggests that caffeine antagonises adenosine, an inhibitory brain chemical that affects norepinephrine, dopamine and serotonin activity. This antagonism may increase neurotransmitter levels, causing psychostimulation.

Causes

People consume caffeine for such reasons as preference of beverage, to 'get going' in the morning, to relieve fatigue or to stay awake for a particular purpose.

Where's the caffeine?

Common sources of caffeine include:

- coffee (brewed) – 40–180 mg per cup
- coffee (instant) – 30–120 mg per cup
- coffee, decaffeinated – 3–5 mg per cup
- tea, brewed – 20–90 mg per cup
- tea, instant – 28 mg per cup
- tea, canned iced – 22–36 mg per 350 ml
- cola and other soft drinks – 36–90 mg per 350 ml
- cola and other soft drinks (decaffeinated) – none
- cocoa – 4 mg per cup
- chocolate milk – 3–6 mg per 30 mg
- chocolate, plain – 25 mg per 30 mg

Over-the-counter preparations that contain caffeine include some cold and flu remedies, paracetamol extra, Pro-plus and guarana.

Risk factors for caffeine dependence or sensitivity to caffeine withdrawal aren't known. Genetic factors, such as differences in the way some people metabolise caffeine or a history of substance abuse or mood disorders, may play a role.

Signs and symptoms

Assessment findings in a service user with caffeine intoxication may include:
- tachycardia
- palpitations
- arrhythmias
- fatigue that worsens during the day
- anxiety, nervousness, irritability and easy excitability
- exaggerated startle response
- disorganised thoughts and speech
- facial flushing
- dehydration (from caffeine's diuretic effect)
- hyperactivity
- gross muscle tremors
- restless leg syndrome (muscle cramping and twitching)
- sleep disturbances, such as insomnia or decreased sleep quality (with grogginess in the morning caused by withdrawal symptoms occurring overnight).

Caffeine withdrawal symptoms
Caffeine withdrawal symptoms may occur with abrupt caffeine cessation or reduction after a long period of daily use. Withdrawal symptoms tend to be worse in heavy caffeine users (those who consume 500 mg/day or more), although people who consume as little as 100 mg/day (equivalent to one cup of coffee) may also experience discomfort.

Headache from hell

Withdrawal symptoms may start within a few hours after the time of normal caffeine consumption, reach a peak within 1 or 2 days, and persist for up to 2 weeks. They may include:
- headache
- nausea or vomiting
- jitteriness, irritability and anxiety
- fatigue
- drowsiness
- depression
- poor concentration or poor performance on mental tasks
- caffeine craving.

Diagnosis

Caffeine blood levels have limited use as a screening tool. Urine drug screening can help uncover associated illicit drug use. Thyroid studies can rule out hyperthyroidism.

Diagnostic criteria: Caffeine intoxication

The diagnosis of caffeine intoxication is confirmed when the person meets these criteria from the *Diagnostic and Statistical Manual of Mental Disorders,* Fourth Edition, Text Revision.

Recent caffeine consumption

- The person recently consumed caffeine, usually in excess of 250 mg (more than two or three cups of brewed coffee).
- During or shortly after caffeine use, the person experienced five or more of the following symptoms:

  - restlessness
  - nervousness
  - excitement
  - insomnia
  - facial flushing
  - diuresis
  - GI disturbances
  - muscle twitching
  - rambling thoughts and speech
  - tachycardia or arrhythmias
  - periods of inexhaustibility
  - psychomotor agitation.

Other features

- The symptoms listed above cause clinically significant distress or impairment in social, occupational or other important areas of functioning.
- These symptoms don't result from a general medical condition and aren't better explained by another mental health disorder (such as an anxiety disorder).

No other specific tests detect caffeine-induced mental health disorders. Cardiac irregularities should be investigated by ECG.

The diagnosis of caffeine intoxication is confirmed if the person meets the criteria established in the *DSM-IV-TR.* (See *Diagnostic criteria: Caffeine intoxication.*)

Treatment

Treatment for caffeine intoxication is the avoidance of caffeine in all forms. Symptoms resolve when the caffeine use stops.

The person should be monitored for caffeine withdrawal. Treatment for withdrawal is symptom based.

Nursing interventions

These nursing interventions may be appropriate for a person with caffeine intoxication:

- Advise the person about the expected symptoms of caffeine withdrawal and the duration of those symptoms.
- Reassure him that the symptoms will subside and are benign.
- If discomfort lasts more than 2 weeks, assess the person for other disorders that cause similar symptoms.

Cannabis abuse

Cannabis is a hemp plant from which marijuana (a tobacco-like substance) and hashish (the plant's resinous secretions) are produced. In Western countries, cannabis is the most widely used illicit drug.

Cannabis may be smoked, consumed as a tea or mixed into foods. Most users smoke marijuana in hand-rolled cigarettes, although some use pipes or bongs (water pipes). Marijuana cigars, called *blunts*, are also popular. To make blunts, users slice open cigars and replace the tobacco with marijuana (which they may combine with crack cocaine or another drug).

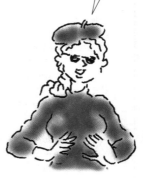

Some people consume cannabis as tea. I'm more of an orange pekoe girl myself.

Nicknames galore

Common street names for cannabis include *pot*, *grass*, *weed*, *mary jane*, *mj*, *roach*, *reefer*, *joints*, *THC*, *blunt*, *herb*, *sinsemilla*, *smoke*, *boo*, *broccoli*, *ace* and *Colombian*. The duration of action is 6–12 hours, with symptoms most pronounced during the first 1–2 hours.

Marijuana as medicine

Medicinal use of cannabis – mainly as an antiemetic in service users undergoing cancer chemotherapy and other types of drug therapy – has been the subject of intense legal and medical debate.

Prevalence
Cannabis is the most frequently used drug – around three million 16- to 59-year-olds have used it in the last year (11%).

But I was only holding it for a friend

In 1999, about 39% of adult males and 26% of adult females who had been arrested tested positive for marijuana. Among juvenile arrestees, marijuana was the most commonly used drug.

How cannabis produces its effects
The most powerful psychoactive substance in cannabis is delta-l-tetrahydrocannabinol (delta-1-THC). When marijuana is smoked, delta-1-THC rapidly passes from the lungs into the bloodstream, which carries it to the brain and other organs.

In the brain, delta-1-THC connects to cannabinoid receptors on neurons, influencing their activity. (See *How cannabis affects the brain*, page 379.)

Health hazards of cannabis use
Cannabis can be addictive and may cause various adverse physiological effects.

Respiratory effects

Marijuana smoke can harm the lungs. The smoke contains carcinogens similar to those found in tobacco smoke. Chronic and heavy cannabis use may increase

How cannabis affects the brain

When marijuana is smoked, its active ingredient attaches to cannabinoid receptors in the brain. The brain areas with many cannabinoid receptors – including the cerebral cortex, hippocampus, basal ganglia and cerebellum – influence pleasure, memory, learning, reward, perception and coordinated movements.

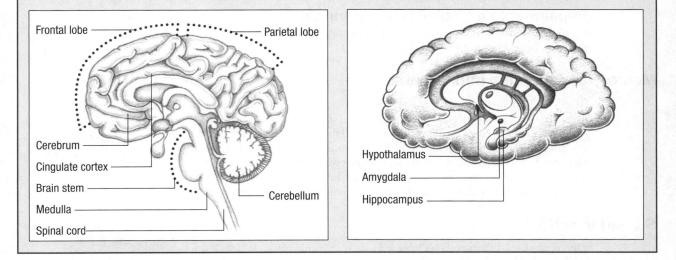

Frontal lobe — Parietal lobe — Cerebrum — Cingulate cortex — Brain stem — Medulla — Spinal cord — Cerebellum

Hypothalamus — Amygdala — Hippocampus

the risk of chronic obstructive lung disease. Also, some studies show that respiratory tumours are more common among habitual marijuana users.

Cardiovascular effects

Acute cannabis intoxication may trigger tachycardia and orthostatic hypotension.

Reproductive effects

In females, cannabis use may increase the number of anovulatory cycles. In males, it may reduce levels of follicle-stimulating hormone, leading to a decrease in testosterone production and, possibly, testicular atrophy.

Although cannabis use has been linked to decreased sperm counts, the drug's effect on fertility remains unclear.

Other health effects

Cannabis may weaken the immune system. In very young teens, it has a profoundly negative effect on development.

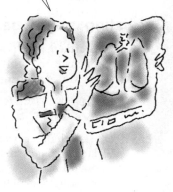

Chronic and heavy cannabis use may raise the risk of chronic obstructive lung disease and respiratory tumours.

Combination drug use

Marijuana may be combined with other substances, such as crack cocaine, phencyclidine (PCP), formaldehyde and codeine cough syrup – sometimes without the user being aware of it. These additional substances compound the risks associated with marijuana use.

Impairments associated with cannabis use

Cannabis use can result in perceptual distortions and impairments in short-term memory, learning ability, judgement and verbal skills.

Memory and learning impairments

Marijuana's adverse impact on learning and memory can last for days or weeks after the acute drug effects wear off. Therefore, someone who smokes marijuana once a day may be functioning at a reduced intellectual level all of the time.

A study of college students found that among heavy cannabis users, critical skills related to attention, learning and memory were impaired significantly even after 24 hours of abstinence. These users had more trouble sustaining and shifting their attention and in registering, organising and using information.

Stoned in school

One study found that students who smoked marijuana seven or more times weekly had significantly lower scores on standardised tests of verbal and mathematical skills. Also, students who smoke marijuana may be more likely to get lower grades and less likely to graduate from high school.

Wasted at work

Problems at work are more common among marijuana-smoking employees. Several studies have linked marijuana use with increased absences, tardiness, accidents, workers' compensation claims and job turnover.

Coexisting mental health disorders

Marijuana use is associated with anxiety, depression and personality disturbances. Research shows that marijuana can cause problems in daily life or worsen existing problems.

Causes

As with other types of substance abuse, the exact causes of cannabis use aren't known. Suggested risk factors include:
- young age
- drug availability (influenced by geographic and cultural factors)

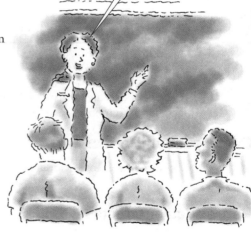

Students who regularly smoke marijuana score lower on standardised verbal and math tests.

- coexisting alcohol abuse or dependence
- coexisting abuse of other drugs.

Signs and symptoms

Assessment findings in a service user under the influence of cannabis include:
- relaxation
- euphoria
- spontaneous laughter
- feelings of well-being or grandiosity
- visual distortions and other perceptual changes
- subjective sense that time is passing more slowly than normal
- tachycardia
- dry mouth
- conjunctival redness
- drowsiness and sluggishness (or paradoxical hyperalertness)
- decreased muscle strength
- poor coordination
- increased hunger (the 'munchies').

With overdose, you may detect signs or symptoms of pulmonary oedema, respiratory depression, aspiration pneumonia or hypotension.

Dysphoric effects

In some people, cannabis intoxication causes a dysphoric reaction, which may manifest as:
- panic and disorientation
- paranoia
- mood swings
- altered perceptions (such as illusions or frank hallucinations)
- depersonalisation
- psychotic episodes.

Findings in chronic cannabis use

Chronic cannabis users may experience a syndrome marked by appetite changes, lack of ambition and energy and reduced social and occupational drive.

Withdrawal symptoms

Although withdrawal symptoms from cannabis are less severe than from other drugs, some users experience restlessness, irritability, appetite loss and sleep difficulties.

Diagnosis

In a chronic marijuana user, urine screening may reveal cannabis presence up to 21 days after use.

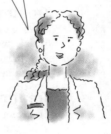

The 'munchies' are but one of many telltale signs of cannabis use.

Memory jogger

WEED is a street name for cannabis – and a quick key to assessing a service user for suspected cannabis use.

W Wacky behaviour (hallucinations, impaired cognition, paranoia, spontaneous laughter)

E Euphoria

E Elevated heart rate (tachycardia)

D Distorted sense of time and self-perception, decreased muscle tone, dry mouth

The diagnosis of cannabis abuse or dependence is confirmed when the person meets the criteria listed in the *DSM-IV-TR*. (See *Diagnostic criteria: Substance abuse*, page 367 and *Diagnostic criteria: Substance dependence*, page 367.)

Treatment

Acute cannabis intoxication usually resolves within 4–6 hours. The person should be moved to a quiet room with minimal stimulation.

Treatment is symptom based. For example, the doctor may prescribe benzodiazepines if the person has marked anxiety.

Treatment of withdrawal symptoms

To ease cannabis withdrawal symptoms, the person may receive a short course of sedatives or tranquilizers to manage insomnia, anxiety and depression. Useful nonpharmacological measures may include psychotherapy, exercise, relaxation techniques and nutritional support.

Treatment of chronic cannabis use

Treatment of cannabis abuse follows the general principles of substance abuse. The goal is total abstinence from all psychoactive substances.

Interventions may include mental health evaluation and counselling, individual or group psychotherapy, occupational and family assessment, self-help groups and lifestyle changes, such as avoiding drug-related situations.

Focused treatment programmes

Few treatment programmes focus solely on marijuana abuse – perhaps because many marijuana users also use other drugs. However, with more people now seeking help to control marijuana abuse, researchers are exploring treatment approaches.

One study of adult cannabis users found comparable benefits from a 14-session cognitive-behavioural group treatment and a two-session individual treatment that included motivational interviewing and advice on ways to reduce marijuana use. After both treatments, cannabis use, dependence symptoms and psychosocial problems diminished for at least 1 year.

Nursing interventions

For general nursing interventions for cannabis intoxication, see *General interventions for acute drug intoxication*, page 370.

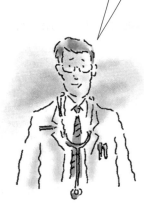

To stay off marijuana, the user must avoid all drug-related situations.

Cocaine abuse

A powerfully addictive narcotic and stimulant, cocaine is one of the oldest known drugs. Coca leaves, the source of cocaine, have been ingested for thousands of years. Cocaine hydrochloride, the pure drug, has been abused for more than 100 years. Cocaine use can range from occasional to repeated or compulsive abuse.

Cocaine's effects occur almost immediately after a single dose and disappear within a few minutes or hours. Taken in small amounts (up to 100 mg), the drug typically makes the user feel euphoric, energetic, talkative and mentally alert – especially to sensations of sight, sound and touch.

Cocaine may temporarily reduce the need for food and sleep. Some users find it helps them perform simple physical and intellectual tasks more quickly, although others experience the opposite effect.

Crystal or crack

Cocaine exists in two chemical forms:
- Cocaine hydrochloride is a fine, white, crystallised powder. It's generally snorted or dissolved in water and injected, with effects lasting 15 minutes to 2 hours.
- Crack or freebase is a chunky, off-white compound that hasn't been neutralised by an acid. It's smoked after being processed with ammonia or sodium bicarbonate and water and then heated to remove the hydrochloride. Crack produces an immediate euphoric high, followed by a 'down' feeling.

By any other name . . .

On the street, cocaine is known as *coke, C, snow, snowball, blow, flake, nose candy, hits, tornado, wicky stick, rock* or *crank*.

Most street dealers dilute cocaine with inert substances, such as cornstarch, talcum powder or sugar; some cut it with procaine or amphetamines. Some users combine cocaine powder or crack with heroin in a 'speedball'.

Snorting, shooting and rubbing

When snorted, cocaine is absorbed into the bloodstream through the nasal tissues. When injected, the drug is released directly into the bloodstream, intensifying its effects. When cocaine is smoked, the vapour is inhaled into the lungs, where it's absorbed into the bloodstream as rapidly as by injection. Cocaine also can be rubbed onto mucous membrane tissues.

Medical uses of cocaine

Doctors sometimes use cocaine for legitimate medical purposes – typically as a local anaesthetic for nasal surgeries, to stop nosebleeds, or as a local anaesthetic for cuts in children.

Prevalence

Cocaine is the third most commonly used illicit drug in the UK. About 198, 000 UK residents are chronic cocaine users. Adults aged 18–25 have a higher rate of cocaine use than any other age group. Men have a higher usage rate than women do.

How cocaine produces its effects

Experts believe cocaine produces pleasurable effects through its action on structures deep within the brain – most notably, a region called the *ventral*

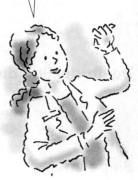

Crack produces an immediate high, followed by a 'down' feeling.

tegmental area (VTA). Neurons originating in the VTA extend to the nucleus accumbens, one of the brain's key pleasure centres. Researchers have found that pleasurable events are accompanied by a significant rise in the amount of dopamine released in the nucleus accumbens by neurons arising from the VTA. (Scientists believe dopamine is involved in the addictive properties of every major drug of abuse.)

Health hazards of cocaine use

Cocaine use can have devastating medical consequences. Absorption of toxic amounts may cause:
- sudden death
- acute cardiovascular problems, such as arrhythmias (particularly ventricular fibrillation), tachycardia, myocardial infarction (MI) and chest pain
- stroke
- seizures
- respiratory failure
- bowel gangrene (with cocaine ingestion).

Death-dealing duo

Combining cocaine with alcohol causes the conversion of the two drugs to cocaethylene, which has a longer duration in the brain and is more toxic than either drug alone. In fact, the mixture of cocaine and alcohol is the most common two-drug combination resulting in drug-related death.

Binge effects

A cocaine binge (taking the drug repeatedly and at increasingly high doses) may cause increasing irritability, restlessness and paranoia. The result may be full-blown paranoid psychosis, in which the person loses touch with reality and experiences auditory hallucinations.

Route-related consequences

Regular cocaine snorting can lead to the loss of the sense of smell, nosebleeds, swallowing difficulty, hoarseness and nasal septum irritation (which may cause a chronically inflamed, runny nose).

Cocaine injection can cause an allergic reaction, either to cocaine or to an additive in street cocaine; in severe cases, death results. Injection also increases the risk for contracting such infections such as human immunodeficiency virus (HIV) and hepatitis.

Fatal first use

In rare instances, sudden death can occur on the first use of cocaine, or unexpectedly thereafter. Cocaine-related deaths commonly result from cardiac arrest or seizures followed by respiratory arrest.

Some users become more sensitive to cocaine's anaesthetic and convulsant effects, even without increasing the dose. This increased sensitivity may explain some deaths resulting from apparently low doses of cocaine.

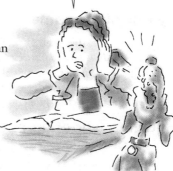

A cocaine binge can bring on paranoid psychosis – complete with auditory hallucinations. Too bad he really is barking that loud!

Advice from the experts

Gathering a history from a drug user

If a service user admits to drug use, try to determine the extent to which his drug abuse interferes with his life. Note whether he expresses a desire to overcome his abuse or dependence.

If possible, obtain a complete drug history. Ask which substances he uses, the amount used, frequency of use and time of his last dose.

What to expect

However, you should expect incomplete or inaccurate responses. Drug-induced amnesia, a decreased level of consciousness or ignorance may distort the service user's recollection of the facts. He may also deliberately fabricate answers to avoid arrest or downplay a suicide attempt. If necessary, interview family members and friends to fill in gaps in the history.

Impairments associated with cocaine use

Cocaine is powerfully addictive. About 10% of people who try cocaine progress to heavy use. After a person tries it, he may have trouble predicting or controlling the extent to which he'll keep using it.

As cocaine use continues, tolerance commonly develops. The person must take higher doses at more frequent intervals, to obtain the same level of pleasure he experienced with initial use.

Causes

A family history of substance abuse may be a risk factor for early cocaine use and rapid cocaine dependence. (See *Gathering a history from a drug user*.)

Some researchers attribute cocaine's addictive properties to the dopamine excess it produces; this excess may be the source of positive reinforcement and addiction. Thus, the drug's dopamine-driven 'rush' reinforces repeated use.

Genetic link?

Researchers have identified a brain process that may help explain addiction to cocaine and other drugs of abuse. Studies have found that repeated cocaine exposure causes a genetic change leading to altered levels of a specific brain protein that regulates dopamine's action.

Signs and symptoms

In a person under the influence of cocaine, general assessment findings may include:
- euphoria
- increased energy
- excitement

- sociability
- reduced hunger
- grandiosity
- sense of increased physical and mental strength
- decreased sensation of pain
- talkativeness or pressured speech
- good humour and laughing
- dilated pupils
- runny nose
- nasal congestion
- nausea and vomiting
- headache
- vertigo.

> Euphoria and laughing are common effects of cocaine use . . . or in my case, watching repeats of *Only Fools and Horses*!

Something bugging you?

Some users experience more pronounced effects (especially with high doses). These effects include flightiness, emotional instability, restlessness, irritability, apprehension, inability to sit still, teeth grinding, cold sweats, tremors, muscle twitching, seizures, violent or bizarre behaviour and hallucinations (cocaine 'bugs' or 'snow lights' as well as voices, sounds and smells). A few experience cocaine psychosis, which resembles paranoid schizophrenia.

Cardiovascular and respiratory findings

Cocaine may raise or lower the blood pressure. It may cause chest pain, tachycardia, ventricular fibrillation or cardiac arrest. Respiratory findings may include tachypnoea; deep, rapid or laboured respirations; or respiratory arrest.

Withdrawal symptoms

Cocaine withdrawal usually isn't as uncomfortable as withdrawal from other drugs. Symptoms may include:
- anxiety, agitation and irritability
- depression
- fatigue
- angry outbursts
- lack of motivation
- nausea and vomiting
- muscle pain
- sleep disturbances
- intense drug craving
- episodes of ST-segment elevation on ECG.

Diagnosis

The diagnosis of cocaine abuse or dependence is confirmed when the person meets the criteria documented in the *DSM-IV-TR*. (See *Diagnostic criteria: Substance abuse*, page 367 and *Diagnostic criteria: Substance dependence*, page 367.)

Memory jogger

CRACK clues you in to some of the symptoms of cocaine use.

C Cardiotoxicity (tachycardia, ventricular fibrillation or cardiac arrest)

R Respiratory arrest

A Auditory, visual and olfactory hallucinations

C Coma and confusion

K Kite-like behaviour (excitability, grandiosity, irritability and psychotic symptoms)

Treatment

A person with acute cocaine intoxication should receive symptomatic treatment. Cardiopulmonary resuscitation is performed, as indicated, for ventricular fibrillation and cardiac arrest. Vital signs should be monitored closely. Propranolol typically is given for tachycardia. Anticonvulsant medications are given for seizures.

If the person has ingested cocaine, induced vomiting or gastric lavage may be performed. If he has snorted cocaine, the residual drug is removed from the mucous membranes.

Depending on the cocaine dosage and time elapsed before admission, additional treatment may include forced diuresis and, possibly, haemoperfusion or haemodialysis.

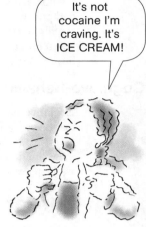

It's not cocaine I'm craving. It's ICE CREAM!

Fluids, food and sleep therapy

Other measures may include fluid replacement therapy and nutritional and vitamin supplements. Sedatives may be given to induce sleep, anticholinergics and antidiarrhoeal agents to relieve GI distress and anxiolytic drugs for severe agitation.

Withdrawal, detoxification and rehabilitation

Treatment of cocaine dependence commonly involves detoxification, short- and long-term rehabilitation and aftercare. The latter means a lifetime of abstinence, usually aided by participation in NA or a similar self-help group.

To ease withdrawal, useful nonpharmacological measures may include psychotherapy, exercise, relaxation techniques and nutritional support. Widespread cocaine abuse has led to extensive efforts to develop treatment programmes for abusers. Cocaine abuse and addiction must address a variety of problems, including psychobiological, social and pharmacological aspects of the service user's drug abuse.

Pharmacological approaches

Currently, there aren't medications available specifically for treating cocaine addiction. However, researchers are testing such agents as selegiline and disulfiram (used to treat alcoholism). Clinical studies have shown that these drugs are effective in reducing cocaine abuse.

Antidepressants may be prescribed to treat the mood changes that some service users experience during the early stages of cocaine abstinence. Sedatives and tranquillisers may be given temporarily to help the service user cope with insomnia and anxiety.

Behavioural interventions

Many behavioural treatments (both outpatient and residential programmes) have been effective in treating cocaine addiction. The treatment regimen should be tailored to the service user's individual needs, with different components added or removed as indicated.

For many cocaine abusers, a treatment called *contingency management* has had positive results. This voucher-based system gives positive rewards for staying in treatment and remaining cocaine-free. Service users earn vouchers based on drug-free urine tests and can exchange them for items that promote healthy living such as joining a gym.

Cognitive-behavioural therapy

Cognitive-behavioural coping skills therapy is a short-term, focused approach that helps cocaine addicts become abstinent. This approach strives to help service users recognise the situations in which they're most likely to use cocaine, avoid these situations and cope more effectively with the problems and behaviours associated with drug abuse.

Therapeutic communities

Service users with more severe problems, such as coexisting mental health problems and criminal involvement, may benefit from a therapeutic community – a residential programme with 6- to 12-month lengths of stay. These communities focus on resocialising the service user to society; some include on-site job rehabilitation and other supportive services.

Nursing interventions

For nursing interventions that may be appropriate during an acute episode or after the episode has resolved, see *General interventions for acute drug intoxication*, page 370.

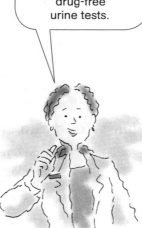

Some cocaine treatment programmes give vouchers to service users who have drug-free urine tests.

Hallucinogen abuse

Hallucinogens (sometimes called *psychedelic drugs*) produce hallucinations or profound distortions in the perception of reality. They may also cause dramatic behavioural changes. Under the influence of hallucinogens, people see images, hear sounds and feel sensations that seem real but don't actually exist. Some hallucinogens also cause rapid, intense emotional swings.

These agents include a wide range of substances, including lysergic acid diethylamide (LSD), Ecstasy, ketamine, dextromethorphan, mescaline and psilocybin. Most are taken orally, but some may be injected.

Most hallucinogens have no known medical use; however, naturally occurring hallucinogens have been used in religious rites for centuries.

The most potent mood- and perception-altering drug known, LSD is a synthetic substance first developed by a pharmaceutical company in 1938. Its street names include *acid*, *green* or *red dragon*, *microdot*, *sugar* and *big D*.

LSD is produced in crystalline form. The pure crystal can be crushed into powder and mixed with binding agents to produce tablets known as microdots or thin gelatin squares called windowpanes. More commonly, it's dissolved, diluted and applied to paper – the most common form of LSD called blotter acid.

Oral doses as small as 30 mcg can produce effects that last 6–12 hours. LSD is 100–200 times more potent than psilocybin and 4,000 times more potent than mescaline.

LSD has dramatic effects on the senses, causing a highly intensified perception of colours, smells, sounds and other sensations. In some cases, sensory perceptions may blend, causing the person to 'see' sounds or 'hear' or 'feel' colours. Hallucinations also distort or transform shapes and movements and may give rise to the perception that time is moving very slowly or that the user's body is changing shape.

Some call it Ecstasy

Ecstasy, or 3,4-methylenedioxymethamphetamine (MDMA), is a synthetic drug with both stimulant and hallucinogenic properties. Available as capsules or tablets, it's taken orally or, rarely, injected or snorted. On the street, it's called *XTC*, *clarify*, *essence* or *Adam*. The Ecstasy experience is sometimes called *rolling*. Ecstasy tablets commonly contain MDMA in addition to other harmful drugs.

Previously used mainly at dance clubs and raves, Ecstasy is now seen in other social settings. Its effects include distortions in time and perception and an amphetamine-like hyperactivity. Like other stimulants, it seems to have addictive potential. Depending on the dosage, acute drug effects typically last 3–6 hours.

Raving over Ketamine

Ketamine distorts perceptions of sight and sound and produces dissociative effects – feelings of detachment from the self and the environment. It's increasingly used as a club drug and distributed at raves and parties.

For therapeutic purposes, ketamine is used mainly in veterinary medicine. Most of the ketamine used illicitly is evaporated to form powder that's snorted, smoked or compressed into tablets. The liquid form of the drug can be injected I.V. or I.M. Street names for ketamine include *K*, *Special K*, *Ket*, *Vitamin K*, *Kit Kat Keller*, *Green*, *Blind Squid* and *cat Valium*.

Odourless and tasteless, ketamine can be added to beverages without being detected; also, it induces amnesia. Because of these properties, the drug sometimes is given to unsuspecting victims to aid in the commission of sexual assault ('drug rape' or date rape).

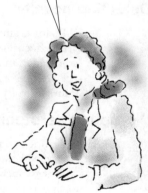

Ketamine induces amnesia and has been used as a date rape drug.

Dextromethorphan daze

Dextromethorphan, sometimes called *DXM* or *robo*, is a cough-suppressing ingredient found in some OTC cold and cough medications. The most common source of abused dextromethorphan is extra-strength cough syrup.

At low doses, the drug has a mild stimulant effect and causes distorted visual perceptions. At much higher doses, it causes dissociative effects similar to those of ketamine. Effects typically last 6 hours.

Mescaline for mind alteration

Found in several cactus species (most notably, *Peyote* and *San Pedro*), mescaline causes hallucinations. Mescaline 'buttons' or 'discs' are cut, then dried and usually swallowed. Sometimes, the drug comes in powdered form and is taken by capsule, injection or smoking.

Mescaline causes visual hallucinations and alters spatial perception. It can produce dizziness, vomiting, tachycardia, increased blood pressure, increased pulse and respiratory rates, sensations of warmth and cold and headache. Effects last approximately 12 hours.

Ecstasy on the upswing

Overall use of hallucinogens by secondary school students has declined since 1998. However, ketamine, LSD and Ecstasy are becoming more widely used at dance clubs and raves by older teens and young adults. A 2005 government survey found that an estimated 332,090 UK residents had used Ecstasy at least once; heaviest use was reported among people aged 18–25.

Most hallucinogens are used experimentally rather than on a regular basis, with users typically reporting only a single use or several uses per year.

How hallucinogens produce their effects

Hallucinogens disrupt the interaction of nerve cells and affect the functioning of serotonin, a neurotransmitter crucial to the regulation of mood, sleep, pain, emotion and appetite.

Detecting novelty

LSD, for example, binds to and activates serotonin receptors in the brain. Drug effects are most prominent in two brain regions – the cerebral cortex (involved in mood, cognition and perception) and the locus ceruleus, which receives sensory signals from all areas of the body and is sometimes called the brain's 'novelty detector'.

Disrupting serotonin

Mescaline and psilocybin are structurally similar to serotonin and produce their effects by disrupting normal functioning of the serotonin system.

Ecstasy increases levels of at least three neurotransmitters – serotonin, dopamine and norepinephrine. By causing excess serotonin release and interfering with serotonin synthesis, Ecstasy leads to serotonin depletion. A single dose of Ecstasy can suppress serotonin levels for up to 2 weeks. At moderate to high doses, users may experience long-term serotonin depletion (which probably accounts for many of the drug's long-lasting behavioural effects).

Redistributing glutamate

Ketamine alters the distribution of glutamate, another neurotransmitter, throughout the brain. Glutamate is involved in memory, pain perception and responses to the environment.

Health hazards of hallucinogen use

Many hallucinogens cause unpleasant and potentially dangerous flashbacks long after the drug was used. Large doses of hallucinogens may cause seizures, ruptured blood vessels in the brain and irreversible brain damage.

LSD intoxication may cause seizures and fatal accidents. Ketamine can result in respiratory depression, heart rate abnormalities, heart failure, inability to move the muscles and insensitivity to pain (which can lead to serious injury).

No ecstasy from these effects

Ecstasy may cause confusion, depression, sleep problems, drug craving, severe anxiety and paranoia (during and sometimes weeks after taking the drug). Physical symptoms may include muscle tension, involuntary teeth clenching, nausea, blurred vision, rapid eye movements, faintness and chills or sweating.

Dance marathon

Ecstasy's stimulant properties may enable users to dance vigorously for extended periods, leading to malignant hyperthermia, dehydration, hypertension and even heart or kidney failure in some people. Typically, the drug causes increased blood pressure and pulse rates.

Other potential complications of Ecstasy include headache, vomiting, panic, anxiety, seizures, MI, exhaustion, dehydration and heat stroke. Death can occur if dehydration and enhanced body temperature aren't controlled.

Impairments associated with hallucinogen use

Hallucinogens can cause short-term impairments in cognition, perception, mood and communication. They may even prevent a person from recognising reality, sometimes resulting in bizarre or dangerous behaviour.

Although hallucinogens are less addictive than most psychoactive drugs, overuse can trigger psychosis in someone with a history of psychosis.

LSD-related impairments

LSD doesn't cause the compulsive drug-seeking behaviour seen with cocaine, heroin or alcohol. However, it can produce tolerance, and those who take it repeatedly may need increasingly higher doses to achieve the desired effects. Because the drug is unpredictable, taking higher doses can be extremely dangerous.

LSD use also produces tolerance for other hallucinogenic drugs, such as psilocybin and mescaline. LSD tolerance is short-lived and fades if the user stops taking the drug for several days.

LSD psychosis

Some LSD users experience devastating psychological effects that persist after the trip has ended, producing a long-lasting psychosis-like state. This persistent psychosis – which may include dramatic mood swings from mania to profound depression, visual disturbances and hallucinations – may last for years.

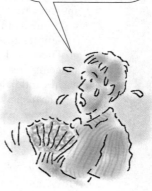

They weren't kidding when they said Ecstasy might make me feel hot.

Bad trips and flashbacks

Many LSD users have 'bad trips' – panic attacks at the height of the drug experience characterised by terrifying thoughts and nightmarish feelings of anxiety and despair. The user may perceive real-world sensations as unreal and even frightening.

Some former LSD users report flashbacks – spontaneous, repeated and sometimes continuous recurrences of the sensory distortions originally produced by LSD. Flashbacks typically consist of visual disturbances, such as seeing false motion on the edges of the field of vision, bright or coloured flashes and halos or trails attached to moving objects.

Flashbacks arise suddenly – commonly without warning – a few days or more than a year after LSD use. They're most common in people who have used hallucinogens chronically or have an underlying personality problem (although otherwise healthy people occasionally have them).

Ecstasy-related impairments

Heavy and prolonged Ecstasy use has been linked to confusion, depression, sleep problems, persistent anxiety, aggressive and impulsive behaviour and selective impairment of working memory and attention. Long-term use may damage the brain's serotonin system, leading to various cognitive and behavioural disturbances, including memory impairment.

Ketamine-related impairments

Ketamine may make the user feel disconnected and out of control. Some users report a terrifying feeling of nearly total sensory detachment, described as a near-death experience.

> Some hallucinogen users seek to transcend the limits of the body or have a spiritual experience, but not me. I'm high on nursing!

Causes

Some people take hallucinogens to enhance bodily sensations and induce sensory gratification. Under the influence of these drugs, music may sound better, colours may seem brighter and sexual orgasm may feel more intense.

Unlocking the doors of perception?

Other people use hallucinogens to try to transcend the limits of the body and the time–space continuum or to have a spiritual or religious experience.

Signs and symptoms

Signs and symptoms of hallucinogen use vary with the drug used. (See *Assessing for hallucinogen use*, page 393.)

Diagnosis

Laboratory studies are rarely useful in diagnosing hallucinogen intoxication. Ecstasy is the only hallucinogen that shows up on standard toxicological screens.

Advice from the experts

Assessing for hallucinogen use

Suspect hallucinogen use if the person has these signs and symptoms.

With LSD or mescaline

A person under the influence of lysergic acid diethylamide (LSD) or mescaline may report a sense of depersonalisation, grandiosity, hallucinations, illusions, distorted perception of time and space or mystical experiences.

GI findings include nausea, vomiting, diarrhoea and abdominal cramps. Cardiovascular findings may include arrhythmias, palpitations, tachycardia and hypertension.

Other signs and symptoms may include:

- chills
- dizziness
- dry mouth
- fever
- sweating
- appetite loss
- hyperpnoea
- increased salivation
- muscle aches.

With psilocybin

Signs and symptoms of psilocybin use include:

- euphoria
- colour distortions
- vivid hallucinations
- 'seeing' music or 'hearing' colour
- dramatic mood swings and personality changes
- increases in blood pressure and body temperature.

With Ecstasy

A person under the influence of Ecstasy may report or exhibit:

- distractibility
- heightened alertness
- irritability or confusion
- euphoria
- enhanced emotional and mental clarity
- increased sensitivity to touch
- enhanced sexuality
- increased energy and motor activity.

Other common findings include:

- increased pulse rate
- elevated blood pressure
- dilated pupils
- perceptual changes
- tightened jaw muscles or jaw grinding or clenching
- increased body temperature, heavy perspiration and dehydration.

At high doses, Ecstasy may cause hallucinations, depression, paranoia and irrational behaviour (including violence).

Ketamine

Ketamine causes dissociative effects and alters visual and auditory perception. At low doses, it causes impairments in attention, learning ability and memory. At higher doses, it may produce delirium, amnesia, impaired motor function, high blood pressure, depression and potentially fatal respiratory problems.

Dextromethorphan

Dextromethorphan use may cause euphoria and a floating sensation, along with increased perceptual awareness and altered time perception. The person may report tactile, auditory or visual hallucinations. Some users experience paranoia and disorientation.

The diagnosis of hallucinogen abuse or dependence is confirmed when the person meets the criteria documented in the *DSM-IV-TR*. See *Diagnostic criteria: Substance abuse*, page 367 and *Diagnostic criteria: Substance dependence*, page 367.)

Treatment

Treatment measures vary with the person's status. A person experiencing a 'bad trip' or an acute panic reaction should be placed in a quiet room with minimal stimuli and reassured that the drug effects will wear off in several hours.

A person who's dangerous to himself or others may need to be restrained physically or chemically. Prolonged or excessive physical restraint should be avoided because it can contribute to hyperthermia and rhabdomyolysis and exacerbate paranoia.

Gastric emptying rarely proves useful because the drug is quickly absorbed. Massive drug ingestion requires supportive care.

> You may need to provide aggressive cooling measures if the person has hyperthermia.

Cool-down phase

A person with marked hyperthermia may require aggressive cooling measures. Benzodiazepines typically are given if the person is anxious or agitated or has hypertension or tachycardia. For severe hypertension or tachycardia, nifedipine or nitroprusside may be indicated. Diazepam is given for seizures.

Treatment for LSD flashbacks

No established treatment exists for LSD flashbacks, although antidepressant drugs may ease symptoms. Psychotherapy may help the person adjust to the visual distraction and ease fears that he's suffering from brain damage or a mental health disorder.

Nursing interventions

For nursing interventions during an acute episode or when the episode has resolved, see *General interventions for acute drug intoxication*, page 370.

Inhalant abuse

Inhalant abuse, commonly called *huffing* or *bagging*, is the deliberate inhalation of chemical vapours to attain an altered mental or physical state (usually a quick 'buzz'). Users inhale vapours from a wide range of substances found in more than 1,000 common household products. Inhalants fall into several general categories. (See *Types of inhalants*, page 395.)

Street names for inhalants include *bang, bolt, boppers, bullet, climax, glading, gluey, hardware, head cleaner, hippie crack, kick, locker room, poor man's pot, poppers, rush* and *snappers*.

Types of inhalants

Inhalants that are abused for their psychoactive effects include aerosols, gases, nitrites and volatile solvents.

Aerosols

Aerosols are sprays containing propellants and solvents such as toluene. Common aerosols include whipping cream, paint, deodorant, hair products, cooking sprays and fabric protector. Silver and gold spray paint are especially popular among inhalant abusers.

Gases

Gases – substances with no definite shape or volume – include refrigerants and medical anaesthetics. Abusers may inhale gases found in propane tanks, butane lighters and air conditioning units as well as those in such medical anaesthetics as ether, chloroform and nitrous oxide (laughing gas). The most commonly abused gas, nitrous oxide is found in whipped cream dispensers and products that boost octane levels in racing cars. It's also sold at raves or drug paraphernalia stores in the form of balloons or as vials called *whippets*.

Nitrites

Such chemicals as amyl nitrite, butyl nitrite and cyclohexyl nitrite are taken mainly to enhance sexual experiences. They're available in adult bookshops and over the Internet. Cyclohexyl nitrite is also found in room deodorisers. Amyl nitrite comes in mesh-covered, sealed capsules that are popped or snapped to release the vapours. Butyl nitrite is sold in small bottles.

Volatile solvents

Volatile solvents are liquids that vaporise at room temperature when left in unsealed containers. They're found in paint thinner, gasoline, correction fluid, felt-tip markers, nail polish and nail polish remover and glue.

By huff or by cuff

Inhalants are breathed in through the nose or mouth in various ways. Users may inhale chemical vapours directly from open containers or may huff fumes from rags soaked in a chemical substance held to the face or stuffed in the mouth.

An aerosol may be sprayed directly into the nose or mouth. Other types of inhalants may be poured onto the collar, sleeves or cuffs and then sniffed repeatedly.

Bagging it

In 'bagging', the user inhales fumes from substances sprayed or deposited inside a paper or plastic bag. Alternatively, the fumes may be discharged into small containers such as soda cans and inhaled from the can. Some users inhale from balloons or other devices.

Prevalence

Inhalant abuse has been increasing steadily. The highest lifetime prevalence of inhalant use is reported by the UK (20%). Least common was the use of inhalants in Portugal, Finland and Turkey (3%). The percentages reported from France and Greece are 6% each and from Spain 3%. In most of the countries the gender differences are very small, i.e. the use of inhalants is about the same among both boys and girls. Essentially it is a group activity with common sites of use being friends' homes, parties and public places. Despite this, recent evidence shows that the majority of users, especially young people, abuse solvents in the home.

Most users are between ages 12 and 17. By the time adolescents reach secondary school, 20% have tried inhalants at least once. Inhalant abuse is roughly equal among males and females.

How inhalants produce their effects

Scientists aren't sure how inhalants produce their effects. Some suggest that the inhaled substance changes the solubility of neurons' cell membranes. Others attribute the effects to potentiation of gamma-aminobutyric acid (GABA), the most important inhibitory neurotransmitter.

Health hazards and impairments associated with inhalants

Inhalants can produce both psychological dependence and physical addiction. Chronic inhalant abuse may lead to serious and possibly irreversible damage to the brain, heart, liver, kidneys and lungs. Brain damage may cause personality changes, diminished cognitive functioning, memory impairment and slurred speech. Impaired judgement may lead to fatal injuries from motor vehicle accidents or sudden falls.

Death can follow within minutes of inhalant use, usually from arrhythmias leading to heart failure. Other possible causes of death include asphyxiation, aspiration or suffocation.

Causes

For most users, the goal of inhalant abuse is a rapid euphoric effect similar to alcohol intoxication, along with loss of inhibitions. After the initial excitation, they experience drowsiness, light-headedness and agitation.

Seeking sexual enhancement

However, nitrite abusers (who tend to be adults rather than adolescents) seek to enhance the sexual experience. Inhaled nitrites dilate blood vessels, increase the pulse rate and produce a sensation of heat and excitement that can last several minutes.

Signs and symptoms

Assessment findings vary with the specific inhalant used. General findings may include:
- loss of muscle control
- slurred speech
- dizziness, drowsiness or loss of consciousness
- hallucinations and delusions

- belligerence
- apathy
- impaired judgement
- drunk or disoriented demeanour
- double vision
- seizures
- nausea
- appetite loss
- red or runny nose
- watery eyes
- sores or rash around the nose or mouth
- arrhythmias
- seizures.

Strong chemical odours on the breath or clothing as well as paint or other stains on the hands, face or clothing strongly suggest inhalant use.

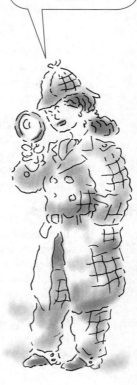

Fetch the scent detector, Watson! Chemical odours may hint at inhalant abuse.

With long-term inhalant use

Long-term inhalant abuse may lead to such signs and symptoms as:
- inflammation, atrophy or perforation of the nasal mucosa
- weight loss
- muscle weakness
- disorientation
- inattentiveness
- irritability
- depression
- permanent ataxia (staggering gait or incoordination)
- peripheral neuropathies.

Withdrawal symptoms

A person undergoing inhalant withdrawal may report or exhibit excessive sweating, headache, rapid pulse, hand tremors, muscle cramps, insomnia, hallucinations, nausea and vomiting.

Diagnosis

In a service user who's known to have used an inhalant, laboratory tests may include:
- serum drug levels (if the particular inhalant is known)
- complete blood count, which may reveal leukocytosis, anaemia, thrombocytopenia, thrombocytosis or platelet defects
- serum electrolyte analysis, which may show hyperchloraemia, hypokalaemia and hypophosphataemia.

The diagnosis of inhalant abuse or dependence is confirmed when the service user meets the criteria documented in the *DSM-IV-TR*. (See *Diagnostic criteria: Substance abuse*, page 367 and *Diagnostic criteria: Substance dependence*, page 367.)

Treatment

Treatment for acute inhalant intoxication is supportive and symptomatic. Haloperidol may be given for severe agitation. A combative service user may require restraints.

Other measures may include:
- fluid replacement therapy
- sedatives to induce sleep
- anticholinergics and antidiarrhoeal agents to relieve GI distress
- anxiolytic drugs for severe agitation.

The person may require continuous ECG monitoring because many inhalants can induce arrhythmias.

Detoxification and rehabilitation

Adequate detoxification is crucial to successful treatment. Regular inhalant abusers may need 30–40 days to detoxify. To ease withdrawal, useful nonpharmacological measures may include psychotherapy, exercise, relaxation techniques and nutritional support.

Relapse blues

Inhalant abusers have high relapse rates, making aftercare and follow-up extremely important. Some may require treatment in an outpatient or residential programme – although few treatment programmes exist specifically for inhalant users. For many users, treatment must continue for an extended period – possibly up to 2 years.

Nursing interventions

For nursing interventions during an acute episode or when the episode has resolved, see *General interventions for acute drug intoxication*, page 370.

> Inhalant abusers have high relapse rates. Some require up to 2 years of treatment.

Nicotine dependence

One of the most frequently used addictive drugs, nicotine is the main psychoactive component found in smoke from tobacco products (cigarettes, cigars and pipes). Smokeless tobacco products, such as snuff and chewing tobacco, also have a high nicotine content.

Cigarette smoking is the most prevalent form of nicotine dependence in the UK. Most cigarettes contain at least 10 mg of nicotine. By inhaling smoke, the average smoker takes in 1–2 mg of nicotine with each cigarette.

Nicotine dependence and withdrawal

Regular nicotine use can result in nicotine dependence. In fact, some experts rank nicotine higher than alcohol, cocaine and heroin in terms of the risk of dependence. A teenager who smokes as few as four cigarettes per day might develop a lifelong addiction to nicotine.

Most smokers use tobacco regularly because they're addicted to nicotine. Although nearly 35 million smokers make a serious attempt to quit each year, less than 7% who try to quit on their own stay abstinent for more than 1 year. Most of them relapse within a few days of trying to quit.

Drawn-out withdrawal

A nicotine-dependent person who stops using nicotine experiences a withdrawal syndrome that may last a month or more. Some people have intense nicotine cravings for 6 months or longer.

Prevalence

Data released by the Office for National Statistics give prevalence estimates of 28% for men and 26% for women. Estimates suggest that the prevalence of smoking in the UK may have been beginning to stabilise in recent years at a level of about one in four adults.

However, inspection of age-specific rates in adults reveals that smoking prevalence has in fact been stable or increasing in recent years amongst most of the younger age groups, particularly in women. Inspection of trends in smoking amongst 15-year-olds in England also shows a progressive increase which is more marked in females. The rate at which new smokers are joining the prevalent smoking population has therefore been increasing for some years, making it likely that unless cessation rates also begin to increase, the overall prevalence of smoking in the UK will soon again begin to rise.

Trends in smoking cessation rates can be inferred from trends in the proportion of ex-smokers amongst UK adults. These have since remained remarkably stable and this suggests that cessation rates are no longer increasing, and that the prevalence of cigarette smoking in the UK is indeed in danger of increasing again over the next few years.

The incidence of smoking is highest among less educated people, and those in lower socioeconomic groups.

How nicotine produces its effects

Absorbed through the skin and mucosal lining of the mouth and nose or by inhalation in the lungs, nicotine activates the brain circuitry that regulates feelings of pleasure (the so-called reward pathways). Specifically, nicotine raises dopamine levels in the brain's reward pathways – a reaction that's thought to underlie the pleasurable sensations that many smokers experience.

Buzzed in 10 seconds

Nicotine's pharmacokinetic properties enhance its abuse potential. Cigarette smoking rapidly distributes nicotine to the brain, with drug levels peaking within 10 seconds of inhalation. Acute effects dissipate in a few minutes, so the smoker must continue to dose throughout the day to maintain pleasurable drug effects and prevent withdrawal. With tolerance comes the need to use progressively higher doses.

Short puffs and long draws

Nicotine can act as both a stimulant and a sedative. Small, rapid doses produce alertness and arousal, whereas long drawn-out doses induce relaxation and sedation.

Epinephrine rush

Nicotine stimulates hypothalamic corticotropin-releasing factor and increases levels of endorphins, adrenocorticotropic hormone and arginine vasopressin. The 'kick' that occurs immediately after exposure results partly from adrenal stimulation and the subsequent epinephrine discharge. The epinephrine 'rush' triggers glucose release, raises blood pressure and speeds the pulse and respiratory rates.

Health hazards of nicotine

Nicotine addiction has a tremendous impact in terms of illness, death and economic costs to society. Cigarette smoking is the single largest avoidable cause of premature death and disability in the UK, and thus presents both the greatest challenge and the greatest opportunity for all involved in improving public health.

Nicotine's ugly aftermath

Tobacco use accounts for approximately one-third of all cancers. Cigarette smoking is linked to nearly 90% of all lung cancers – the leading cause of cancer deaths in both men and women. Additionally, it's associated with cancers of the mouth, pharynx, larynx, oesophagus, stomach, pancreas, cervix, kidney, ureter and bladder. Overall death rates from cancer are twice as high among smokers as nonsmokers.

Smoking also causes lung diseases, such as chronic bronchitis and emphysema, and can exacerbate asthma symptoms. It may also heighten the risk for peptic ulcers, GI disorders, maternal and foetal complications and other disorders.

Cardiovascular disease

Smoking dramatically increases the risk of cardiovascular disease, including coronary artery disease, myocardial infarction, stroke, vascular problems and aneurysms. Smoking accounts for nearly 20% of deaths from heart disease.

Passive smoking and its consequences

Second-hand smoke (passive smoking) causes approximately 3,000 lung cancer deaths yearly in nonsmokers and contributes to as many as 40,000 deaths from cardiovascular disease.

Exposure to tobacco smoke in the home increases the severity of asthma in children and contributes to childhood asthma.

Causes

Scientists suspect that certain genes make some people more susceptible to nicotine addiction and cigarette smoking. Studies involving twins suggest that genes account for 50–70% of the risk of becoming a smoker.

Some researchers believe that as many as 50 genes are involved in nicotine addiction. Genetic factors must be distinguished from environmental factors that contribute to smoking.

Susceptible teens

Among adolescents, risk factors for cigarette smoking include:
- use of alcohol and other drugs
- attention deficit disorder
- depression
- peer influences
- urge to experiment
- disruptive behaviour
- failing to perceive the risks of smoking
- having friends who abuse substances
- having family members who smoke
- divorce or family conflict.

Signs and symptoms

Nicotine withdrawal symptoms may begin within a few hours after the last cigarette – and can quickly drive the smoker back to tobacco use. Usually, symptoms peak within the first few days and subside within a few weeks. For some people, however, increased appetite and nicotine cravings last for months.

Nicotine withdrawal symptoms include:
- depressed mood
- insomnia
- irritability, frustration or anger
- anxiety
- difficulty concentrating
- restlessness
- increased appetite or weight gain
- desire for sweets
- increased coughing
- nicotine craving.

Diagnosis

The diagnosis of nicotine dependence is confirmed when the person meets the criteria documented in the *DSM-IV-TR*. (See *Diagnostic criteria: Substance dependence*, page 367.)

Treatment

Various behavioural and pharmacological treatments have proven to be effective in treating nicotine dependence. For people who are motivated to quit smoking, a combination of behavioural and pharmacological treatments can double the success rate over placebo treatments.

Pharmacological therapies for smoking cessation include nicotine replacement, antagonist therapy, aversive therapy, nicotine-mimicking agents and nonnicotine medication. Nonpharmacological therapies include sensory replacement and acupuncture. To remain abstinent, many people require behavioural therapy.

Nicotine replacement

Used to relieve withdrawal symptoms and nicotine craving, nicotine replacement products include nicotine gum, transdermal patches, nasal spray and inhalers.

These products cause milder physiological changes than tobacco-based cessation systems and generally provide lower overall nicotine levels than tobacco. Also, they have little abuse potential because they don't cause the pleasurable effects of tobacco. Additionally, they don't contain the carcinogens and gases found in tobacco smoke.

Respectable track record

All nicotine replacement products seem to be equally effective. OTC availability of many of the products partly accounts for an estimated 20% rise in successful smoking cessation each year. Since nicotine gum and transdermal patches were introduced, approximately 1 million people have been successfully treated for nicotine addiction.

Antagonist therapy

Nicotine antagonist therapy is used to prevent the positive reinforcing and subjective effects of cigarette smoking. Antagonist agents include mecamylamine (a noncompetitive blocker of CNS and peripheral nicotinic receptors) and naltrexone (a long-acting form of the opioid antagonist naloxone).

Aversive therapy

Aversive therapy typically involves silver acetate, which combines with sulphides in tobacco smoke to produce a bad taste.

Nicotine-mimicking agents

Agents that mimic nicotine's effects include clonidine and anxiolytics (such as diazepam), antidepressants, stimulants and anorectic agents (such as fenfluramine and phenylpropanolamine, used to suppress appetite and prevent weight gain).

Nonnicotine medication

Bupropion, a prescription antidepressant (marketed as Zyban for smoking cessation), was introduced for nicotine addiction in 1996. It's the first drug approved for smoking cessation that's taken in pill form and the first that doesn't contain nicotine.

Sensory replacement

Sensory replacement agents, such as black pepper extract, capsaicin, denicotinised tobacco, flavourings and regenerated (denicotinised) smoke, can be used to decrease nicotine cravings or withdrawal or to substitute for satisfaction from cigarettes.

Acupuncture

Some people undergo acupuncture treatment for smoking cessation and nicotine withdrawal. However, studies don't support claims that acupuncture is as effective as other types of smoking cessation treatments.

Behavioural treatments

Behavioural interventions can play a key role in treating nicotine dependence. Such methods help people identify high-risk relapse situations, create an aversion to smoking, self-monitor their smoking behaviour and establish alternative coping responses. Identifying and removing environmental cues that influence the person to smoke (such as cigarettes, lighters and ashtrays) are crucial.

Nicotine fade-out

Some behavioural therapists use a technique in which the person, if willing to do so, rapidly smokes without inhaling. Another technique is nicotine fading, in which the person smokes the same number of cigarettes but the amount of nicotine is reduced.

Combination approach

Although pharmacological and behavioural treatments can be successful when used alone, integrating both types of treatments is the most effective approach to smoking cessation. For example, the nicotine patch is often combined with a behavioural technique.

Adjunctive measures

The single most important factor in nicotine abstinence may be learning and using coping skills that aid both short- and long-term relapse prevention. Social support can also influence the outcome of a smoking cessation programme. Ideally, the person should avoid smokers and smoking environments and receive support from family and friends. (See *Improving the service user's coping skills*, page 404.)

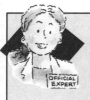

Advice from the experts

Improving the service user's coping skills

Many service users who abuse drugs exhibit ineffective coping and need help in identifying and using available support systems. To enhance your service user's coping skills, use these nursing interventions:

- Spend uninterrupted periods of time with the service user. Encourage him to express his feelings; accept what he says.
- Try to identify factors that cause, exacerbate or reduce the service user's inability to cope, such as the fear of health problems or losing his job.
- Encourage the service user to make decisions about his care to increase his sense of self-worth and mastery over his current situation.
- Praise him for making decisions and performing activities to reinforce coping behaviours.
- Encourage him to use support systems that can help him to cope.
- Help him evaluate his current situation and coping behaviours to encourage a realistic view of his crisis.
- Encourage the service user to try alternative coping behaviours. A service user in crisis tends to accept interventions and develop new coping behaviours more easily.
- Ask the service user for feedback about behaviours that seem to work. This encourages him to evaluate the effect of these behaviours.

Other helpful measures include self-help materials, educational and supportive groups, exercise, hypnosis, 12-step programmes, biofeedback, family therapy, interpersonal therapy and psychodynamic therapies.

Nursing interventions

These nursing interventions may be appropriate for a service user with nicotine dependence:
- Teach the service user about the dangers of smoking and ways to stop.
- Provide emotional support for the service user's attempts to stop smoking.
- Explain how to use nicotine replacement devices, antagonist or aversive medications, or other prescribed drugs.
- As indicated, refer the service user to a smoking cessation programme.

Opioid abuse

Opioids are narcotics that can produce euphoria. They have a high potential for abuse and dependence. Naturally occurring opioids include morphine and codeine. Partially synthetic morphine derivatives include heroin, oxycodone

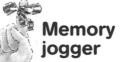

Memory jogger

During nicotine withdrawal, a service user NEEDS CARE.

N Nervousness

E Extreme fatigue

E Excited cardiovascular system

D Difficulty concentrating

S Sleep disturbances

C Cravings

A Anxiety

R Restlessness

E Excessive appetite

and oxymorphone. Synthetic opioids include fentanyl, alfentanil, levorphanol, meperidine, methadone and propoxyphene.

Opioids are used medically as analgesics. Some agents have additional uses. Codeine, for example, is used as an antitussive; opium, as an antidiarrhoeal.

Opioids produce relaxation with an immediate 'rush', but also have initial unpleasant effects, such as restlessness and nausea. With a typical dose, effects last 3–6 hours.

Codeine and morphine may be ingested, injected or smoked. Heroin (whose street names include *junk*, *horse* and *H*) may be injected, inhaled or smoked. Opium (known as *O*, *ope* or *OP*) may be ingested or smoked.

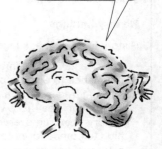

Opioid drugs stimulate opioid receptors in the brain. Injecting them I.V. causes an initial 'rush' of pleasure.

Prevalence

The lifetime prevalence of opioid use in people aged 12–17 is just over 2%. Lifetime prevalence is slightly higher in people aged 35–44 because of peak heroin use during the 1960s and 1970s.

How opioids produce their effects

Opioids stimulate opioid receptors in the CNS and surrounding tissues. CNS effects of opioids include euphoria and sedation, followed by elation, relaxation and, then, sedation or sleep.

Causes

Because of their euphoric and anxiolytic effects, opioids are strong reinforcing agents. For example, when taken I.V., heroin causes a 'rush' of pleasure or an orgasmic feeling.

Behavioural theory proposes that basic reward–punishment mechanisms perpetuate addictive behaviour. Rapid development of physical dependence and a prolonged withdrawal syndrome can make abstinence difficult.

Genetic, social and psychological factors also play a role in opioid abuse and dependence.

Genetic factors

Some evidence shows that identical twins have similar opioid use patterns. Also, several studies support the theory that genetically transmitted vulnerability predisposes a person to drug dependence.

Social factors

Easy drug availability and social acceptance of drug use promote drug experimentation. Drug use rates are higher in urban areas with poor parental functioning, greater drug exposure and higher crime and unemployment rates.

Psychological factors

Opioid abuse sometimes follows the use of prescribed opioids to relieve pain. Some users are motivated by the desire to manage uncomfortable emotions, such as anxiety, guilt and anger.

When to suspect drug abuse

Many people try to hide their drug abuse – especially if they inject drugs. If you suspect a person is abusing drugs, carefully review his medical history and perform a physical assessment.

History findings

History findings that suggest drug abuse include:

- use of a fictitious name and address
- reluctance to discuss previous hospitalisations
- seeking treatment at a medical facility across town rather than near his own home
- history of a drug overdose
- high tolerance for potentially addictive drugs
- history of hepatitis or human immunodeficiency virus infection
- amenorrhoea
- complaints of a painful injury or chronic illness – but refusal to a diagnostic investigation
- feigned illnesses, such as migraine headache, myocardial infarction or renal colic, in an attempt to obtain drugs
- claims of an allergy to over-the-counter analgesics
- requests for a specific medication.

Physical findings

Physical findings that hint at drug abuse include:

- fever (from stimulant intoxication, withdrawal or infection caused by I.V. drug use)

- needle marks or tracks (from I.V. drug use)
- attempts to conceal or disguise injection sites with tattoos
- use of inconspicuous injection sites, such as under the nails or tongue
- cellulitis or abscess from self-injection
- puffy hands (a late sign of thrombophlebitis or of fascial infection caused by self-injection on the hands or arms)
- dental conditions (from poor oral hygiene associated with chronic drug use)
- excoriated skin (from scratching induced by formication, a sensation of bugs crawling on the skin)
- refractory acute-onset hypertension or cardiac arrhythmias (stimulant use)
- liver enlargement, with or without tenderness (from hepatitis caused by sharing contaminated needles).

Behavioural clues

A hospitalised drug abuser is likely to be uncooperative, disruptive or even violent. He may experience mood swings, anxiety, impaired memory, sleep disturbances, flashbacks, slurred speech, depression and thought disorders.

To obtain drugs, some users resort to plays on sympathy, bribery or threats. They may try to manipulate caregivers by pitting one staff member against another.

Signs and symptoms

A person who abuses opioids – or other drugs, for that matter – may try to hide drug use from family, friends, coworkers and health care professionals. However, even if the person isn't forthcoming, you can check for certain telltale signs. (See *When to suspect drug abuse*.)

Also check for these signs and symptoms of opioid use:

- constricted pupils, bloodshot eyes and drooping eyelids
- slurred speech
- sweating
- clammy skin
- anorexia
- respiratory depression
- hypotension
- sweating

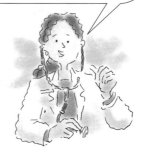

A person who has taken opioids may have respiratory depression, with slow or shallow breathing.

Advice from the experts

Identifying I.V. drug abuse

Needle marks or tracks are an obvious sign of I.V. drug abuse. Some I.V. drug abusers try to conceal or disguise injection sites with tattoos or by selecting an inconspicuous injection site such as under the nails.

Be aware that self-injection sometimes causes cellulitis or abscesses, especially in service users who are also chronic alcoholics. Puffy hands may be a late sign of thrombophlebitis or of fascial infection caused by self-injection on the hands or arms.

- impaired judgment
- euphoria
- drowsiness
- decreased level of consciousness
- sense of tranquillity
- detachment from reality
- indifference to pain
- lack of concern
- nystagmus
- seizures
- constipation
- haemorrhoids.

Some people experience nausea and vomiting, hypotension and arrhythmia. Severe opioid intoxication can lead to delirium and coma.

Tale of the tracks

With I.V. use, the user may have visible needle marks or tracks, skin lesions or abscesses, soft tissue infection and thrombosed veins. (See *Identifying I.V. drug abuse*.)

Findings in opioid withdrawal

Opioid withdrawal can be quite unpleasant. For general findings, see *Evaluating for opioid withdrawal*.

Heroin withdrawal symptoms resemble a bad case of the flu. They generally begin 12–14 hours after the last dose, peak within 36 and 72 hours and may last 7–14 days.

Opioid overdose

With opioid overdose, auscultation may reveal bilateral crackles and rhonchi caused by opiate overdose. Other cardiopulmonary findings may include pulmonary oedema, respiratory depression, aspiration pneumonia and hypotension.

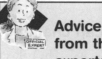

Advice from the experts

Evaluating for opioid withdrawal

Signs and symptoms of opioid withdrawal include:

- abdominal cramps, nausea or vomiting
- anorexia
- fever or chills
- profuse sweating
- dilated pupils
- hyperactive bowel sounds
- irritability
- nausea
- panic
- piloerection (goose flesh)
- runny nose
- tremors
- watery eyes
- yawning
- bone pain
- diffuse muscle aches
- drug craving.

Diagnosis

A doctor who suspects opioid abuse or dependence may order a urine drug screen. (See *Toxicology screening*.)

For service users with clinical or historical evidence of I.V. drug abuse, the doctor may order:

- liver function tests
- rapid plasma reagin test for syphilis
- hepatitis viral testing
- HIV testing
- lung X-rays (to check for pulmonary fibrosis).

To evaluate for opioid withdrawal, the doctor may order serum electrolyte studies and a complete blood count.

Narcan challenge

The naloxone challenge test assesses for physical dependence on opioids. A positive result consists of typical withdrawal signs and symptoms (usually lasting 30–60 minutes) after I.V. or I.M. naloxone administration. This test can be valuable before starting an opioid antagonist for maintenance therapy.

The diagnosis of opioid abuse or dependence is confirmed if the person meets the criteria documented in the *DSM-IV-TR*. (See *Diagnostic criteria: Substance abuse*, page 367 and *Diagnostic criteria: Substance dependence*, page 367.)

Treatment

For opioid intoxication or overdose, general supportive measures include ensuring an adequate airway and ventilation (with ventilatory support if needed) and supporting cardiovascular function.

Other treatments depend on symptoms, the specific opioid and administration route. If the drug was ingested, vomiting is induced or gastric lavage is performed.

I.V. fluids and nutritional and vitamin supplements may be given. An opioid antagonist such as naloxone may be administered. (See *Naloxone for opioid reversal*, page 409.)

The doctor also may prescribe:

- sedatives, to induce sleep
- anticholinergics and antidiarrhoeal agents, to relieve GI distress
- anxiolytic drugs, for severe agitation.

Depending on the opioid dosage and time elapsed before admission, additional treatments may include forced diuresis and haemoperfusion or haemodialysis.

Withdrawal and detoxification

For withdrawal, the person should receive a sufficient amount of opioids on the first day to decrease symptoms, followed by gradual withdrawal of the abused drug over 5–10 days.

Toxicology screening

A blood or urine screen may detect drugs that are present in concentrations above 5 μg/ml. Current methods quantitate only drugs detected in the blood.

Toxicology screening commonly is done in the emergency department or on admission. It may require a legal chain of custody in which precautions are taken to prevent anyone from tampering with the specimens.

Meds matters

Naloxone for opioid reversal

Naloxone hydrochloride (Narcan) is an opioid antagonist used to reverse the effects of opioids. It works by displacing opioids from their receptors in the central nervous system (CNS).

Naloxone is administered I.V., I.M. or subcutaneously every 2–3 minutes, as needed. It rapidly reverses opioid-induced CNS depression and increases the respiratory rate within 1–2 minutes. Side effects include nausea, vomiting, diaphoresis, tachycardia, CNS excitement and increased blood pressure.

Relapse and respiratory peril

Because the opioid's duration of action may exceed that of naloxone, the service user may relapse into respiratory depression. Be sure to monitor respiratory rate and depth. Be prepared to provide oxygen, ventilation and other resuscitation measures.

Treatment of withdrawal symptoms may include antidiarrhoeals, decongestants for runny nose and nonopioid analgesics for pain. Clonidine, an alpha-2 adrenergic agonist, decreases sympathetic nervous system overactivity and produces sedation. Buprenorphine, a partial opioid agonist and potent antagonist, may be given once per day to block withdrawal symptoms.

Substitution strategy

For detoxification, the abused opioid usually is replaced with a drug that has a similar action but a longer duration. Gradual substitution controls withdrawal effects, reducing discomfort and associated risks. Depending on which drug the person has abused, detoxification may be managed on an inpatient or outpatient basis.

Ultrarapid detox

In an ultrarapid (1-day) detoxification programme, the person is placed under heavy sedation or general anaesthesia and is given I.V. naloxone or oral naltrexone; acute withdrawal takes place during an unconscious state.

Maintenance therapy

For maintenance, the person typically receives an opioid agonist as a substitute for the abused drug. The goal of maintenance is to replace the abused drug with one that's available legally, can be taken orally and requires only a once-daily dose.

> Methadone, given in an oral liquid, is the most common drug used in opioid detox.

The methadone file

Methadone is the most commonly used opioid agonist in opioid detoxification. Methadone treatment reduces drug cravings, improves the person's functioning, promotes stability, reduces illicit drug use and other criminal behaviour and improves productive social behaviour.

Given once per day as an oral liquid, methadone has nearly all the physiological properties of heroin. Three-quarters of the service users who take methadone for maintenance are likely to stay heroin-free for 6 months or more.

Levomethadyl acetate hydrochloride (ORLAAM), a methadone derivative, may also be used. Longer acting than methadone, ORLAAM can be taken just two or three times per week. Clinical studies have found ORLAAM to be as effective as methadone.

Antagonist approach

Some service users may prefer opioid antagonist therapy to methadone or ORLAAM. Naltrexone, the antagonist usually chosen, blocks the 'high' produced by opioids. The service user must be free of opioids for at least 5 days before starting naltrexone therapy.

Naltrexone therapy has had mixed success. Only 10–20% of service users who try naltrexone take it for 6 months or longer.

Acupuncture

An acupuncture technique called *auriculotherapy* is gaining popularity in treating opioid abuse. Needles are inserted in each ear and are connected to a constant-current electrical stimulator. The efficacy of this approach hasn't been established.

Psychotherapy

Detoxification alone, without ongoing psychotherapy, isn't sufficient to manage a service user with opioid dependence. To remain abstinent, he should receive standard drug counselling along with cognitive-behavioural, dynamic or group therapy. (Some service users may prefer aversion therapy, in which aversive stimuli are paired with cognitive images of opioid use.)

Cognitive-behavioural therapy focuses on the service user's thoughts and behaviours. It helps him learn specific skills for resisting drug abuse as well as coping skills to reduce problems related to drug use.

Dynamic psychotherapy is based on the concept that all symptoms arise from underlying unconscious psychological conflicts. The goal is to make the service user aware of these conflicts and develop better coping mechanisms and healthier ways of resolving intrapsychic conflicts.

An opioid-dependent service user needs psychotherapy in addition to detox.

Group sobriety

Group therapy targets the social stigma attached to drug abuse. The presence of other group members who acknowledge their abuse problem has

> ### Advice from the experts
> # Reducing impaired social interaction
>
> Impaired social interaction is common among service users who abuse substances. Appropriate nursing interventions can help the service user improve social interaction skills in both one-on-one and group settings.
>
> - If delusions and hallucinations occur, don't focus on them. Instead, provide reality-based information, and reassure the service user that he's safe.
> - Provide additional time with the service user on each shift (besides the time spent on caregiving) to encourage social interaction. Start with one-on-one interaction and increase to group interaction when the service user's social skills indicate that he's ready.
> - Give positive reinforcement for appropriate and effective interaction behaviours (both verbal and nonverbal). This helps the service user recognise progress and enhances feelings of self-worth.
> - Assist the service user and his family or close friends in progressive participation in care and therapies. This reduces feelings of helplessness and enhances the service user's feeling of control and independence.

a therapeutic effect in helping the service user develop alternative methods of staying sober. (See *Reducing impaired social interaction*.)

Nursing interventions

These nursing interventions may be appropriate for a service user with acute opioid intoxication:

- Provide extra blankets or a hypothermia blanket, for hypothermia.
- Reorient the service user to time, place and person.
- Monitor breath sounds for evidence of pulmonary oedema.
- Frequently monitor vital signs and cardiopulmonary status until opioids have cleared from the system.
- Monitor for withdrawal symptoms.

For other interventions during an acute episode or when the episode has resolved, see *General interventions for acute drug intoxication*, page 370.

Phencyclidine abuse

A dissociative drug, PCP was developed in the 1950s as an I.V. anaesthetic. It was used in veterinary medicine but never approved for human use.

Today, PCP is manufactured illegally in laboratories. On the street, it's available as tablets, capsules and powders, and it's sold as *angel dust, wack, ozone, love boat, superweed, hog, peace pill, embalming fluid, elephant tranquilliser* and *rocket fuel*. The combination of PCP and marijuana is called a *killer joint* or *crystal supergrass*.

PCP can be snorted, smoked or eaten. For smoking, it's typically applied to a leafy material, such as parsley, oregano or marijuana. Some users ingest PCP by snorting the powder or by swallowing it in tablet form.

Numb but quarrelsome

PCP makes the user feel disconnected and out of control. It also has a numbing effect on the mind and can cause unpredictable and often violent behaviour. Repeated use may result in psychological dependence and craving.

Many people have bad reactions to PCP. Some users have flashbacks long after they stop using it. Memory loss and depression may last for up to 1 year after a chronic user stops taking PCP.

Prevalence

PCP use isn't widespread. It's most common in older teenagers and in young adults.

How PCP produces its effects

PCP's primary sites of action are glutamate receptors known as *N*-methyl-D-aspartate (NMDA) receptors. PCP acts as an NMDA antagonist, lowering the glutamate levels in the brain.

PCP also increases levels of GABA, an inhibitory neurotransmitter. Increased GABA levels probably explain the inhibition of pain seen in PCP users. In addition, PCP also alters the action of dopamine, which is responsible for the euphoria and 'rush' associated with many psychoactive drugs.

Health hazards of PCP

At low to moderate doses, PCP's physiological effects include increased body temperature, marked rises in blood pressure and pulse, shallow respirations, flushing and profuse sweating.

At high doses, PCP decreases blood pressure and slows the pulse and respiratory rates. Cardiac arrest, hypertensive crisis, renal failure and seizures may occur.

Feeling no pain

Other dangerous effects include violent or suicidal behaviour, seizures, decreased awareness of pain, coma and death. (However, death more commonly results from accidental injury or suicide during PCP intoxication.)

In adolescents, PCP may interfere with the learning process and with hormones related to normal growth and development.

Rhabdomyolysis blues

PCP sometimes leads to rhabdomyolysis – breakdown of muscle fibres, with the leakage of potentially toxic cellular contents into the systemic circulation. This life-threatening condition can result in muscle pain

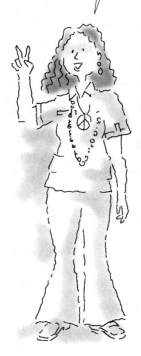

Some people call PCP the peace pill. But from what I hear, taking it is anything but peaceful.

and weakness, malaise, fever and nausea and vomiting. Complications of rhabdomyolysis include:

- compartment syndrome (causing vessel and nerve compressions)
- hypovolaemia
- hyperkalaemia
- metabolic acidosis
- cardiac arrest and arrhythmias
- disseminated intravascular coagulation
- acute renal failure.

Causes

As with other drugs, the precise causes of PCP abuse aren't known. Some people may use PCP because it provides a feeling of strength, power and invulnerability.

In young people, drug abuse commonly follows experimentation with drugs stemming from peer pressure. Risk factors for PCP use include male gender and young adulthood (ages 20–29).

Signs and symptoms

A person under the influence of PCP may report numbness of the arms and legs and may exhibit poor muscle coordination. Psychological effects include changes in body awareness, resembling those caused by alcohol intoxication.

Other physical findings may include:

- sparse, garbled speech
- blurred vision
- blank stare
- drooling
- nausea and vomiting
- loss of balance
- dizziness
- decreased deep tendon reflexes
- fever
- gait ataxia
- nystagmus
- hyperactivity
- increased vital signs
- tachycardia.

Mental status mayhem

Mental status findings may vary greatly – even in the same service user. The service user may seem normal one moment, then exhibit apparent psychotic symptoms and homicidal or suicidal ideation the next.

Other mental status findings may include:

- euphoria
- amnesia

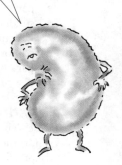

PCP sometimes causes rhabdomyolysis, a dangerous condition that may lead to kidney failure.

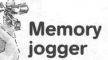

Memory jogger

Each letter in ANGEL DUST stands for a sign or symptom of phencyclidine (PCP) use.

A Amnesia

N Nystagmus

G Gait ataxia

E Euphoria

L Loopiness (poor perception of time and distance)

D Delusions and distortions

U Unpredictable effects

S Sudden behavioural changes

T Tachycardia

- delusions and hallucinations
- poor perception of time and distance
- distorted sense of sight, hearing and touch
- decreased awareness of pain
- distorted body image
- excitation
- panic
- sudden behavioural changes
- violent behaviour
- stupor or coma
- paranoia
- disordered thinking.

Withdrawal symptoms

Research suggests that with repeated or prolonged PCP use, a withdrawal syndrome may occur when drug use is stopped. Some users experience dysphoria and an intense drug craving.

Diagnosis

The doctor typically orders a urine drug screen if PCP use is suspected. Because PCP may cause rhabdomyolysis, serum enzyme levels (especially creatine kinase) may be useful.

The diagnosis of PCP abuse or dependence is confirmed when the person meets the criteria documented in the *DSM-IV-TR*. (See *Diagnostic criteria: Substance abuse*, page 367 and *Diagnostic criteria: Substance dependence*, page 367.)

Treatment

A person with acute PCP intoxication should be placed in a quiet room with minimal stimulation. If he's violent, restraints may be needed.

Induced vomiting or gastric lavage may be performed, followed by the administration of activated charcoal. Other drug therapy may include:
- benzodiazepines (such as diazepam), to ease seizures, agitation, aggressiveness, psychotic symptoms, hypertension and tachycardia
- haloperidol, for agitation or psychotic behaviour
- diuretics, to force diuresis
- anticholinergics and antidiarrhoeal agents, to relieve GI distress
- propranolol, for hypertension or tachycardia
- nitroprusside for severe hypertensive crisis
- I.V. fluids.

Treatment of PCP overdose

Because PCP has anticholinergic properties, physostigmine, an acetylcholinesterase inhibitor, may be used as a partial antidote. (See *Fighting PCP with physostigmine*, page 415.)

> Someone with a history of prolonged PCP use may experience dysphoria and drug craving during withdrawal.

Meds matters

Fighting PCP with physostigmine

Physostigmine (Antilirium) is an acetylcholinesterase inhibitor that enhances acetylcholine's effects. It's sometimes used to reverse central nervous system (CNS) toxicity associated with toxic doses of phencyclidine (PCP) and other drugs with anticholinergic effects.

Usually, physostigmine is given I.M. or I.V. and repeated as needed until a desired response or adverse cholinergic effects occur.

Nursing actions

If the person is receiving physostigmine, take the following actions:

- Monitor closely for adverse reactions – particularly seizures, bradycardia, bronchospasm and respiratory paralysis.
- Raise the side rails if the person becomes restless.
- Monitor vital signs closely, especially respirations. Provide respiratory support as needed.

With a large overdose, treatment (such as induced emesis, gastric lavage or activated charcoal) aims to support respiratory function and decrease drug absorption.

Treatment of PCP-induced psychosis

For a person with PCP-induced psychosis, treatment must address the high risk of violence. The person may require seclusion or restraint, and suicide and assault precautions should be instituted.

If psychosis persists, the doctor may prescribe an antipsychotic, such as haloperidol or risperidone. The person usually needs mental health follow-up care and chemical dependency treatment. Most people with PCP-induced psychosis can be weaned from antipsychotics within 6 months.

Nursing interventions

For appropriate measures, see *General interventions for acute drug intoxication*, page 370.

Sedative, hypnotic or anxiolytic abuse

Sedative, hypnotic and anxiolytic drugs produce sedation, ease anxiety and relax muscles. Most are classified as benzodiazepines. Typically, benzodiazepines act as hypnotics in high doses, anxiolytics in moderate doses and sedatives in low doses. Besides the main indications described above, they're used to prevent seizures or help people withdraw from alcohol.

Benzodiazepines from A to T

Benzodiazepines include:

- alprazolam
- chlordiazepoxide
- clonazepam
- clorazepate
- diazepam
- flurazepam
- halazepam
- lorazepam
- midazolam
- oxazepam
- quazepam
- temazepam
- triazolam.

Forging for drugs

Abusers maintain their drug supply by getting prescriptions from several doctors, forging prescriptions or buying the drugs on the street. Street names for benzodiazepines include *dolls*, *green and whites*, *roaches* and *yellow jackets*.

Benzodiazepines are ingested or injected. Their duration of action ranges from 4 to 8 hours.

Mixed motives

Some people use benzodiazepines to get intoxicated; others take intentional or accidental overdoses. Heroin users may use benzodiazepines when they can't get heroin, when they want to enhance heroin's effects or when they're trying to stop using heroin. Amphetamine and Ecstasy users may take benzodiazepines when 'coming down' from a high or to induce sleep.

Prevalence

In the UK, 1 million people appear to have used benzodiazepine hypnotics or tranquillisers regularly for 12 months or over; 50% of these for 5–10 years or more. A high proportion of these users must be assumed to be at least to some degree dependent on benzodiazepines.

How benzodiazepines produce their effects

Like alcohol, heroin and cannabis, benzodiazepines are depressants that slow CNS activity. They work by potentiating the activity of GABA, causing sedation, relaxing muscles, easing anxiety and have anticonvulsant properties. In the peripheral nervous system, stimulation of GABA receptors may decrease cardiac contractility and enhance perfusion.

Health hazards of benzodiazepines

In addition to causing tolerance and physical dependence, repeated use of large benzodiazepine doses can lead to amnesia, hostility, irritability and vivid or disturbing dreams. Concurrent use with alcohol or other depressants can be life threatening.

The risky business of injection

Some people inject benzodiazepines for an enhanced 'high' or to increase the effects of other drugs. This practice can lead to severe health effects, such as:

- collapsed veins
- red, swollen, infected skin
- necessity for limb amputation (because of poor circulation)
- stroke
- cardiac and respiratory arrest
- death.

Sharing needles, syringes and other injecting equipment greatly increases the risk of contracting hepatitis and HIV.

Impairments associated with benzodiazepine use

At low to moderate doses, benzodiazepines can produce drowsiness, fatigue, lethargy, dizziness, vertigo, blurred or double vision, slurred speech, stuttering, mild impairment of memory and thought processes, feelings of isolation and depression.

A booze-like wooziness

At high doses, these drugs may induce oversedation, sleep or effects similar to alcohol intoxication – confusion, poor coordination, impaired memory and judgement, difficulty thinking clearly, blurred or double vision and dizziness. Mood swings and aggressive outbursts may also occur. As the high dose wears off, the user may feel jittery and excitable.

Benzodiazepine overdose can cause coma. When combined with alcohol, death may occur.

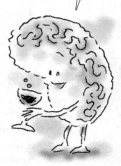

Benzodiazepines and alcohol make for a killer combination.

Causes

Some people may have a genetic tendency towards drug dependence or addiction. Environmental factors also play a significant role. Drug availability and prescriber dispensing practices may contribute to benzodiazepine abuse.

Signs and symptoms

A person under the influence of benzodiazepine may exhibit:

- ataxia (poor muscle coordination)
- drowsiness
- hypotension
- increased self-confidence
- relaxation
- slurred speech.

Findings in benzodiazepine overdose

Assessment findings in a person with a benzodiazepine overdose may include:

- dizziness
- altered mental status, ranging from confusion and drowsiness to unresponsiveness or coma

- blurred vision
- anxiety and agitation
- nystagmus
- ataxia
- hallucinations
- slurred speech
- hypotonia (reduced skeletal muscle tone)
- weakness
- impaired cognition
- amnesia
- respiratory depression
- hypotension.

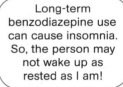

Expect low blood pressure in a person who has taken a benzodiazepine overdose.

Findings in chronic abuse

Long-term benzodiazepine use (more than several weeks) may result in:

- drowsiness
- lack of motivation
- clouded thinking
- memory loss
- changes in personality and emotional responses
- anxiety
- irritability
- aggression
- insomnia
- disturbing dreams
- nausea
- headache
- skin rash
- menstrual problems
- sexual problems
- increased appetite
- weight gain
- increased risk of accidents (including falls in older adults).

Withdrawal symptoms

Benzodiazepine withdrawal resembles that of alcohol withdrawal. It can be severe and may necessitate hospitalisation.

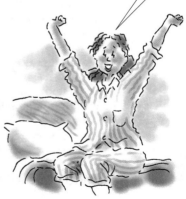

Long-term benzodiazepine use can cause insomnia. So, the person may not wake up as rested as I am!

Rough withdrawal

Withdrawal symptoms usually develop 3–4 days after the drug is stopped; however, they may arise earlier with shorter-acting agents or later with longer-acting agents. Symptoms can last a few weeks or months; some people have them for 1 year – or even longer.

Withdrawal symptoms may include:

- headache
- sweating

- confusion
- seizures
- nervousness
- tension
- anxiety and panic attacks
- hypertension
- dizziness
- poor appetite
- nausea, vomiting and abdominal pain
- inability to sleep properly
- depression
- feelings of isolation and unreality
- delirium and paranoia.

Diagnosis

The diagnosis of benzodiazepine substance abuse or dependence is confirmed if the person meets the criteria documented in the *DSM-IV-TR*. (See *Diagnostic criteria: Substance abuse*, page 367 and *Diagnostic criteria: Substance dependence*, page 367.)

Treatment

Treatment of benzodiazepine intoxication depends on which drug was taken, how much and when. The service user may need supportive care and monitoring, including cardiac monitoring, I.V. fluid administration, pulse oximetry and vital sign monitoring. Respiratory depression may necessitate assisted ventilation. (See *Dealing with drug overdose*, page 420.)

Detoxification

For detoxification, single-dose activated charcoal is recommended if the person ingested the drug within the past 4 hours. Alternatively, gastric lavage may be considered. (Ipecac is contraindicated because of the risk of CNS depression and subsequent aspiration of emesis.)

The only specific benzodiazepine antidote is flumazenil, a GABA antagonist. Given I.V., flumazenil reverses sedation, memory and psychomotor impairments and respiratory depression produced by benzodiazepines. However, it's usually reserved for severe poisoning because it can cause withdrawal and seizures in chronic benzodiazepine abusers. (See *Drug detoxification programmes*, page 421.)

Treatment of chronic abuse

Treatment of chronic benzodiazepine abuse usually is done on an outpatient basis or at a drug rehabilitation centre. However, service users who have been using high doses of sedatives or hypnotics, have a history of withdrawal seizures or DTs, or have concurrent medical illnesses should undergo withdrawal in an inpatient setting.

Advice from the experts

Dealing with drug overdose

Whether intentional or accidental, a drug overdose is life threatening. In very high doses, some drugs cause central nervous system (CNS) depression, ranging from lethargy to coma. Others cause CNS stimulation, ranging from euphoria to violent behaviour.

Depending on the specific drug and the extent of damage, other symptoms of overdose may include hallucinations, respiratory depression, seizures, abnormal pupil size and response or nausea and vomiting.

Diagnosing overdose

Arterial blood gas analysis and blood and urine screening tests help detect drug use and guide treatment.

Treatment

A person with signs of respiratory depression receives oxygen, or intubation and mechanical ventilation. He's attached to a cardiac monitor, and a 12-lead electrocardiogram is taken. Urine, blood and vomitus specimens are obtained for toxicology screening. Restraints may be applied to prevent him from harming himself or others.

Emergency nursing interventions

- Take appropriate steps to stop further drug absorption. If the person ingested the drug, induce vomiting or use gastric lavage, as ordered. You may administer activated charcoal to help adsorb the substance, and use a saline cathartic to speed its elimination.
- Frequently reassess the person's airway, breathing and circulation. Keep oxygen, suction equipment and emergency airway equipment nearby. Be prepared to perform cardiopulmonary resuscitation, if necessary.
- When possible, find out which drug the person took, how much and when. Did he combine several drugs or take a drug along with alcohol? Question the person's family, friends or rescue personnel thoroughly.
- Watch for complications. Stay alert for shock, indicated by decreased blood pressure and a faint, rapid pulse. Reassess respiratory rate and depth, and auscultate breath sounds frequently. Know that dyspnoea and tachypnoea may warn of impending respiratory complications, such as pulmonary oedema or aspiration pneumonia. A person with crackles who's pale, diaphoretic and gasping for air may have pulmonary oedema. A person with rhonchi or decreased breath sounds probably has aspiration pneumonia.
- Carefully monitor heart rate and rhythm. Because the person's neurological status may change as his body metabolises the drug, frequently assess neurological function.
- You may detect hypothermia or hyperthermia, so expect to use either extra blankets and a hyperthermia mattress or an antipyretic and a hypothermia mattress, as ordered.
- If the overdose was accidental, recommend a rehabilitation programme for substance abuse. If it was intentional, refer the person to crisis intervention for psychological counselling.

Replacement therapy

The first step involves gradual reduction of the drug to prevent withdrawal and seizures. The benzodiazepine may be replaced gradually with another drug that has a similar action. A long-term benzodiazepine abuser with severe withdrawal symptoms (such as elevated vital signs or delirium) should receive an agent with a rapid onset, in doses sufficient to suppress withdrawal symptoms. I.V. lorazepam or diazepam are commonly given for their immediate results.

Drug detoxification programmes

Designed to help people achieve abstinence, drug detoxification programmes offer a relatively safe alternative to self-withdrawal after prolonged dependence on alcohol or drugs. These programmes, offered in outpatient centres or in special units, provide symptomatic treatment as well as counselling or psychotherapy on an individual, group or family basis.

Be aware that deeply motivated people with strong support systems are most likely to overcome their substance abuse.

Replacing the abused drug

To help the person through withdrawal, the doctor gradually lowers the dosage of the abused drug or substitutes a drug with similar action. For example, he may substitute methadone for heroin, or treat cocaine addiction with bromocriptine or naltrexone. If these options aren't available, treatment is supportive and symptomatic.

Urine and blood samples are obtained for alcohol and drug screening to provide information on the most recent ingestion. Medical and psychosocial evaluations help determine appropriate treatment as well as whether it should be provided on an inpatient or outpatient basis.

After withdrawal from alcohol or drugs, the person needs rehabilitation to prevent recurrence of abuse. Rehabilitation may include supportive counselling or individual, group or family psychotherapy. For the drug abuser, rehabilitation may include psychotherapy.

Nursing actions

- Know that caring for a person undergoing detoxification requires skill, compassion and commitment.

- Because substance abusers have low self-esteem and commonly try to manipulate people, you'll need to control your natural feelings of anger and frustration.
- If the person is undergoing opioid withdrawal, detoxify him by administering methadone, as prescribed.
- To ease withdrawal from opioids, depressants and other drugs, provide nutritional support, suggest mild exercise and teach relaxation techniques. If appropriate, administer sedatives or tranquillisers to help the person cope with anxiety, depression or insomnia.
- Encourage the person's participation in rehabilitation programmes and self-help groups. Be alert for continued substance abuse after admission to the detoxification programme. Carefully administer prescribed medications to prevent hoarding by the person, and closely monitor visitors, who might bring him drugs or alcohol from the outside.
- Be aware that a person who returns to a social setting in which others are abusing drugs will probably have a relapse. Encourage professional and family support after the person leaves the detoxification programme.
- Emphasise the benefits of joining an appropriate self-help group, such as Alcoholics Anonymous or Narcotics Anonymous. Recommend that the person's spouse or mature children accompany him to group meetings. Also refer his family to a support group, if necessary. Stress to the person that he ultimately must accept responsibility for avoiding abused substances.

When stabilised, the service user is switched to an equivalent dose of a long-acting agent (such as phenobarbital), which causes milder withdrawal symptoms. He's tapered off this long-acting agent slowly over 2–6 months.

For mild benzodiazepine withdrawal symptoms, anticonvulsants that aren't cross dependent with sedative-hypnotics (such as carbamazepine and valproate) have been used successfully.

Recovery phase

After withdrawal comes a prolonged recovery and rehabilitation phase, in which the service user attempts to stay drug-free. The service user needs social support and involvement of his family and friends during this difficult stage.

Rehabilitation programmes are available for both inpatients and outpatients. They usually last a month or longer and may include individual, group and family psychotherapy. During and after rehabilitation, participation in a drug-oriented self-help group may be helpful.

Nursing interventions

Nursing interventions for a service user who abuses benzodiazepine are described in *General interventions for acute drug intoxication*, page 370.)

Quick quiz

1. Expected effects of a disulfiram reaction include:
    A.   chest pain, chills and hypertension.
    B.   slow pulse, chills and excitation.
    C.   slow pulse, slow respiratory rate and hypertension.
    D.   chest pain, headache and hypotension.

Answer: D. A person who consumes alcohol up to 2 weeks after taking disulfiram will experience a reaction that includes shortness of breath, chest pain, nausea, vomiting, facial flushing, headache, red eyes, blurred vision, sweating, tachycardia, hypotension and fainting.

2. A service user admits to taking 'crystal'. This drug is classified as:
    A.   a depressant.
    B.   a stimulant.
    C.   a hallucinogen.
    D.   an antidepressant.

Answer: B. 'Crystal' is a street name for methamphetamine, a stimulant. Other amphetamines include amphetamine sulphate and dextroamphetamine.

3. The assessment finding that most strongly suggests I.V. drug abuse is:
    A.   skin lesions.
    B.   gastritis.
    C.   tachycardia.
    D.   tachypnoea.

Answer: A. Self-injection of drugs can cause skin lesions or abscesses.

4. To treat tachycardia induced by cocaine, the doctor may prescribe:
    A.   buprenorphine.
    B.   digoxin.
    C.   lidocaine.
    D.   propranolol.

Answer: D. Propranolol is typically given to treat tachycardia caused by cocaine use.

5. The effects of LSD typically last:
    A. 4–6 hours.
    B. 6–8 hours.
    C. 8–12 hours.
    D. 14–16 hours.

Answer: C. The duration of effect of LSD and most other hallucinogens is 8–12 hours.

6. An antagonist that's administered for narcotic overdose is:
    A. disulfiram.
    B. naloxone.
    C. diazepam.
    D. bupropion.

Answer: B. Naloxone is a narcotic antagonist that displaces previously administered narcotic analgesics from CNS receptors.

Scoring

✩✩✩ If you answered all six items correctly, mind blowing! Your comprehension of substance abuse has given us quite a rush.

✩✩ If you answered four or five items correctly, far out! One more hit of this chapter may be all you need to achieve euphoria.

✩ If you answered fewer than four items correctly, don't get weirded out! Just abstain from all other activities until you complete a thorough review of this chapter.

12 Sleep disorders

Just the facts

In this chapter, you'll learn:

◆ sleep stages and circadian rhythms

◆ types of sleep disorders and their causes

◆ assessment findings in people with sleep disorders

◆ special procedures used to diagnose sleep disorders

◆ treatments and nursing interventions for people with sleep disorders.

A look at sleep disorders

Sleep is a natural state of rest during which muscle movements and awareness of the surroundings diminish. Sleep restores energy and well-being, allowing us to function optimally the next day. Unlike other states resembling sleep (such as coma), sleep is easily interrupted – or prevented – by noise, light and other external stimuli. Internal factors, such as stress and anxiety, can also decrease the amount and quality of sleep.

Many people have long-term sleep disorders, whilst we all have occasional sleeping problems. Nearly one-third of people seen in primary care settings complain of occasional sleep difficulties.

This chapter discusses the major sleep disorders – breathing-related sleep disorders, circadian rhythm sleep disorders, narcolepsy, primary hypersomnia and primary insomnia.

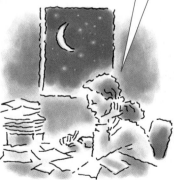

All of this research on sleep disorders is making me sleepy.

Causes

Sleep disorders may be primary or may arise secondary to a medical or mental health disorder, substance use or environmental factors. Medical conditions that can cause sleep disorders include Parkinson's disease, Huntington's disease, viral encephalitis, brain disease, thyroid disease and hormonal imbalances.

Mental health disorders, such as depression and anxiety, are the most common cause of chronic insomnia. High levels of stress also may contribute to sleep disorders.

Substances that can disrupt sleep include alcohol, caffeine and prescription medications – most notably, antihistamines, corticosteroids and central nervous system (CNS) drugs.

High levels of stress may contribute to sleep disorders. I guess I won't be getting much sleep tonight!

Impact of sleep disorders

Sleep disorders can lead to sleep deprivation, which can seriously interfere with a person's family life, occupation, driving ability and social activities.

Chronic sleep deprivation can cause or contribute to accidents, social and marital disruption and mental health disturbances. It's also an independent risk factor for cardiovascular and GI disorders.

Driving while drowsy

Sleepy drivers and equipment operators cause many accidents. Experts believe sleepy drivers pose an even greater safety threat than alcoholic drivers.

At work, someone who isn't well rested can't perform at his best. Poor work performance can lead to corrective action and even job dismissal.

Dangerous deprivation

Sleep-deprived health care professionals are more likely to use poor judgement and make potentially life-threatening mistakes. Sleep-deprived factory workers may cause injury to themselves or others as well as contribute to the manufacture of defective products. Major environmental incidents linked to lack of sleep include the near-nuclear disaster of Three Mile Island in 1979, the nuclear meltdown at Chernobyl in 1986 and the oil spill of the Exxon Valdez in 1989.

Sleep occurs in five stages, growing progressively deeper with each stage.

Fuel for family feuds

Someone who doesn't sleep well is likely to feel tense, unhappy and even depressed. These feelings can compromise healthy family relationships.

Sleep disturbances can have a direct impact on other family members' sleep patterns. For example, snoring may awaken the person's spouse or prevent the spouse from falling asleep in the first place.

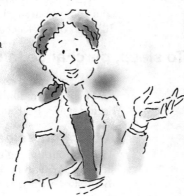

Sleep stages

Sleep occurs in five stages. With each stage, sleep becomes deeper and brain waves grow progressively larger and slower, as shown by electroencephalography (EEG).

Stage 1
The lightest stage of sleep, stage 1 occurs as a person falls asleep. The muscles relax and brain waves are fast and irregular. Called *theta waves*, these spikelike waves have a low-medium amplitude and occur three to seven times per second. Stage 1 accounts for approximately 5% of an adult's total sleep time.

Stage 2

During stage 2, a relatively light stage of sleep, theta waves continue but become interspersed with sleep spindles (sudden increases in wave frequency) and K complexes (sudden increases in wave amplitude). Stage 2 comprises approximately 50% of total sleep time.

Stages 3 and 4

Stages 3 and 4 are the deepest stages of sleep. Delta waves – large, slow waves of high amplitude and low frequency, appear on the EEG. Stage 3 and stage 4 differ only in the percentage of delta waves seen: during stage 3, delta waves account for less than 50% of brain waves, whereas during stage 4, they account for more than 50%.

Conserve as you sleep

Arousing a sleeper from stage 3 or 4 is harder than during any other stage. Because these stages are marked by decreased body temperature and metabolism, researchers believe they function to conserve energy. They account for 10–20% of total sleep time.

As night fades into morning, stages 3 and 4 get progressively shorter. During the last few cycles of the sleep period, no delta-wave sleep occurs at all.

Stage 5

Stage 5 is a deep sleep called *rapid-eye-movement (REM) sleep*. During this stage, the sleeper shows darting eye movements, muscle twitching and short, rapid brain waves resembling those seen during the waking state. (See *Sleep stages and brain waves*, page 427.)

REM sleep usually begins about 90 minutes after sleep onset. Over the course of the night, REM periods lengthen. Overall, REM sleep accounts for 20–25% of total sleep time.

To sleep, perchance to dream

Most storylike dreams take place during REM sleep. People awakened from REM sleep commonly report vivid dreams. In contrast, people awakened during stages 1 through 4 rarely report vivid dreams.

Alternating sleep cycles

Throughout the night, REM (stage 5) and non-REM (NREM) (stages 1 to 4) sleep alternate in cycles of about 90 minutes each. Stages 3 and 4 occur during the first one-third to the first one-half of the night. REM sleep increases towards the morning.

Functions of REM and NREM sleep

Scientists believe REM and NREM sleep serve different biological functions, although they don't know exactly what these functions are. REM sleep may stimulate brain growth or consolidate memory.

REM is my friend! Scientists think REM sleep may stimulate brain growth.

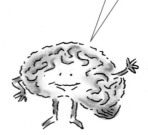

Sleep stages and brain waves

Each sleep stage generates distinctive brain waves, as measured by EEG.

During stage 1, which occurs as a person falls asleep, fast, irregular brain waves called *theta waves* appear on the EEG.

During stage 2, theta waves are interspersed with wave phenomena called *sleep spindles* and *K complexes*.

During stages 3 and 4, the EEG shows large, slow, high-amplitude waves called *delta waves*.

During stage 5, called *rapid-eye-movement (REM) sleep*, short, rapid brain waves appear.

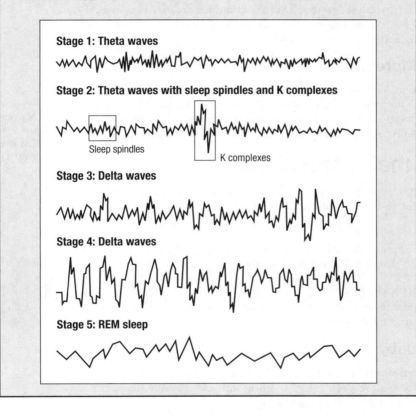

Stage 1: Theta waves

Stage 2: Theta waves with sleep spindles and K complexes

Sleep spindles

K complexes

Stage 3: Delta waves

Stage 4: Delta waves

Stage 5: REM sleep

A person deprived of REM sleep tends to have longer REM cycles during the next sleep episode. These longer REM cycles are more intense, with more eye movements per minute.

Make-up sleep

Similarly, people deprived of NREM sleep have longer NREM sleep during the next sleep period – and the 'make-up' NREM sleep produces different EEG patterns than normal NREM sleep.

Neurological regulation of sleep stages

The various sleep stages are influenced by different parts of the brain. REM sleep is controlled by the pons (a part of the brainstem) and adjacent portions of the midbrain. Chemical stimulation of the pons may induce long periods of REM sleep, while damage to the pons may reduce or prevent REM sleep.

Paralysis and the pons

During REM sleep, neurons in the pons and midbrain that control muscle tone show various levels of activity: Some are active while others aren't. Reflecting this variable activity, certain body muscles remain inactive during REM sleep – especially those of the back, neck, arms and legs. As a result, the sleeper is effectively paralysed so that he can't act out his dreams. However, if these regulatory neurons malfunction, the sleeper may be more active during dreams, thrashing about or becoming violent.

Baths and the basal forebrain

The basal forebrain, located in front of the hypothalamus, controls NREM sleep. Damage to this region of the brain may cause difficulty falling or staying asleep. Some neurons in the basal forebrain are activated by heat, which may explain the sleep-promoting benefits of taking a warm bath in the evening.

Factors that affect sleep

Factors affecting sleep quality and quantity include the person's age, lifestyle, sleep environment and medication use.

Age

Amounts and patterns of sleep differ at each major stage of the life cycle. Both REM and NREM sleep periods decrease with age.

Newborns and toddlers

Newborns sleep the most, averaging 17–18 hours a day, with REM accounting for roughly half of total sleep time.

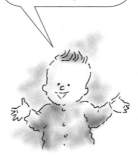

My homies and I just love to sleep! On average, we sleep 17–18 hours a day.

Go to sleep-y, little baby

At first, a newborn sleeps in episodes of 3–4 hours. Gradually, by about age 3 or 4 months, he gets more sleep at night. A 6-month-old typically sleeps 12 hours a night and naps 1–2 hours each day.

Toddlers sleep about 11 or 12 hours a night, with a 1- to 2-hour nap after lunch. Nap requirements vary, with some children taking naps up to age 5.

By age 5, children typically sleep 10–12 hours a day, with REM sleep accounting for about 20% of the total.

Tweens and teens

Preadolescents need about 10 hours of sleep. Adolescent requirements aren't well defined. Many teenagers get too little sleep because of their busy schedules and academic pressures.

Myth busters

Sleep requirements of older adults

Another misconception about elderly adults bites the dust.

Myth: Older adults need much less sleep than younger adults.

Reality: Sleep requirements increase in the elderly because they tend to get decreased amounts of deep sleep and suffer frequent sleep interruptions.

Young adults

A typical young adult needs about 8 hours of sleep, though the requirement varies widely. Some young adults need as little as 6 or 7 hours, while others may need 9 or 10 hours to function optimally. Lifestyle choices make this group vulnerable to sleep disturbances.

Middle-aged adults

In middle-aged adults, sleep requirements may remain unchanged from those of the young adult years. Typical sleep disturbances during middle age may stem from hormonal changes in women, breathing-related disorders and insomnia.

Older adults

Sleep problems are common among older adults. Besides taking longer to fall asleep, they spend less time in deep NREM sleep, so their sleep is more easily interrupted or fragmented. (See *Sleep requirements of older adults.*)

Bathroom breaks

Early awakening is also common and may result from an earlier rise in body temperature. Finally, many older people have trouble falling back to sleep after awakening to urinate.

Environment

The sleep environment can greatly affect sleep quality. Environmental influences on sleep include noise, bright lights or sunlight, excessive activity and an uncomfortable room temperature. When these influences are prominent, sleep can be difficult even for someone who's sleepy. Removing such stimuli produces an environment that's more conducive to sleeping.

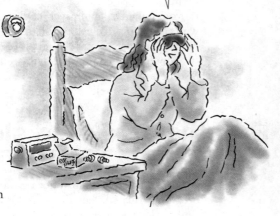

Darkness, silence and a comfortable room temperature promote sleep.

Lifestyle

Travel, shift work, stress and anxiety can greatly influence sleep. A person who travels through different time zones may suffer jet lag, which is worse when travelling west to east. A 'jet-setter' typically tries to sleep when he isn't tired (travelling west to east) and tries to stay awake when it's daylight (travelling east to west).

Night-shift blues

Up to 20% of night-shift workers experience sleep problems resulting from the disruption of the body's natural rhythms.

Medications and substances

Medications of any kind may alter sleep patterns. Prescription drugs may cause somnolence (drowsiness) at inappropriate times; some may cause insomnia. Illicit drugs may also disturb established sleep patterns.

Alcohol

Alcohol's effect on sleep varies with the amount and time of consumption. In nonalcoholics, alcohol may have a sedative effect, increasing the amount of slow-wave sleep for the first 4 hours after sleep onset. After alcohol's effects wear off, sleep may be disrupted, with an increased amount of REM sleep and anxiety-causing dreams.

Alcoholics may have trouble falling asleep and staying asleep. Many have REM sleep disturbances.

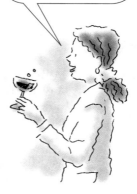

Although alcohol initially may increase the amount of slow-wave sleep, it later causes sleep disruptions.

Withdrawal woes

During alcohol withdrawal, sleep deprivation is common. When sleep occurs, it's usually fragmented and accompanied by nightmares and anxiety-causing dreams.

Approach to assessment

The most important symptoms of sleep disturbances are insomnia at night (the most common symptom) and sleepiness during waking hours. A thorough medical and psychological history should be obtained from a person who complains of sleep problems. The family may also need to be questioned because the person may be unaware of his sleep behaviour.

Sometimes, a physical examination is also warranted. Because sleep disorders are commonly linked to mood disorders, psychological tests may be administered as well.

Breathing-related sleep disorders

Breathing-related sleep disorders are marked by abnormal breathing during sleep. Obstructive sleep apnoea syndrome (OSAS) is the most common breathing-related sleep disorder. Other disorders in this category include central sleep apnoea syndrome and central alveolar hypoventilation syndrome.

Airway obstruction during sleep apnoea

In a person with obstructive sleep apnoea, the airway is blocked by increased tissue of the soft palate or tongue, increased amounts of fat around the pharynx or a small or receding jaw that leaves too little room for the tongue.

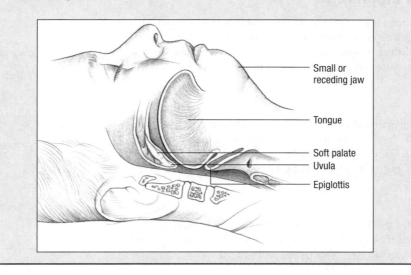

Small or receding jaw

Tongue

Soft palate
Uvula
Epiglottis

Breathing blockade

In OSAS, the upper airway becomes blocked during sleep, impeding airflow. Reduced airway muscle tone and the pull of gravity in the supine position further limit airway size during sleep. As tissue collapse worsens, the airway may become completely obstructed. (See *Airway obstruction during sleep apnoea*.)

With either partial or complete airway obstruction, the person struggles to breathe. Blockage of airflow lasts 10 seconds to 1 minute and arouses the person from sleep as the brain responds to decreased blood oxygen levels. (However, arousal is commonly partial and goes unrecognised by the person.)

Snoring, then silence

This pattern causes disturbed and fragmented sleep, with periods of loud snoring or gasping when the airway is partly open alternating with silence when the airway is blocked. (However, not everyone who snores has OSAS.)

With arousal, the muscle tone of the tongue and airway tissues increases, causing the person to awaken just enough to tighten the upper airway muscles and open the windpipe. However, when he falls back to sleep, the tongue and soft tissue relax again – and the cycle begins anew. This cycle may be repeated hundreds of times each night.

Complications

Repetitive cycles of snoring, airway collapse and arousal may lead to cardiovascular problems – high blood pressure, arrhythmias and even myocardial infarction or stroke. In some high-risk people, sleep apnoea may lead to sudden death from respiratory arrest during sleep.

Drowsy, irritable and indifferent

Frequent awakenings leave the person sleepy during the day and can cause irritability or depression. The person may suffer morning headaches, decreased mental functioning and a reduced sex drive. People with severe, untreated sleep apnoea have two to three times the risk of motor vehicle accidents.

Prevalence

OSAS affects approximately 2–3% of the population. Incidence rises with age – especially after age 50. It's most common in overweight, middle-aged men but can affect females and males of any age. In women, menopause is a significant precipitating factor.

Causes

Most people with OSAS are overweight with a short, thick neck and fat infiltration around the pharynx that increases the risk of airway blockage. Some have an unusually large soft palate and tongue.

Apnoea and anatomy

In people who aren't overweight, OSAS typically results from a small or receding jaw that leaves insufficient room for the tongue. Other structural causes of OSAS include malformations of the oropharynx or jaw and tumours and other growths that narrow the airway. Among older adults, loss of muscle tone may contribute to the condition.

Rotational forces

People with rotating work schedules may be at higher risk for OSAS. The use of alcohol or sedatives may increase the frequency and length of apnoeic periods.

Signs and symptoms

People with OSAS typically report chronic daytime sleepiness. Some also report snoring, which may be pronounced enough to disturb the sleep of other household members. In fact, the person himself may not be aware of his heavy snoring and nocturnal arousals, so you may need to question family members about these symptoms.

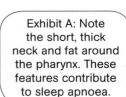

I hear a symphony . . . of snoring. That person needs to be checked for sleep apnoea.

Exhibit A: Note the short, thick neck and fat around the pharynx. These features contribute to sleep apnoea.

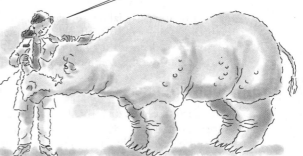

Other complaints in a person with OSAS include:
- frequent headaches
- general feeling of tiredness and fatigue
- frequent daytime naps (which usually aren't effective in restoring energy)
- irritability
- difficulty paying attention
- learning or memory problems
- depression
- excessive urination at night
- impotence
- heartburn or acid indigestion (suggesting oesophageal reflux).

Body reconnaissance

During the physical examination, stay alert for:
- obesity
- hypertension
- jaw malformation
- signs and symptoms of tumours or other tissue abnormalities
- reduced chest excursion (from obesity)
- indications of cardiovascular and cerebrovascular conditions.

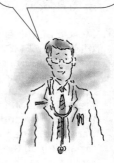

Polysomnography is a sleep study used to evaluate people for sleep disorders.

Diagnosis

Polysomnography, a sleep study performed in a sleep laboratory, is the gold standard for diagnosing OSAS. However, this test is expensive and not widely available. Home sleep studies are cheaper – but less accurate. (See *Polysomnography: It knows when you're asleep*, page 434.)

The diagnosis of a breathing-related sleep disorder is confirmed when the person meets the criteria listed in the *Diagnostic and Statistical Manual of Mental Disorders*, Fourth Edition, Text Revision (*DSM-IV-TR*). (See *Diagnostic criteria: Breathing-related sleep disorder*, page 435.)

Treatment

Treatments for OSAS include lifestyle changes, continuous positive airway pressure (CPAP) therapy and dental devices that modify tongue or jaw position. For selected people, upper airway and jaw surgical procedures may be appropriate; however, their invasiveness and expense restrict their use.

Lifestyle changes

Lifestyle changes – especially weight loss – are the simplest treatments for OSAS. Weight loss reduces the amount of excess tissue in and around the airway. Decreasing the body mass index to 30 or less significantly reduces the frequency of obstructive sleep episodes. However, even small weight reductions can improve the person's condition.

Polysomnography: It knows when you're asleep

Polysomnography is an overnight sleep study, performed in a special laboratory or a sleep centre, that measures various physiological functions related to sleep and wakefulness. Sensor leads and other detectors are placed on the person to gather the following information:

- Brain wave activity, recorded by EEG. The EEG reveals the stage of sleep that the person is in during any given period.
- Eye movements, recorded by electro-oculography (EOG). EOG determines when the person is experiencing rapid-eye-movement sleep. Along with the EEG, it also helps determine how long it takes him to fall asleep, his total sleep time, time spent in each sleep stage and the number of arousals from sleep.
- Muscle movements, measured by electromyography (EMG). The EMG recording helps document wakeful periods, arousal or spastic movements.
- Respiratory effort, which determines chest and abdominal excursion during breathing. Velcro bands are placed around the person's chest and around the abdomen and connected to a piezo crystal transducer. The force of chest and abdominal expansion on the bands stretches the transducer and alters the signal to a recorder.
- Oxygen saturation, recorded by a pulse oximeter probe placed on the finger, earlobe or other appropriate site, to determine oxygen starvation during an apnoeic episode.
- Electrocardiography (ECG), which can reveal whether low oxygen saturation during apnoeic episodes leads to arrhythmias. The ECG also alerts the technician to any emergency condition.
- Airflow, recorded by a thermistor secured to the person's nose. The thermistor detects the amount of air moving into and out of the airways, thus revealing apnoeic or hypopnoeic (inadequate breathing) episodes.
- Blood pressure, to detect dangerous blood pressure elevations (sometimes caused by apnoeic episodes).

Optional monitoring includes core body temperature, penile tumescence and the pressure and pH at various oesophageal levels. Information gathered from all the leads and sensors is fed into a computer and transformed into a series of waveform tracings.

Smile for the camera

The person may be videotaped as he sleeps so that the technician can determine whether any abnormal waveforms were caused by an actual arousal, a period of wakefulness or normal movement in bed. Sound recordings may be made to evaluate snoring.

Sleep latency testing

The day after polysomnography, the person may undergo a multiple sleep latency test (MSLT) to evaluate excessive daytime sleepiness or narcolepsy. The MSLT records sleep patterns (including napping) throughout the day.

The MSLT usually involves five testing periods spaced about 2 hours apart. For each testing period, the person is taken to a 'sleeping' room, where electrodes are attached to the face and scalp to record eye movements, muscle tone and brain waves.

Then the lights are turned off and the person is asked to sleep for 15–20 minutes. Recordings are taken as he sleeps. The technician awakens the person after the testing period. Even if the person can't sleep during the test, the information can be useful. Altogether the MSLT takes about 8 hours.

Supine is not sublime

Sleeping on the side rather than in a supine (back-lying) position may reduce apnoeic episodes. Avoiding alcohol and sleeping pills can decrease the number and duration of these episodes.

Diagnostic criteria: Breathing-related sleep disorder

The diagnosis of a breathing-related sleep disorder is confirmed if the person meets these criteria from the *Diagnostic and Statistical Manual of Mental Disorders*, Fourth Edition, Text Revision.

- The person experiences sleep disruption (causing excessive sleepiness or insomnia) that's judged to stem from a sleep-related breathing condition (such as obstructive or central sleep apnoea or central alveolar hypoventilation syndrome).
- The sleep disturbance isn't better explained by another psychiatric disorder.
- It doesn't result from direct physiological effects of a substance or another medical condition (other than a breathing-related disorder).

Continuous positive airway pressure

CPAP therapy during sleep is the most common and effective treatment for OSAS. Positive pressure splints the airway open, preventing its collapse. The desired level of pressure varies with the type of CPAP device used. The person wears either a full facial mask or a nasal mask.

Dental devices

Oral appliances worn during sleep may help to relieve airway obstruction. However, they may be uncomfortable for some people and may cause excessive salivation.

Surgery

Surgical procedures used to correct OSAS include:
- tonsil and adenoid removal, which increases the size of the pharynx
- removal of any growths or nasal polyps obstructing the airway
- correction of jaw abnormalities
- uvulopalatopharyngoplasty – surgical revision of the uvula, tonsils, soft palate and soft tissues of the oropharynx
- laser-assisted uvulopalatoplasty – surgical revision of the uvula, tonsils and soft palate using a laser.

Unfortunately, these procedures have a relatively high failure rate.

Nursing interventions

These nursing interventions may be appropriate for a person with OSAS:
- Remember that the person is likely to be tired and irritable. Be helpful and supportive.
- If the person reports associated symptoms, such as oesophageal reflux, nocturia or impotence, refer him for appropriate treatment.
- Assist the person in a weight loss programme, if indicated.
- Urge him to stop smoking, if indicated.
- Encourage him to avoid alcohol and illicit drug use.
- Help family members deal with issues related to the person's snoring.

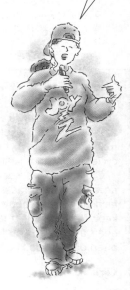

If he's tubby and crabby, and snores when he naps, you can betcha he's apnoeic – make way for CPAP!

Circadian rhythm sleep disorder

In circadian rhythm sleep disorder, the person's internal sleep–awake pattern is out of synch with the demands of his work schedule, travel requirements or social activities. The result is insomnia and sleepiness.

The body's internal clock governs the sleep–awake cycles and many other body functions.

Circadian lullaby

Circadian refers to biological rhythms with a cycle of about 24 hours. (*Circadian* comes from the Latin phrase 'circa diem', meaning 'about a day'.) The circadian rhythm functions as the body's internal 'clock', regulating the 24-hour sleep–awake cycle and other body functions, such as body temperature, hormones and heart rate. (See *Tick tock, it's the body clock*.)

The body's internal clock can reset itself to help a person adjust to such disturbances as seasonal changes, transitions to or from daylight saving time or the start of a new working week. However, it can't always overcome longer-lasting disruptions resulting from shift work or jet lag (air travel across time zones).

Weirded-out rhythms

Disruption of circadian rhythms may cause sleep difficulties, fatigue, a short attention span, impaired cognitive abilities (such as poor judgement and decision-making) and even GI disorders.

Tick tock, it's the body clock

The human body has an internal 'clock' that follows a 24-hour cycle of wakefulness and sleepiness. This clock runs on circadian rhythms, which are linked to nature's cycle of light and darkness.

Critical organs, such as the heart, liver and kidneys, have their own 'clocks' that work in a coordinated fashion with the body's master clock. Researchers know, for example, that certain cardiac events, such as heart attacks and sudden cardiac death, occur more often during specific times of the circadian cycle.

Lark vs. owl

The body's clock keeps us alert during daylight hours and makes us sleepy when night falls. All of our physiological functions are geared towards being active during the day and resting at night. The desire to sleep is strongest between 12 and 6 a.m.

Nonetheless, individual patterns of alertness vary, explaining why some people are relatively more alert during the day ('larks') while others are more alert at night ('night owls').

Mighty melatonin

The body's internal clock is regulated by melatonin, a hormone that causes sleepiness. Melatonin is secreted by the pineal gland, a structure located in the roof of the brain's third ventricle. Influenced by light, the pineal gland slows melatonin production during daylight hours to promote alertness and increases production when darkness falls, causing sleepiness.

With age, the body produces less melatonin. Not surprisingly, many older adults suffer from sleep disorders.

Types of circadian rhythm sleep disorders

The main types of circadian rhythm sleep disorders include the delayed sleep phase, jet lag and shift work disorders.

Delayed sleep phase sleep disorder

In delayed sleep phase sleep disorder, the person sleeps according to a delayed clock time, relative to the light–dark cycle and social, economic and family demands. Typically, he has trouble falling asleep until the early hours of morning and ends up sleeping through much of the day. This disorder often begins in childhood and is relatively common among adolescents.

Jet lag sleep disorder

The jet lag sleep disorder results from rapid travel across more than one time zone. Until the body clock fully adjusts to the new time zone, the person feels sleepy or alert at an inappropriate time of day relative to local time. Jet lag often requires a recovery period of 1 day for every time zone passed over.

Shift work sleep disorder

In the shift work sleep disorder, night-shift work or frequently changing shift work causes insomnia during the major sleep period or excessive sleepiness during the major awake period. The person typically suffers chronic sleep disruption.

Asleep on the job

Few, if any, night workers regularly get restful restorative day sleep. An estimated 10–20% report falling asleep on the job, usually during the second half of the shift.

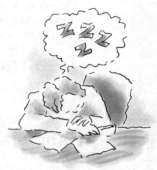

Prevalence

A circadian rhythm sleep disorder is diagnosed in 7–10% of people who complain of insomnia.

Causes

A circadian rhythm sleep disorder results from intrinsic factors such as delayed sleep phases or extrinsic factors such as jet lag or shift work.

Signs and symptoms

Assessment findings vary with the type of circadian rhythm sleep disorder.

Findings in delayed sleep phase sleep disorder

People with delayed sleep phase sleep disorder may report:
- inability to fall asleep until the early hours of the morning
- difficulty awakening in the morning
- feeling of being sleep deprived

- significant social or work impairment
- need for multiple means to awaken (several alarm clocks, other people, telephone wake-up calls or a combination of these).

Findings in jet lag sleep disorder

People with jet lag sleep disorder complain of grogginess and a general malaise, which may last for up to 1 week (especially after travelling west to east). Jet lag may impair the person's work performance.

Findings in shift work sleep disorder

People with shift work sleep disorder commonly report:
- sleepiness while performing their jobs, especially if they work nights
- insufficient daytime sleep because of family or social demands or environmental disturbances
- significant social or work impairment.

Diagnosis

The person's history may suggest a circadian rhythm sleep disorder. The diagnosis is confirmed if the person meets the criteria listed in the *DSM-IV-TR*. (See *Diagnostic criteria: Circadian rhythm sleep disorder*.)

Treatment

Various treatments have been used for circadian rhythm disorders.

Diagnostic criteria: Circadian rhythm sleep disorder

The diagnosis of circadian rhythm sleep disorder is confirmed when the person meets these criteria from the *Diagnostic and Statistical Manual of Mental Disorders*, Fourth Edition, Text Revision.

Sleep disturbance pattern

- The person experiences a persistent or recurrent pattern of sleep disruption that leads to excessive sleepiness or insomnia. This pattern is caused by a mismatch between the person's circadian sleep–awake pattern and the sleep–awake schedule required by his environment.
- The sleep disturbance leads to clinically significant distress or impairment in social, occupational or other important areas of functioning.
- The disturbance doesn't occur only during the course of another sleep disorder or another psychiatric disorder.
- The disturbance doesn't result from direct physiological effects of a substance or a general medical condition.

Types of circadian rhythm sleep disorder

- *Delayed sleep phase:* The person experiences a persistent pattern of late sleep onset and late awakening times, with inability to fall asleep and awaken at a desired earlier time.
- *Jet lag:* After repeated travel across more than one time zone, the person is sleepy and alert at inappropriate times of day relative to local time.
- *Shift work:* Because of night-shift work or frequently changing shift work, the person experiences insomnia during the major sleep period or excessive sleepiness during the major wakefulness period.

(*Note:* An unspecified type of circadian rhythm sleep disorder also exists.)

Chronotherapy

Chronotherapy involves manipulating the person's sleep schedule by progressively delaying bedtime by 1 or more hours each night, until the person can go to sleep and wake up at appropriate times. It is most commonly used to treat delayed sleep phase sleep disorder.

Luminotherapy

Luminotherapy is the use of bright light to manipulate the circadian system. Typically administered with light boxes, it's safe and effective when used according to recommendations.

Here comes the sun

For people with delayed sleep phase sleep disorder, some doctors recommend exposure to bright light on awakening. Sunlight exposure for night-shift workers or jet travellers at their destination may help reset the circadian clock to environmental time.

> Sunlight exposure can help a night-shift worker or jet-setter adjust her body clock.

Chronopharmacotherapy

Chronopharmacotherapy involves the use of drugs to induce sleep or promote wakefulness when desired. Short-acting sedative-hypnotic drugs may be used to promote sleep, especially in jet lag sleep disorder.

Many night-shift workers use caffeine to keep themselves awake on the job. However, some become tolerant to caffeine's effects over time.

Mellowing out with melatonin

Supplemental melatonin therapy has been studied recently as a treatment for circadian rhythm sleep disorders. However, it hasn't been proven safe or effective in long-term use. Also, because melatonin is a hormone, it may have unpredictable effects.

Bypassing jet lag

To prevent jet lag, some experts suggest travellers try to reach their destination by early evening and go to sleep around 10 p.m. local time. To prepare their bodies for the change, they should go to sleep at the new bedtime for a few days before the trip. Avoiding alcohol and caffeine in flight may help minimise jet lag.

Nursing interventions

These nursing interventions may be appropriate for a person with a circadian rhythm sleep disorder:
• To promote his compliance with sleep interventions, review the required procedures with the person. Assess his understanding of these procedures.
• If the person is using chronotherapy, make sure that he understands how to adjust his bedtime correctly.

- Teach the person about the purpose, administration and side effects of prescribed drugs such as sedative-hypnotics. Monitor for side effects.
- Caution the person about the dangers of using unproved treatments.
- If the person is taking melatonin, inform him that this product isn't always manufactured under quality-controlled conditions.

Narcolepsy

Narcolepsy is characterised by sudden, uncontrollable attacks of deep sleep lasting up to 20 minutes. These 'sleep attacks' come on without warning and may be accompanied by paralysis and hallucinations. Although the brief sleep is refreshing, the urge to sleep soon returns.

Sleep paralysis and hallucinations typically occur during sleep onset (hypnagogic hallucinations) or during the transition from sleep to wakefulness (hypnopompic hallucinations). Mostly visual, these hallucinations are intense, dreamlike images commonly involving the immediate environment.

It doesn't take a fortune-teller to predict that a narcoleptic will experience cataplexy after a strong emotion, like anger or surprise.

A confounding cataplexy

It's believed around one in 2,000 people has narcolepsy. Men and women are affected in equal numbers. It most often begins between the ages of 15 and 30.

About 70% of people with narcolepsy experience attacks of cataplexy – sudden loss of muscle tone and strength. (In more subtle forms of cataplexy, the person's head may drop or his jaw may slacken.)

Cataplexy is commonly triggered by emotions – for example, the knees may buckle after the person laughs, gets angry or feels elated or surprised. Cataplexy typically lasts just a few seconds, and the person remains alert during the episode. However, in severe cases, the person falls down and becomes completely paralysed for up to several minutes.

Complications

Narcoleptic sleep attacks may occur at any time of day. All too often, they occur during activities that call for undivided attention, such as driving.

Image problems

Besides causing accidents, narcolepsy can be disabling, impairing work performance and disrupting leisure activities and interpersonal relationships. Coworkers may perceive the person as lazy; an employer may suspect him of illegal drug use. In one study, 24% of narcoleptic people had to give up work and 18% had been fired because of the disease.

Jeers from their peers

In children, narcolepsy impairs school performance and social relationships and invites ridicule from peers. Teenagers with the disorder are at increased risk for road traffic accidents.

Prevalence and onset

Narcolepsy is relatively common, occurring in up to 1.6 of every 1,000 people (although it may be underdiagnosed). One study found that the mean number of years between symptom onset and diagnosis was 14 years.

Narcolepsy is the second leading cause of daytime sleepiness diagnosed in sleep centres. (OSAS is the most common.) The disorder affects males and females equally. The usual onset is during young adulthood, but the condition has been reported in children as young as age 3.

Causes

The cause of narcolepsy is unknown. Scientists suspect it may involve a neuroimmune interaction or a genetic predisposition. First-degree relatives have a 10–40 times greater risk than the general population. Narcolepsy isn't related to the amount of sleep a person gets.

Signs and symptoms

Assessment findings in narcolepsy include:
- excessive daytime sleepiness, even during active states, such as eating and talking
- cataplexy
- brief episodes of sleep paralysis (inability to move or speak when falling asleep or waking up)
- dreamlike hallucinations at sleep onset or when awakening from sleep
- disturbed night-time sleep, such as tossing and turning, leg jerks, nightmares, frequent awakenings and abnormal REM sleep.

Diagnosis

A history of excessive daytime sleepiness, uncontrollable sleep and observed cataplexy strongly suggests narcolepsy. However, other possible causes of excessive daytime sleepiness – heart disease, brain tumours, anaemia and depression, to name a few – must be ruled out.

Napping on demand

Overnight polysomnography and a multiple sleep latency test (MSLT) may be performed. During the MSLT, the person tries to take four to five 20-minute naps every 2 hours throughout the day as his EEG, electro-oculogram and chin electromyogram are recorded. After these naps, the time he required to fall asleep (sleep latency) is averaged. In narcolepsy, sleep latency usually is less than 8 minutes.

The diagnosis of narcolepsy is confirmed when the person meets the criteria listed in the *DSM-IV-TR*. (See *Diagnostic criteria: Narcolepsy*, page 442.)

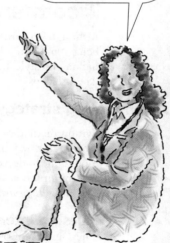

If someone you know is a narcoleptic, you might see him with his arm raised like this after suffering from an episode of sleep paralysis.

Diagnostic criteria: Narcolepsy

The diagnosis of narcolepsy is confirmed when the person meets these criteria from the *Diagnostic and Statistical Manual of Mental Disorders*, Fourth Edition, Text Revision.

- The person experiences irresistible daily attacks of refreshing sleep for a period of at least 3 months.
- One or both of the following criteria are present:
  - cataplexy (brief episodes of sudden bilateral muscle tone loss, most often associated with intense emotion)
  - recurrent intrusions of rapid-eye-movement sleep into the transition between sleep and wakefulness (indicated by hallucinations either during sleep onset or awakening from sleep or during sleep paralysis at the beginning or end of sleep episodes).
- The disturbance doesn't result from direct physiological effects of a substance or another general medical condition.

Treatment

Although no cure exists for narcolepsy, symptoms can be controlled with behavioural and pharmacological interventions. Behavioural interventions include lifestyle adjustments, such as regulating sleep schedules and taking daytime naps.

A stimulating strategy

Symptomatic treatment is focused on excessive somnolence and cataplexy. The doctor may prescribe CNS stimulants (such as methylphenidate or modafinil) to decrease daytime sleepiness and antidepressants (such as clomipramine or fluoxetine) to reduce cataplectic attacks. (See *Modafinil: Narcolepsy treatment*, page 443.)

Nursing interventions

These interventions may be appropriate for a person with narcolepsy:
- Review recommended lifestyle changes.
- Help the person plan and maintain a regular sleep schedule.
- Teach him about the purpose, administration and side effects of prescribed drugs.
- Monitor for side effects.

Primary hypersomnia

Primary hypersomnia is a condition of excessive sleepiness characterised by either prolonged sleep periods at night or daytime sleep episodes occurring nearly every day. During long periods of drowsiness, the person may exhibit

Meds matters

Modafinil: Narcolepsy treatment

A central nervous system stimulant that promotes wakefulness and alertness, modafinil is used to prevent excessive daytime sleepiness in people with narcolepsy. When taken as directed, it doesn't interfere with night-time sleep.

Modafinil seems to be safe, effective and well tolerated. It's less likely than traditional stimulants (such as amphetamines and methylphenidate) to cause jitteriness, anxiety, excessive motor activity or a rebound effect. The drug may cause mild psychological dependence.

How it works

Modafinil is a central alpha-1 adrenergic agonist that induces wakefulness partly through its action in the brain's hypothalamus. It acts selectively through the brain's sleep–awake centre, stimulating the person only when stimulation is required and avoiding the highs and lows caused by other stimulants such as amphetamine.

How it's given

The standard dosage is 200 mg/day, given as a single dose in the morning.

Side effects typically are mild and may include headache, anxiety, nervousness, insomnia, nausea and infection.

Nursing considerations

- Teach the person about the drug, including the dosage, purpose, administration and side effects.
- Monitor the person for side effects.
- Instruct the person not to drive or operate other complex machinery until he knows how the drug affects his ability to function.
- Advise him to avoid alcohol while using this drug.
- Tell him to call the doctor if he develops a skin rash, hives or an allergic reaction.
- Know that people with severe hepatic impairment should receive one-half of the standard dosage.
- Be aware that elderly people may need a decreased dosage.
- Don't give this drug to people who have a history of cardiovascular disease or are taking oral contraceptives, cyclosporine, theophylline, diazepam, phenytoin, warfarin or propranolol.

Even after 12 hours of sleep, a person with hypersomnia may feel drowsy during the day.

automatic behaviour, acting in a semicontrolled fashion. He may have trouble meeting morning obligations, frequently arriving late.

Symptomatic categories

Primary hypersomnia can be monosymptomatic or polysymptomatic.
- In the *monosymptomatic* form, the person has isolated excessive daytime sleepiness unrelated to abnormal nocturnal awakenings.
- The *polysymptomatic* form involves abnormally long night-time sleep and signs of sleep 'drunkenness' (difficulty awakening completely, confusion, disorientation, poor motor coordination and slowness)

Kleine–Levin syndrome

Kleine–Levin syndrome refers to recurrent episodes of hypersomnia, or excessive sleep. This condition is characterised by periods of hypersomnia that last from days to weeks and recur several times a year. Between episodes, the person has normal sleep requirements without excessive daytime sleepiness.

Interesting accompaniments

Some people with Kleine–Levin syndrome experience hypersexuality, compulsive overeating, irritability, impulsive behaviour, depersonalisation, hallucinations, depression and confusion. The cause of this rare disorder isn't known.

on awakening. Usually, the person falls asleep easily at night and is able to stay asleep – but seems out of sorts or even combative on awakening in the morning.

Teenage Rip van Winkles

A recurrent form of hypersomnia called *Kleine–Levin syndrome* affects mostly adolescents. (See *Kleine–Levin syndrome*.)

Prevalence

The prevalence of primary hypersomnia in the general population isn't known. In sleep disorder clinics, an estimated 5–10% of people are diagnosed with this disorder.

Primary hypersomnia usually affects adolescents and young adults between ages 15 and 30.

Causes

Based on the underlying cause of the disorder, experts have identified three possible subgroups of primary hypersomnia.

Family history and autonomic dysfunction

People with subgroup 1 have a family history of hypersomnia, along with clinical findings that suggest autonomic nervous system dysfunction – headache, syncope, orthostatic hypotension and peripheral vasoconstriction (indicated by cold hands and feet).

Viral infection with neurological symptoms

People with subgroup 2 have a history of a viral infection that causes neurological symptoms, such as Guillain–Barré syndrome, infectious mononucleosis or atypical viral pneumonia. Even after the infectious disease resolves, they continue to need significantly more night-time sleep and to feel very tired.

A viral infection with neurological symptoms has been linked to some cases of hypersomnia.

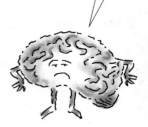

Viral lassitude

Although initially fatigued, people subsequently have trouble differentiating fatigue from sleepiness. To fight tiredness, they nap and eventually complain of excessive daytime sleepiness. Cerebrospinal fluid analysis often shows a moderate increase in the number of lymphocytes, along with protein elevations.

Unknown cause

People with subgroup 3 lack a history of viral infection or a family history of the disorder. The cause of their hypersomnia isn't known.

Signs and symptoms

In people with primary hypersomnia, assessment findings typically include:
- excessive sleepiness on a daily basis
- daytime napping without feeling refreshed
- long night-time sleeping (8–12 hours).

Many people also complain of irritability, mild depression, memory loss, headache, poor concentration, impaired performance, fainting episodes and dizziness on standing (from orthostatic hypotension). A few report hypnagogic hallucinations and sleep paralysis.

Diagnosis

Physical examination, a complete blood cell count and thyroid-stimulating hormone tests may rule out other possible causes of excessive sleepiness or prolonged nocturnal sleep, including:
- OSAS
- circadian rhythm sleep disorders
- narcolepsy
- thyroid abnormalities
- chronic pain
- CNS disorders, damage or malfunction
- viral infection
- primary depression
- medication withdrawal
- adverse drug effects.

Out like a light

Polysomnography typically reveals a short sleep latency, long sleep duration and a normal sleep pattern.

The diagnosis of primary hypersomnia is confirmed if the person meets the criteria listed in the *DSM-IV-TR*. (See *Diagnostic criteria: Primary hypersomnia*, page 446.)

Diagnostic criteria: Primary hypersomnia

The diagnosis of hypersomnia is confirmed when the person meets these criteria from the *Diagnostic and Statistical Manual of Mental Disorders*, Fourth Edition, Text Revision.

Sleep disturbance pattern

- The person's predominant complaint is excessive sleepiness lasting at least 1 month (or less if recurrent), indicated by prolonged sleep episodes or daytime sleep episodes that occur almost daily.
- Excessive sleepiness causes clinically significant distress or impairment in social, occupational or other important areas of functioning.

Other features

- Excessive sleepiness isn't better explained by insomnia or an inadequate amount of sleep. Also,

it doesn't occur only during the course of another sleep disorder.
- The disturbance doesn't occur solely during the course of another psychiatric disorder.
- It doesn't result from direct physiological effects of a substance or a general medical condition.

Recurrent hypersomnia is diagnosed if the person has periods of excessive sleepiness lasting at least 3 days, several times a year for at least 2 years.

Treatment

Treatment focuses on relieving symptoms and may include behavioural approaches, sleep hygiene techniques and pharmacological interventions.

Awake and wired

Drugs used to treat primary hypersomnia include antidepressants and stimulants (such as pemoline, modafinil, methylphenidate and dextroamphetamine). Stimulants are the only drugs that have brought relief (although it's only partial). Typically, the person is maintained on daily stimulants, with the dosage titrated so that he can stay alert during the day.

Java jolt therapy

Self-medicating with caffeine is probably the most commonly tried treatment. Caffeine temporarily improves psychomotor performance and increases alertness.
- Teach the person about prescribed drugs; include their purpose, administration and side effects.
- Caution him about driving or using dangerous machinery when drowsy. Help him develop an alternate plan, such as taking public transportation or car-pooling.
- Inform the person that excessive caffeine may cause anxiety, irritability, jitteriness and tolerance.

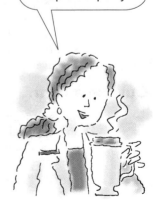

Many people with hypersomnia rely on caffeine to keep them perky.

Primary insomnia

The most common sleep disorder, primary insomnia encompasses many types of problems – difficulty falling asleep, sleeping too lightly, frequent awakenings during the night, inability to fall back to sleep once awakened and waking up in the early morning and being unable to fall back to sleep. These problems aren't attributable to another sleep disorder or mental health disorder, a general medical condition or substance use.

Obsessing over insomnia

It is important to know that nearly everyone has problems sleeping at some time or other and it is thought that a third of people in the UK have bouts of insomnia.

Insomnia can be acute or chronic. With chronic insomnia, the person may become preoccupied with getting enough sleep. The more he tries to sleep, the greater his sense of frustration and distress – and the more elusive sleep becomes.

Consequences

Insomnia commonly leads to daytime drowsiness that causes poor concentration, memory impairments, difficulty coping with minor problems and reduced ability to enjoy family and social relationships.

You snooze, you lose

Insomniacs are more than twice as likely as the general population to have a fatigue-related motor vehicle accident. Those who sleep less than 5 hours per night may have a higher death rate, too.

Prevalence

The condition is diagnosed in approximately 15% of people who are referred to sleep disorder centres after other conditions have been ruled out. Prevalence increases with age and is greater in women.

Causes

Acute insomnia often stems from a specific event – a physical or emotional stressor (such as illness), a significant life change (such as divorce) or an environmental disturbance that makes sleep difficult (such as noise, unwanted light or an uncomfortable room temperature).

You booze, you may not snooze

Chronic insomnia may result from either a single factor or multiple factors. Everyday stress and anxiety, caffeine consumption and alcohol use are the biggest culprits.

Risk factors for developing chronic insomnia include:
• history of being a light sleeper
• tendency towards easy arousal at night

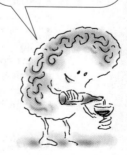

Alcohol, caffeine and anxiety are the main culprits in chronic insomnia.

Memory jogger

Typical findings in people with INSOMNIA

I   Intermittent wakefulness

N   Not able to fall asleep easily

S   Stressed by the inability to fall asleep

O   Overly concerned with the consequences of not sleeping

M   May medicate with inappropriate drugs

N   Needs frequent daytime naps

I   Irritable

A   Attention and concentration problems

• inability to fall asleep or stay asleep after an initial stressful situation is resolved
• conversion of feelings into physical symptoms rather than expressing them outright or dealing with them constructively.

Signs and symptoms

A person with primary insomnia may report or exhibit:
• difficulty falling asleep
• difficulty staying asleep
• waking up too early in the morning
• inability to fall back to sleep once awakened
• nonrefreshing sleep
• daytime fatigue and lack of energy
• haggard appearance
• irritability
• short attention span
• poor concentration
• anxious concern over his health
• interpersonal, social or occupational problems stemming from anxiety over sleeplessness
• inappropriate use of sedative-hypnotic drugs, alcohol or caffeine.
   (See *Key questions to ask when assessing for insomnia*, page 449.)

Diagnosis

Primary insomnia may be diagnosed from the person's history and physical findings. Polysomnography can rule out other sleep disorders such as

Advice from the experts

Key questions to ask when assessing for insomnia

When assessing a person who complains of insomnia, ask the following questions:

- When did the problem begin?
- Do you have a medical or mental health problem that might affect your ability to sleep?
- What's your sleep environment like? Is it dark? Quiet? Bright? Noisy? Does it have a comfortable room temperature?
- What time do you usually go to bed?
- What time do you usually get up in the morning on weekdays? On weekends?
- Do you drink alcohol or smoke? Are you taking prescribed medications? Nonprescription preparations? Street drugs?
- What's your typical work schedule?
- How do you feel the day after a poor night's sleep?

Family inquiries

If possible, ask the person's spouse or other family members if the person snores or has unusual limb movements when he sleeps.

OSAS. In primary insomnia, polysomnography usually shows increased stage 1 sleep and decreased slow-wave sleep.

Depression must also be ruled out because insomnia is a common symptom of depression.

Sleep scribblings

To aid diagnosis, the doctor may ask the person to keep a sleep diary for 1–2 weeks. (See *Dear Sleep Diary*, pages 450 and 451.)

The diagnosis of insomnia is confirmed if the person meets the criteria listed in the *DSM-IV-TR*. (See *Diagnostic criteria: Primary insomnia*, page 452.)

Treatment

Treatment for primary insomnia may involve relaxation techniques, improved sleep hygiene, behavioural interventions, cognitive therapy, alternative and complementary measures or pharmacological options.

Nipping it in the bud

With acute insomnia, the need for treatment is based on the severity of daytime symptoms and duration of the episode. A person who suffers brief episodes of insomnia should be monitored for prolonged negative effects because untreated acute insomnia can lead to a chronic condition.

Recording bedtimes, awakening times and other sleep-related information can help the doctor diagnose a person with insomnia.

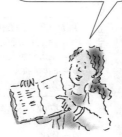

Dear Sleep Diary

A sleep diary, such as the sample one shown here, can aid the diagnosis and treatment of insomnia. The diary provides a night-by-night account of the person's sleep schedule and perception of sleep and serves as a baseline for monitoring treatment efficacy. In the diary, the person records such information as:

- bedtime of the previous night
- total sleep time
- time elapsed before sleep onset

- number of awakenings
- morning awakening time
- total time awake

- use of sleep medications
- subjective rating of sleep quality and daytime symptoms.

Sample sleep diary

Name: *Willa Selby*

	Date	Mon 5/12	Tues 5/13
Complete in a.m.	**Bedtime (previous night)**	11:00 p.m.	10:45 p.m.
	Awakening time	7:30 a.m.	7:45 a.m.
	Estimated time to sleep onset (previous night)	45 minutes	1 hour
	Estimated number of awakenings and total time awake (previous night)	6 times/total of 3 hours	5 times/total of 4 hours
	Estimated amount of sleep obtained (previous night)	4 1/2 hours	5 hours
Complete in p.m.	**Naps (time and duration)**	4:00 p.m. for 30 minutes	4:30 p.m. for 30 minutes
	Alcoholic drinks (number and time)	2 drinks at 8:00 p.m.	1 drink at 9:00 p.m.
	Stresses experienced today	Car wouldn't start, argued with boss	none
	Rate how you felt today 1—Very tired/sleepy 2—Somewhat tired/sleepy 3—Fairly alert 4—Wide awake	1	2
	Irritabiliy 1—Not at all 5—Very	5 (very)	3
	Medications	Benadryl	Benadryl

Encourage the person to complete the diary each morning, using estimates rather than exact times to make the process less disruptive to sleep.

Wed 5/14	Thu 5/15	Fri 5/16
11:00 p.m.		
7:30 a.m.		
30 minutes		
6 times/total of 3 hours		
4 1/2 hours		
4:00 p.m. for 45 minutes		
2 drinks at 8:00 p.m.		
argued with a friend		
1		
4		
Benadryl		

Diagnostic criteria: Primary insomnia

The diagnosis of primary insomnia is confirmed when the person meets these criteria from the *Diagnostic and Statistical Manual of Mental Disorders*, Fourth Edition, Text Revision.

- The person's predominant complaint is difficulty falling or staying asleep or nonrestorative sleep, lasting at least 1 month.
- The sleep disturbance or associated daytime fatigue causes clinically significant distress or impairment in social, occupational or other important areas of functioning.
- The disturbance doesn't occur only during the course of narcolepsy, breathing-related sleep disorder, circadian rhythm sleep disorder or a parasomnia (such as sleepwalking, night terrors or bed-wetting).
- It doesn't occur exclusively during the course of another psychiatric disorder.
- The disturbance doesn't result from direct physiological effects of a substance or a general medical condition.

Relaxation techniques

Because many insomniacs display high levels of physiological and cognitive arousal (both at night and during the day), relaxation-based interventions may provide relief. Techniques that help deactivate the arousal system include progressive muscle relaxation, abdominal or deep breathing, biofeedback and imagery training.

Sleep hygiene

For some people, insomnia responds well to simple lifestyle changes, sometimes called *sleep hygiene*. Such changes include going to bed at the same time every night, optimising sleeping conditions and avoiding naps during the day. (See *Getting hygienic about sleep*, page 453.)

Behavioural interventions

Behavioural interventions aim to change maladaptive sleep habits, reduce autonomic arousal and alter dysfunctional beliefs and attitudes. A wide range of behavioural techniques may be used to treat chronic primary insomnia.

Stimulus control

Stimulus control centres on the theory that insomnia represents a learned response to bedtime and bedroom cues.

Bedroom behaviour

Give the person these instructions:
- Go to bed only when sleepy.
- Use the bed and bedroom only for sleep (or sex).
- If you can't fall asleep or stay asleep, get out of bed and go to another room. Return to bed only when you feel sleepy.

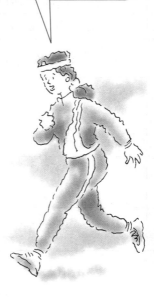

A person who's using paradoxical intention does the opposite of what she would usually do to get to sleep – like jogging.

Advice from the experts

Getting hygienic about sleep

For most people with insomnia, simple lifestyle measures – termed *sleep hygiene* – are used first. When teaching a person about sleep hygiene, cover the following do's and don'ts.

Sleep-promoting measures

- Use the bed only for sleep and sex – not for reading, watching television or working.
- Establish a regular bedtime and a regular time for getting up in the morning. Stick to these times even on weekends and on holiday.
- Exercise in the evening. Energy levels bottom out a few hours after exercise, promoting sleep at that time.
- Take a hot bath 90 minutes to 2 hours before bedtime. This alters core body temperature and helps you fall asleep more easily.
- During the 30 minutes before bedtime, do something relaxing, such as reading, meditating or taking a leisurely walk.
- Keep the bedroom quiet, dark, relatively cool and well ventilated.
- Eat dinner 4–5 hours before bedtime. At bedtime, a light snack (low in sugar and calories) may promote sleep.
- Spend 30 minutes in the sun each day. (However, be sure to take precautions against overexposure.)
- If you don't fall asleep after 15 or 20 minutes, get up and go into another room. Read or perform a quiet activity, using dim lighting, until you feel sleepy.
- If your bed partner distracts you, consider moving to another bedroom or the sofa for a few nights. (One

study showed that sleeping alone is more restful than sleeping with another person.)

What not to do

- Don't use the bedroom for work, reading or watching television.
- Avoid large meals before bedtime.
- Don't look at the clock. Obsessing over time makes it harder to sleep.
- Avoid naps, especially in the evening.
- Don't drink a large amount of fluid after dinner, or the need to urinate may disturb your sleep.
- Avoid exercising close to bedtime because this may make you more alert.
- Avoid alcohol and caffeine in the evening.
- Don't take a bath just before bedtime because this could increase your alertness.
- Don't engage in highly stimulating activities before bed, such as watching a frightening movie or playing competitive computer games.
- Quit smoking because nicotine's effects may contribute to sleep loss.
- Avoid tossing and turning in bed. Instead, get up and read or listen to relaxing music. However, don't watch television because it emits too bright of a light.

- Awaken and get out of bed at the same time every morning regardless of how much sleep you got.
- Avoid naps.

Paradoxical intention

In paradoxical intention, the person does the opposite of what he wants, sometimes taking it to an extreme. For instance, instead of going through activities that promote sleep, he prepares himself for staying awake and doing something energetic. If worry is a factor in insomnia, he may deliberately intensify the worrying.

Biofeedback

In biofeedback, the person is connected to a device that measures brain waves and other body functions. Then he's given feedback so that he can learn to recognise certain states of tension or sleep stages – and either avoid or repeat these states voluntarily.

Sleep restriction

Sleep restriction creates a mild state of sleep deprivation, which may promote more rapid sleep onset and more 'efficient' sleep. The person limits the amount of time spent in bed so as to increase the percentage of time spent asleep.

Bedtime amendments

To maintain a consistent sleep–awake pattern, he usually alters his bedtime rather than his rising time. However, time in bed shouldn't be reduced to less than 5 hours a day. Naps aren't allowed (except in older adults).

Cognitive therapy

Cognitive therapy helps the person identify his dysfunctional beliefs and attitudes about sleep (such as 'I'll never fall asleep') and replace them with positive ones. Changing beliefs and attitudes can decrease the anticipatory anxiety that interferes with sleep. Cognitive therapy also focuses on actions intended to change behaviour.

Alternative and complementary therapies

Alternative and complementary therapies that may be used to treat insomnia include acupressure, acupuncture, aromatherapy, massage, biofeedback, chiropractic, homoeopathy, light and dark therapy, meditation, reflexology, visualisation and yoga.

A mouthful of electromagnetic waves

Another technique, low-energy emission therapy, delivers electromagnetic waves through a mouthpiece. Early studies suggest that it may benefit some people.

Supplements to sleep by

Some people use herbal preparations (such as St. John's wort and chamomile), nutritional substances and other nonprescription preparations to treat insomnia. However, few of such products have been demonstrated to be safe and effective.

Dietary supplements sometimes recommended for insomnia relief include vitamins B_6, B_{12} and D. Some practitioners also recommend calcium and magnesium. Tryptophan may relieve insomnia in some people, but the person must be monitored for side effects. Melatonin may increase sleepiness and is currently undergoing clinical studies.

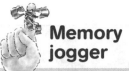

Memory jogger

Help your client DISCOVER ways to overcome sleep disorders.

D Define what may be causing the problem

I Identify changes in the person's sleep pattern

S State his understanding of 'good' sleep

C Calculate how many hours of sleep he needs

O Offer assistance on ways to promote sleep

V Venting his feelings about sleep problems can be therapeutic

E Educate the person about how sleep patterns change throughout life

R Review the negative effects of stress on sleep

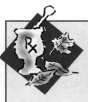

Meds matters

Pharmacological therapy for sleep disorders

This chart highlights several drugs used to treat sleep disorders. A person with insomnia may receive a benzodiazepine, such as temazepam or a nonbenzodiazepine hypnotic, such as zolpidem.

Drugs	Side effects	Contraindications	Nursing interventions
Temazepam	• Dizziness • Drowsiness • Lethargy • Orthostatic hypotension	• Pregnancy	• Teach the person about the drug's action, dosage and side effects. • Instruct the person not to take other medications unless the doctor approves. • Caution the person not to drink alcohol, drive a motor vehicle or operate machinery while under the influence of this drug. • Advise the person to change position slowly to avoid dizziness. • Inform the person that prolonged use isn't recommended.
Zolpidem	• Abdominal pain • Daytime drowsiness • Dizziness • GI disturbances • Headache • Nightmares	• Breast-feeding • Hepatic impairment • Pregnancy	• Teach the person about the drug's action, dosage and side effects. • Advise him not to take the drug with or immediately after a meal. • Caution the person against taking other medications unless the doctor approves. • Advise the person not to drink alcohol, drive a motor vehicle or operate machinery while under the influence of this drug. • Inform the person that tolerance may occur if this drug is taken for more than a few weeks.

Pharmacological options

If insomnia persists despite other measures, the doctor may recommend drug therapy. The most commonly prescribed drugs are short-acting sedative-hypnotics (primarily benzodiazepines), antidepressants and antihistamines. (See *Pharmacological therapy for sleep disorders*.)

Knockout pills

Sedative-hypnotics – usually temazepam and zolpidem – are commonly prescribed for short-term management of insomnia.

Both prescription and nonprescription antihistamines can be used for short-term management of insomnia. Side effects include daytime sedation, cognitive impairment and anticholinergic effects (for example, dry mouth, constipation or urinary retention). Tolerance may also occur.

Antidepressants may be given in low dosages – especially if the person has related mental health disorders or a history of substance abuse. However, some antidepressants can exacerbate other disorders, such as mania or restless leg syndrome, so the person should be monitored closely.

Nursing interventions

These nursing interventions may be appropriate for a person with primary insomnia:

• Provide teaching about prescribed medications, including the drug's purpose, administration and side effects. Inform the person that taking these drugs for more than a few weeks may lead to tolerance and withdrawal, making it even more difficult to sleep when he stops taking the drug.

• Monitor the person for drug side effects.

• Instruct the person in good sleep hygiene, such as maintaining regular bedtime and awakening times, avoiding naps and eliminating caffeine, alcohol and nicotine.

• Encourage him to practise relaxation routines, such as progressive muscle relaxation or meditation.

• Caution him about the possible dangers of using unproven therapies.

• Advise him to move the alarm clock away from the bed if it's distracting.

Memory jogger

Cover these basic TEACHING points to help your client get better sleep.

T Take prescribed sleep medications appropriately

E Eliminate caffeine, alcohol and nicotine at least 4 hours before bedtime

A Attend to adequate sleep hygiene

C Consider the effects of foods and fluids on sleep

H Have a consistent bedtime routine

I Initiate relaxation strategies before bedtime

N Nightmares and dreams that disrupt sleep must be addressed

G Get family support, as needed

Quick quiz

1. REM sleep is characterised by:
   A. light sleep.
   B. paralysis of the muscles.
   C. restricted eye movements.
   D. nonvivid dreams.

Answer: B. During REM sleep, many muscles are effectively paralysed so that the sleeper won't act out dreams. Eye movements are rapid.

2. NREM sleep is regulated by the:
   A. pons.
   B. hypothalamus.
   C. basal forebrain.
   D. amygdala.

Answer: C. The basal forebrain controls NREM sleep. The pons and the midbrain control REM sleep.

3. A classic feature of OSAS is:
   A. snoring.
   B. sneezing.
   C. early morning awakening.
   D. bursts of energy.

Answer: A. Snoring is a hallmark of OSAS. Sneezing, bursts of energy and early morning awakening aren't common in this disorder.

4. Primary treatments for circadian rhythm sleep disorders include all of the following except:
   A. chronotherapy.
   B. short-acting sedative-hypnotics.
   C. relaxation techniques.
   D. luminotherapy.

Answer: C. Relaxation techniques aren't used as primary treatments for circadian rhythm sleep disorders.

5. Cataplexy is a symptom of:
   A. REM sleep.
   B. primary hypersomnia.
   C. OSAS.
   D. narcolepsy.

Answer: D. Cataplexy – a condition marked by sudden attacks of bilateral muscle tone loss – occurs in narcolepsy.

6. 'Sleep drunkenness' is a common finding in people with:
A. primary insomnia.
B. primary hypersomnia.
C. narcolepsy.
D. alcoholism.

Answer: B. 'Sleep drunkenness' (difficulty awakening completely, confusion, disorientation and poor motor coordination) on awakening occurs in primary hypersomnia.

7. Information typically gathered in a sleep diary includes:
A. usual bedtime.
B. foods consumed before bedtime.
C. daily weights.
D. fluid consumption.

Answer: A. In a sleep diary, the person records sleep-related items, such as usual bedtime and awakening times, time elapsed before sleep onset, number of nightly awakenings and total time spent in sleep. Food and fluid consumption and daily weights aren't relevant.

Scoring

☆☆☆ If you answered all seven items correctly, stupendous! Your study of snoozing and snoring has succeeded beyond our wildest dreams!

☆☆ If you answered five or six items correctly, remarkable. Your solid grasp of sleep disorders should make for a sweet slumber tonight.

☆ If you answered fewer than five items correctly, consider this your wake-up call. Read the chapter again – but try not to doze off this time.

13 Sexual disorders

Just the facts

In this chapter, you'll learn:

♦ stages of sexual development

♦ phases of the sexual response cycle

♦ categories and definitions of sexual disorders

♦ causes, diagnosis and treatment of sexual disorders

♦ nursing interventions for service users with sexual disorders.

A look at sexual disorders

Sexuality is expressed not just in a person's appearance but also in his attitude, behaviours and relationships. Influenced by ongoing biophysical and psychosocial factors, sexuality starts to take shape during early childhood and is reshaped throughout life.

A sexual disorder can cause distress and anxiety for an individual who has it and strife in his intimate relationships. In 1999, a survey of people aged 18–59 found that 31% of the men and 43% of the women had experienced sexual dysfunction at some time.

Scrolling through sexual disorders

Sexual disorders described in the *Diagnostic and Statistical Manual of Mental Disorders*, Fourth Edition, Text Revision (*DSM-IV-TR*), include:
* paraphilias (such as exhibitionism and fetishism)
* sexual dysfunctions (such as orgasmic disorder and premature ejaculation)
* sexual pain disorders (such as dyspareunia)
* gender identity disorder.

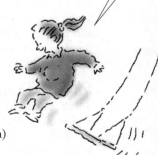

Dad's not gonna want to hear this, but my sexuality is already starting to take shape. Cowabunga!

Defining 'abnormal' sexual behaviour

The definition of 'abnormal' sexual behaviour depends largely on the cultural and historical context. Accepted norms of sexual behaviour and attitudes vary greatly within and among different cultures.

In the past, many people believed that the only 'normal' sexual behaviour was intercourse between heterosexual partners for procreation. Even masturbation was widely seen as a perversion and a potential cause of mental disorders. Until the 1970s, psychiatrists officially described homosexuality as abnormal.

Today, a much broader range of attitudes towards sexuality exists. Homosexuality is now widely regarded as a normal variant of sexuality, and masturbation is accepted as a normal sexual activity.

Other opinions on abnormality

Some authorities classify abnormal sexual behaviour as any behaviour that causes personal distress. Others view sexuality on a continuum from adaptive to maladaptive; in their view, normal sexuality is adaptive, whereas abnormal sexuality is maladaptive.

For example, sexual behaviour is maladaptive for an individual if it prevents him from reaching his goals and adapting to life's demands. It's maladaptive to society if it interferes with or disrupts social group functioning.

> Lighten up! Psychiatrists no longer consider homosexuality abnormal.

Stages of sexual development

Human beings progress through various phases of sexual and psychosexual development, which begins in infancy. Characteristic physical attributes and feelings related to sex develop during each phase.

Parents and puritans

Crucial factors affecting sexual development include early role models, religious and cultural teachings, early sexual experiences and parental attitudes towards sex. A parent's puritanical rejection of sexuality, for example, can produce guilt and shame in a child, subsequently inhibiting his capacity to enjoy sex and develop healthy relationships as an adult. Similarly, a child who's treated with cruelty, hostility or rejection may become sexually maladjusted.

Infancy to age 5

The combination of the mother's X chromosome and the father's X or Y chromosome creates either a male or a female child. Gender assignment of a healthy infant is reinforced by family members' interactions with the infant, which influence and reinforce either masculine or feminine behaviour. For example, an infant girl may be rocked gently while an infant boy is played with more roughly. Young girls receive dolls as gifts; boys receive sports-related items and toy cars. By age 2, most children have a clear sense of their gender identity. (See *Components of sexual identity*, page 461.)

Components of sexual identity

Sexual identity encompasses four components – biosexual identity, gender role, gender identity and sexual orientation or preference.

Biosexual identity

Biosexual identity is the physical state of being either male or female. It results from genetic and hormonal influences.

Gender role

Gender role is the outward expression of one's gender – the behaviours, feelings and attitudes appropriate for either a male or female. Labels attached to gender role include masculine or feminine, traditional or conforming, and gender-neutral. Learned by the individual, gender role is influenced by culture, religion, schools, peers and social messages.

Gender identity

Gender identity is a person's private experience of gender – the sense of oneself as being male, female or ambivalent. It's usually based on physical features, parental attitudes and expectations and psychological and social pressures.

Various theories explain how gender identity develops.

- Biological theory proposes that gender identity develops in utero and contributes to the foetus's anatomic development.
- Psychodynamic theory sees gender identity as evolving from role-modelling, during which the child learns to identify with the same-sex parent.
- Social learning theory holds that gender identity is learned and reinforced by environment and social expectations.
- Cognitive theory holds that a child can mentally construct male or female behaviour and tell these behaviours apart.

Sexual orientation or preference

Sexual orientation or preference refers to a person's feelings about his or her sexual attraction and erotic potential.

- Heterosexuality is marked by sexual arousal from or sexual activity with people of the opposite gender.
- Homosexuality refers to sexual arousal from or sexual activity with people of the same gender.
- Bisexuality is characterised by sexual arousal from or sexual activity with both males and females.

Age of discovery

Between ages 1 and 3, children start to observe body differences and show an interest in bathroom habits. Sexual discovery starts between ages 3 and 5. Curious and explorative, young children commonly ask where babies come from and what their sex organs are for. They're accepting and straightforward about sex, and may comment on the differences between genders. At this age, they learn that touching feels good. They also may receive nonverbal messages about sex.

A topic apart

Towards the end of this stage, children pick up cues from others that sex is a 'different' topic. They may become shy, ask fewer questions about sex and show a desire for privacy about their bodies.

Ages 5–10

Children aged 5–10 may think in terms of 'good' and 'bad' parts of their bodies. Aware of bodily functions and how these relate to sex, they're same-sex oriented.

Outwardly, they may seem unconcerned about sex or uncomfortable or apprehensive about discussing it. However, they're actually quite interested in it.

Kids educating each other

Children receive verbal or nonverbal cues from the adults around them that they shouldn't talk about sex, so they may avoid the topic. However, many of them exchange information about sex with their peers. Also, masturbation and sexual exploration are common at this stage.

Ages 10–14

Puberty begins at about age 11 for girls and age 12 for boys. Young adolescents may be confused, embarrassed and self-conscious about their bodily changes and may be uncomfortable with, or unaware of, their social roles.

Sexual responsiveness develops during this stage, as does the ability to reproduce. In response to peer pressure and other influences, some young adolescents become sexually active.

Ages 14 and older

From age 14 onwards, children become more adult physically, emotionally and socially – but they're easily influenced by peer pressure and media messages. They want to be in control of themselves and are forming their identities and self-concepts.

Active but uncertain

Approximately one-half of adolescents over age 14 are sexually active or experienced; however, they're still uncertain about sex. They may feel that it's a part of the adult world.

Adults

By adulthood, sex and sexuality are a part of a person's life. An estimated 90% of adults are sexually active. Adults hold views on sexuality that have been influenced by society and its standards of normal behaviour.

Human sexual response cycle

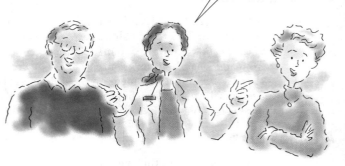

The sexual response cycle refers to the progressive mental, physical and emotional changes that occur during sexual stimulation. Although the sexual response is highly individualised, nearly everyone experiences certain basic physiological changes.

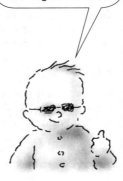

Mum and Dad better get their answers ready! When I turn 3, I'm gonna start asking where babies come from and what my sex organs are for.

By adulthood, sex and sexuality are a part of a person's life. An estimated 90% of adults are sexually active.

The sex scientists

Different researchers have proposed various models of the sexual response cycle, describing three, four or five distinct phases. For example, Helen Singer Kaplan's model encompasses three stages – desire, excitement and orgasm. William Masters and Virginia Johnson describe four phases – excitement (arousal), plateau, orgasm and resolution. Using instruments that monitor changes in heart rate and muscle tension, Masters and Johnson identified the physiological changes that take place during each phase.

Currently, many experts conceptualise a five-phase cycle that begins with desire.

Desire phase

The desire phase is marked by a strong urge for sexual stimulation and satisfaction, either by oneself or with another person. Cultural and societal values affect the range of stimulation that provokes sexual desire.

Potential sexual partners may communicate desire either verbally or through behaviour and body language (for example, flirting). Such communication may be subtle and easily misread. (See *Flirting across cultures*.)

Desire is mental, not physical. Without further mental or physical stimulation, the desire phase may not progress to sexual excitement.

Nice – but not always needed

Desire doesn't have to be present for sex to occur. For example, a couple trying to conceive a child may have intercourse even on days when they lack sexual desire. Also, a person can respond to a partner's sexual advances even if he or she doesn't feel desire to begin with.

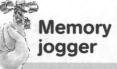

Memory jogger

Think DEAR to remember the main phases of the sexual response cycle.

D Desire

E Excitement

A Attains orgasm

R Resolution

Bridging the gap

Flirting across cultures

In different cultures, behaviours meant to communicate sexual desire may vary greatly along gender lines. Some cultures disapprove of women expressing overt communication of their sexual desire – but expect such communication from men. In other cultures, women have more leeway to be flirtatious.

Culturally defined behaviours can also influence perceptions of what is – and what isn't – flirting. In some cultures, especially Latin American, Southern European and Arabian cultures, people tend to stand relatively close to each other and make frequent physical contact. British people might misinterpret this behaviour as flirting.

In other cultures, such as the American, Australian and East Asian cultures, people tend to stand farther away and make less physical contact. Someone who isn't aware of these social customs might misconstrue them as a lack of romantic interest – even when such interest is present.

Excitement or arousal phase

The excitement or arousal phase prepares both partners for intercourse. Muscle tension increases, the heart rate quickens, the skin becomes flushed or blotchy (called *sexual flush*) and the nipples grow hard or erect.

Congested, lubricated and swollen

Vasocongestion begins during this phase, causing the female's clitoris, vagina and labia minora to swell. The vaginal walls start to produce a lubricating fluid, the uterus and breasts enlarge and the pubococcygeal muscle surrounding the vaginal opening tightens.

In the male, the penis becomes erect, the testes become elevated and swollen, the scrotal sac tightens and the Cowper's glands secrete a lubricating fluid.

Plateau

With continued stimulation (especially stroking and rubbing of the erogenous zones or sexual intercourse) during full arousal, the plateau stage may be reached. Actually, a person may achieve, lose and regain a plateau several times without orgasm occurring.

During the plateau stage, the heart and respiratory rates and blood pressure rise further, sexual flush deepens and muscle tension increases. A sense of impending orgasm occurs. In the female, the clitoris withdraws, vaginal lubrication increases, the labia continue to swell and the areolae enlarge. The lower vagina narrows and tightens.

In the male, the ridge of the glans penis becomes more prominent, the Cowper's glands secrete pre-ejaculatory fluid and the testes rise closer to the body.

Orgasm phase

The orgasm phase is the peak of sexual excitement. Physiological changes include involuntary muscle contractions, elevated heart rate and blood pressure, rapid oxygen intake, sphincter muscle contraction and sudden, forceful release of sexual tension.

Describing the indescribable

Orgasm is the shortest phase of the sexual response cycle, typically lasting just a few seconds. (It may be slightly longer in women.) For men, orgasm usually climaxes with the ejaculation of semen. For women, orgasm involves rhythmic muscle contractions of the uterus, which puts pressure on the penis and promotes male orgasm. Unless a sexual dysfunction is present, orgasm is intensely pleasurable for both sexes.

It's getting hot in here! I'm glad I'm wearing clothes so that no one can see my sexual flush.

If this were an old movie, you'd see a volcano erupting or a wave crashing on the beach right about now.

Resolution phase

During the resolution phase, the body returns to its normal, unexcited state. The heart and respiratory rates slow, blood pressure decreases and muscle tone slackens. Swollen and erect body parts return to normal, and skin flushing disappears. Some of these changes occur rapidly, whereas others take longer. This phase is marked by a general sense of well-being and enhanced intimacy.

Refractory period

For a male, the resolution phase includes a refractory period during which he can't reach orgasm – although he may be able to maintain a partial or full erection. This period lasts a few minutes to several days, depending on such factors as age and frequency of sexual activity.

Phase fluctuation

Many females, in contrast, can return rapidly to the orgasmic phase with minimal stimulation. Some, in fact, may experience continued orgasms for up to 1 hour.

Paraphilias

Paraphilias are complex psychosexual disorders marked by sexual urges, fantasies or behaviours that centre on:

- inanimate objects (such as clothing)
- suffering or humiliation
- children or other nonconsenting individuals.

Certain unusual psychosexual behaviours are similar to paraphilias but aren't officially designated as such. (See *Paraphilia-related disorders*.)

Paraphilia-related disorders

Some sexual behaviours are similar to paraphilias but don't fall into the main classifications of the *Diagnostic and Statistical Manual of Mental Disorders*, Fourth Edition, Text Revision. These behaviours include:

- *compulsive masturbation*, in which masturbation is the primary sexual outlet, even if the person has a stable intimate relationship
- *protracted promiscuity*, a pattern of repeated sexual conquests in which the person can't maintain a monogamous relationship despite a desire to do so
- *pornography dependency*, a repetitive pattern involving the use of pornographic materials, such as magazines, videos and pornographic websites
- *telephone sex*, a dependence on discussing sex over the telephone to achieve arousal
- *severe sexual desire*, in which a person's excessive sexual demands burden the partner and interfere with intimate relationships
- *use of sexual accessories*, marked by the repetitive use of sex 'toys' (such as vibrators) or, in some cases, drugs (such as cocaine or nitrate inhalants) exclusively for sexual arousal.

Myth busters

Puncturing some paraphilia myths

Like other sexual topics, paraphilias aren't well understood by the public – and even by some health care professionals. Here are some examples.

Myth: Exhibitionism is the act of masturbating in front of peers or family members.

Reality: Exhibitionism is an intense sexual urge to expose one's genitals to an unsuspecting person. Masturbation may occur during an exhibitionist act.

Myth: Paedophilia is defined as exhibitionism in front of a prepubescent child.

Reality: Paedophilia is defined as having sexually arousing fantasies, sexual urges or behaviours involving sexual activity with a prepubescent child.

Myth: Most sexual assaults on children are committed by strangers.

Reality: A study conducted from 1999 to 2001 found that nearly one-half of sexual assaults on children were committed by relatives and the other one-half by acquaintances (such as a neighbour or teacher). Only 4% were committed by strangers.

Forbidden fruits

All paraphilias involve an attraction to a nonsanctioned source of sexual satisfaction. The source may be a behaviour, as with exhibitionism or sadism, or a forbidden object of attraction, as with paedophilia or fetishism.

Paraphilias commonly involve sexual arousal and orgasm, usually achieved through masturbation and fantasy. (See *Puncturing some paraphilia myths*.) In most people with these disorders, the paraphiliac urge, fantasy or behaviour is always present, though its frequency and intensity may vary. Usually, a paraphilia is chronic and lifelong, although it may diminish with age.

Like other mental disorders, paraphilias may worsen during times of increased psychological stress, when other mental disorders are present, or when opportunities to engage in the paraphilia become more available.

Pinning down prevalence

Reliable statistics on the prevalence of paraphilias are hard to come by. These disorders are rarely diagnosed in clinical settings – most likely because people with paraphilias are secretive about them. Although some experts believe paraphilias are relatively rare, large commercial markets in paraphiliac pornography and paraphernalia suggest otherwise.

In clinics specialising in paraphilia treatment, the most commonly seen disorders include paedophilia, voyeurism and exhibitionism. Sexual masochism and sexual sadism are much less common.

The majority of paraphiliacs are males. Sexual masochists are the exception; female masochists outnumber male masochists by 20 to 1.

> For some people, the paraphilia is destined to diminish as they get older.

Criminal compulsions

Some paraphilias are crimes in many jurisdictions. Those that involve or harm another person – particularly paedophilia, exhibitionism, voyeurism, frotteurism and sexual sadism – are commonly considered criminal acts, leading to arrest and possible imprisonment.

Exhibitionists, paedophiles and voyeurs make up the majority of apprehended sex offenders. Sex offences against children, as in paedophilia, constitute a significant portion of reported criminal sex acts.

Specific paraphilias

The *DSM-IV-TR* recognises eight paraphilias. This chapter discusses four of them in detail. For information on the other four, see *Learning about other paraphilias*, page 468.

Exhibitionism

One of the most common paraphilias, exhibitionism is marked by sexual fantasies, urges or behaviours involving surprise exposure of the male genitals to strangers – primarily female passersby in public places. The behaviour is usually limited to genital exposure, with no harmful advances or assaults made towards the victim. The exhibitionist is considered more of a nuisance than an actual danger.

Exhibitionism has three characteristic features:
• It's typically performed by men for unknown women.
• It occurs in a place where sexual intercourse is impossible such as a crowded shopping centre.
• It's meant to be shocking; otherwise, it loses its power to produce sexual arousal in the paraphiliac.

Exhibitionism is the most prominent sexual offence leading to arrest, accounting for approximately one-third of sexual crimes.

Post-40 fadeout

Exhibitionism usually begins during adolescence and continues into adulthood. Although it may be a lifelong problem if untreated, it commonly becomes less severe by about age 40.

Fetishism

Fetishism is characterised by sexual fantasies, urges or behaviours that involve the use of a fetish – a nonhuman object or a nonsexual part of the body – to produce or enhance sexual arousal.

Fetishism may involve a partner. Sometimes, focusing on certain parts of the body, such as the feet, hair or ears, can become a fetish. In some cases, the person can achieve sexual gratification only when using the fetish. Usually, fetishes begin during adolescence and persist into adulthood.

Learning about other paraphilias

In addition to the paraphilias described in this chapter, the *Diagnostic and Statistical Manual of Mental Disorders, Fourth Edition, Text Revision* (*DSM-IV-TR*), provides diagnostic criteria for four other paraphilias – frotteurism, sexual masochism, sexual sadism and voyeurism. Rare paraphilias also exist.

Frotteurism

A person with frotteurism becomes sexually aroused from touching or rubbing against a nonconsenting person. For example, he may rub his genitals against a woman's thigh or fondle her breasts. The behaviour frequently occurs in crowded places, where it's easier to avoid detection. Frotteurism is most common between ages 15 and 25.

Sexual masochism

With sexual masochism, a person gets sexual gratification from being physically or emotionally abused. The term masochism comes from Leopold von Sacher-Masoch, a 19th-century writer whose novels describe a man who becomes a slave to a woman and encourages her to treat him in progressively more degrading ways.

Infantilism, another form of sexual masochism, is a desire to be treated as a helpless infant, including wearing nappies.

One dangerous form of sexual masochism, called sexual hypoxyphilia, relies on oxygen deprivation to induce sexual arousal. The person uses a noose, mask, plastic bag or chemical to temporarily decrease brain oxygenation. Equipment malfunction or other mistakes can cause accidental eath.

Sexual sadism

With sexual sadism, a person achieves sexual gratification by inflicting pain, cruelty or emotional abuse on others. The term dates back to an 18th-century French writer and libertine, Donatien Alphonse François. Known as the Marquis de Sade, he engaged in violent and scandalous behaviour and published erotic writings.

The sexual sadist may verbally humiliate his partner and abuse her physically through torture, whipping, cutting, binding, beating, burning, stabbing or rape.

Both sadism and masochism may start in adolescence or early adulthood. The behaviours are chronic and usually grow more severe over time.

Voyeurism

The voyeur derives sexual pleasure from looking at sexual objects or sexually arousing situations, such as an unsuspecting couple engaged in sex. He may experience an orgasm during the voyeuristic activity or later, in response to the memory of what he witnessed.

The onset of voyeurism occurs before age 15. The disorder tends to be chronic.

Rare paraphilias

Rare paraphilias not included in the *DSM-IV-TR* include:

- coprophilia – sexual attraction to faeces
- emetophilia – sexual attraction to vomit
- hybristophilia – sexual arousal by people who have committed crimes, particularly cruel or outrageous crimes
- klismaphilia – sexual pleasure from enemas
- necrophilia – sexual attraction to corpses
- plushophilia – sexual attraction to stuffed toys
- urolagnia – sexual attraction to urine
- zoophilia – sexual attraction to animals.

Forms of fetishism

Fetishism can take one of two forms. The first form involves a partner and associates sexual activity with some object such as a woman's knickers. It's relatively harmless if the action is taken playfully and if the partner accepts it.

Velvet infatuation

In the extreme form of fetishism, a nonliving object completely replaces a human partner. The object may be underwear, boots, shoes or a sumptuous fabric, such as velvet or silk. The person achieves orgasm when alone and fondling the object.

Transvestic fetishism

In transvestic fetishism, a heterosexual male dresses in female clothes (called *cross-dressing*) to produce or enhance sexual arousal. He may only wear a single item of clothing, such as a garter or stockings, under masculine clothing. Alternatively, he may dress entirely as a woman, including full make-up and a feminine hairstyle to achieve a female appearance.

Dressing like Mrs Doubtfire

Transvestites believe they have both male and female personalities. Cross-dressing allows them to display their feminine side. When not cross-dressing, they may behave in a stereotypical – or even exaggerated – masculine fashion. (See *The truth about transvestites*.)

Transvestic fetishism is commonly accompanied by masturbation and mental images of other men being attracted to them as a 'woman'.

> Cross-dressing allows a man to display the feminine side of his personality.

Myth busters

The truth about transvestites

Let's lay to rest some common myths about transvestites – that is, people with transvestic fetishism.

Myth: Transvestites are homosexuals.

Reality: Most transvestites – by some estimates, 90% – are heterosexual. (In fact, *only* heterosexual males qualify for the official diagnosis established in the *Diagnostic and Statistical Manual of Mental Disorders*, Fourth Edition, Text Revision.) Many are or have been married. Only a small minority are bisexual or exclusively homosexual.

Myth: Transvestites act like women even when wearing men's clothes.

Reality: Because many transvestites fear they'll be discovered, they consciously try to act as traditionally masculine as possible when not cross-dressing. For most, this isn't difficult because they're 'masculine' men.

Myth: Transvestites are effeminate.

Reality: Transvestites are no more effeminate than any other males. While wearing men's clothes, most don't stand out from the crowd. In fact, out of fear that others will discover their secret, some transvestites adopt exaggerated masculine mannerisms and may appear extremely macho when not cross-dressing.

Myth: Transvestites want to be women.

Reality: Few transvestites wish to change sexes. Although both transvestites and transsexuals (people with gender identity disorder, who wish to live as or become the opposite gender) cross-dress, their motives differ. Transvestites gain sexual gratification from dressing as women, but always revert back to and maintain their male gender identity. They identify primarily as males and usually feel and behave like normal males.

Myth: Transvestites cross-dress because they were dressed as girls when they were children.

Reality: Although many transvestites first experienced cross-dressing as young children, in many cases they initiated these experiences themselves to play out fantasies involving their gender role. Typically, their parents strongly disapproved of cross-dressing.

Commonly, transvestic fetishism has its onset during childhood or adolescence and tends to be chronic. Open cross-dressing – if it occurs at all – begins much later.

Paedophilia

Paedophilia is marked by sexual fantasies, urges or activity involving a child, usually age 13 or younger. (In adolescent paedophiles, the child is 5 years younger than the adolescent is.) The paedophile (almost always a man) is erotically aroused by children and seeks sexual gratification with them. This urge is his preferred or exclusive sexual activity, although some paedophiles are also attracted to adults.

Activity agenda

During sexual activity with a child, the paedophile may:
- undress the child
- encourage the child to watch him masturbate
- touch or fondle the child's genitals
- forcefully perform sexual acts on the child.

Preferred victims

Prepubertal children are the most common targets of paedophiles. Attraction to girls is almost twice as common as attraction to boys. The paedophile may sexually abuse his own children or those of a friend or relative.

Behaviour profile

Many paedophiles probably never come to the attention of authorities. Relatively few engage in violent behaviour. Even more rarely, they kidnap or murder their victims – probably to prevent the victims from reporting their predatory behaviour.

More typically, the paedophile behaves seductively, showering the child with money, gifts, drugs or alcohol. He may be quite attentive to the child's needs to gain loyalty and prevent the child from reporting the encounters.

Causes

The specific cause of paraphilias is unknown, but experts have proposed behavioural, psychoanalytical, biological and learning theories to explain these disorders. Behavioural models suggest that a child who was the victim or observer of inappropriate sexual behaviours learns to imitate such behaviour and later gains reinforcement for it. Biological models, on the other hand, focus on the relationship among hormones, behaviour and the central nervous system (CNS) – especially the role of aggression and male sexual hormones.

Contributing factors

Based on common personal history findings, some experts have identified factors that may contribute to paraphilia. For example, many paraphiliacs come from dysfunctional families marked by isolation and sexual, emotional or physical abuse. Some have concurrent mental disorders, such as psychoactive substance use or personality disorders.

Other factors that may contribute to paraphilias include:
- closed head injury
- CNS tumours
- history of emotional or sexual trauma
- lack of knowledge about sex
- neuroendocrine disorders
- psychosocial stressors.

Signs and symptoms

The person's history reveals the particular pattern of abnormal sexual fantasies, urges or behaviours associated with one of the eight recognised paraphilias.

General assessment findings may include:
- anxiety
- depression
- development of a hobby or an occupation change that makes the paraphilia more accessible
- disturbance in body image
- guilt or shame
- ineffective coping
- multiple paraphilias at the same time
- purchase of books, videos or magazines related to the paraphilia or frequent visits to paraphilia-related websites
- recurrent fantasies involving a paraphilia
- sexual dysfunction
- social isolation
- troubled social or sexual relationships.

Diagnosis

Penile plethysmography may measure the person's sexual arousal in response to visual imagery. However, the results of this procedure can be unreliable.

The diagnosis of paraphilia is confirmed if the person meets the criteria established in the *DSM-IV-TR*. (See *Diagnostic criteria: Paraphilias*, page 472.)

Treatment

Paraphiliacs seldom seek help because of their guilt, shame and fear of social ostracism and legal problems. Those who encounter the health care system usually do so only at the behest of their family or when forced to by legal authorities. Treatment is mandatory if the person's sexual behaviour is harmful to others.

Some paraphiliacs enter the health care system only because they're forced to by legal authorities.

Diagnostic criteria: Paraphilias

The diagnosis of a paraphilia is confirmed when the person's symptoms meet the criteria established in the *Diagnostic and Statistical Manual of Mental Disorders*, Fourth Edition, Text Revision. The criteria below apply to the specific paraphilias discussed in this chapter.

Exhibitionism

- Over a period of at least 6 months, the person has experienced recurrent, intense, sexually arousing fantasies, urges or behaviours involving the exposure of his genitals to an unsuspecting stranger.
- These fantasies, urges or behaviours cause clinically significant distress or impairment in his social, occupational or other areas of functioning.

Fetishism

- Over a period of at least 6 months, the person has experienced intense, recurrent, sexually arousing fantasies, urges or behaviours involving the use of nonliving objects (such as female undergarments).
- The fetish objects aren't limited to items of female clothing used in cross-dressing or devices used for tactile genital stimulation (for instance, a vibrator).
- The person's fantasies, urges or behaviours cause clinically significant distress or impairment in his social, occupational or other important areas of functioning.

Transvestic fetishism

- Over a period of at least 6 months, a heterosexual male has experienced recurrent, intense, sexually arousing fantasies, urges or behaviours involving cross-dressing (dressing in feminine clothing).
- These fantasies, urges or behaviours cause clinically significant distress or impairment in his social, occupational or other important areas of functioning.

Transvestic fetishism occurs with gender dysphoria if the person has persistent discomfort with his gender identity or role.

Paedophilia

- Over a period of at least 6 months, the person has experienced recurrent, intense, sexually arousing fantasies, urges or behaviours involving sexual activity with one or more prepubescent children (generally age 13 or younger).
- The person has acted on these urges, or the urges or fantasies cause marked distress or interpersonal difficulty.
- The person is at least age 16 and at least 5 years older than the child or children who are the object of his fantasies, urges or behaviours. (*Note:* A person in his late teens who's involved in an ongoing sexual relationship with a 12- or 13-year-old *isn't* considered a paedophile.)

Subtypes

- A paedophile may be sexually attracted to males, females or both.
- The paedophilia may be limited to incest.
- The paedophilia may be of the exclusive type, in which the person is attracted only to children, or of the nonexclusive type, in which he's also attracted to adults.

Depending on the specific paraphilia, treatment may involve a combination of psychotherapy, cognitive therapy, behavioural therapy, pharmacotherapy and surgery.

Shock treatment

In behavioural therapy, the person may be subjected to aversive stimuli, such as bad odours or electric shocks, when he engages in the paraphiliac behaviour.

To succeed, treatment should include teaching the person alternatives to the forbidden behaviours. The effectiveness of treatment varies. In nearly all cases, treatment must be long term to be effective.

Improving social skills

Some people with paraphilias (especially paedophilia) have deficient social skills, which are required to obtain sexual satisfaction with consenting adults. Thus, social skills training is an essential part of treatment.

Treatment programs for sex offenders

Treatment for paraphiliacs who are sex offenders may include:
- a specialised sex offender programme
- group therapy
- a 12-step sexual addiction or compulsion recovery programme
- a rational thinking group
- a structured sexual disorder process group
- educational sessions focusing on the offender's psychological factors, victim impact and human sexuality
- therapeutically structured recreational activities, adventure-based programming, arts and crafts, team sports and experimental games
- resident and parent participation in treatment reviews
- alcohol and drug awareness programmes
- values clarification
- independent living skills
- vocational exploration.

Pharmacological therapy

Certain drugs may be used to reduce the compulsive thinking associated with paraphilias. Occasionally, hormones are prescribed if the person experiences intrusive sexual thoughts or urges or demonstrates frequent abnormal sexual behaviours.

Hormones may be used to treat paraphiliacs with intrusive sexual thoughts or urges or frequent abnormal sexual behaviours.

Nursing interventions

For nursing actions appropriate for people with paraphilias, see *Nursing interventions for people with sexual disorders*, pages 474 and 475.

Sexual dysfunctions

Sexual dysfunctions are characterised by pain during sex or by a disturbance in one of the phases of the sexual response cycle. (See *Sexual pain disorders*, pages 475 and 476.)

These dysfunctions may cause marked distress and interpersonal problems. They can impair intimate relationships by reducing the enjoyment of normal sex or preventing the normal physiological changes of the sexual response cycle.

Advice from the experts

Nursing interventions for people with sexual disorders

You can use the general interventions below when caring for a person with any sexual disorder.

Ensure a therapeutic relationship

- Arrange to spend uninterrupted time with the person. Encourage him to express his feelings, and accept what he says.
- Explain all treatments and procedures, and answer the person's questions to allay his fear and help him regain a sense of control.
- Never say anything that would make the person feel ashamed. It's his needs and feelings – not your opinions – that matter.
- Realise that treating the person with empathy doesn't threaten your sexuality.

Promote self-knowledge

- Initiate a discussion about how the need for self-esteem, respect, love and intimacy influence a person's sexual expression. This helps the person understand his disorder.
- Encourage the person to identify feelings – such as pleasure, reduced anxiety, increased control or shame – associated with his sexual behaviour and fantasies.
- Help the person distinguish between practices that are distressing because they don't conform to social norms or personal values and those that may place him or others in emotional, medical or legal jeopardy. Doing this reinforces the need for him to stop behaviours that could harm himself or others.
- Encourage him to express his sexual preferences as well as his feelings about them.

Increase the level of interaction

- Spend specific, non-care-related time with the person during each shift to encourage social interaction. Start with one-on-one interaction and increase to group interaction when his social skills indicate he's ready.

Increasing social interaction gradually eases his feeling of being overwhelmed and minimises sensory input that may renew cognitive or perceptual disturbances.
- Give positive reinforcement for appropriate and effective interaction behaviours, both verbal and nonverbal.

Promote participation in care

- Encourage the person to take decisions about his care, to enhance his self-esteem and to increase his sense of mastery over the current situation.
- Assist the person and his family or close friends in progressive participation in care and therapies.
- Have the person increase his self-care performance levels gradually so that he can progress at his own pace.
- Initiate or participate in multidisciplinary person-centred conferences to evaluate progress and plan discharge. These conferences should involve the person and his family in a cooperative effort to individualise his care plan.

Improve coping skills

- Encourage the person to use support systems to assist with coping, thereby helping to restore psychological equilibrium and prevent crises.
- Try to identify factors that cause or exacerbate poor coping ability, such as a fear of being fired.
- Help the person look at his current situation and evaluate various coping behaviours to encourage a realistic view of the crisis.
- Urge the person to try new coping behaviours. A person in crisis tends to accept interventions and develop new coping behaviours more readily than at other times.
- Request feedback from the person about behaviours that seem to work. This encourages him to evaluate the effect of these behaviours.
- Praise the person for taking decisions and performing activities, to reinforce coping behaviours.

Nursing interventions for people with sexual disorders *(continued)*

Provide referrals

- Refer the person for professional psychological counselling. If his maladaptive behaviour has high crisis potential, formal counselling can help ease your frustration, increase your objectivity and foster a collaborative approach to service user care. As appropriate, refer the person to a physician, nurse, psychologist, social worker or counsellor trained in sex therapy.

Other actions

- Be aware that whenever possible, a primary nurse should be assigned to the person to ensure continuity of care and promote a therapeutic relationship.
- Initially, allow the person to depend partly on you for self-care because he may regress to a lower developmental level during the initial crisis phase.
- If the person poses a threat to himself and others, institute safety precautions, according to facility protocol.
- Identify and reduce unnecessary environment stimuli.

Sexual pain disorders

The two main types of sexual pain disorders are dyspareunia and vaginismus.

Dyspareunia

With dyspareunia, which can occur in both males and females, unexplained genital pain occurs before, during or after intercourse. The condition may be mild – or may be severe enough to restrict the enjoyment of sex.

Causes

Physical conditions that can cause dyspareunia include:

- acute or chronic infections of the genitourinary tract
- allergic reactions (as from diaphragms, condoms or other contraceptives)
- benign or malignant reproductive system growths or tumours
- deformities or lesions of the vagina or its opening
- disorders of the surrounding viscera (including the residual effects of pelvic inflammatory disease and disease of the adnexal and broad ligaments)
- endometriosis
- genital, rectal or pelvic scar tissue

- insufficient lubrication (as from medications, oestrogen loss or radiation to the genital area)
- intact hymen
- local trauma (such as hymenal tears or bruising of the urethral meatus)
- retroversion of the uterus.

Psychological causes of dyspareunia include a history of sexual abuse and problems in intimate relationships.

Treatment

When dyspareunia has a physical cause, treatment may include:

- creams and water-soluble jellies for inadequate lubrication
- medications for infections
- excision of hymenal scars
- gentle stretching of painful scars at the vaginal opening
- a change in coital position to reduce pain on deep penetration.

When the condition has a psychological cause, interventions may include psychotherapy or sensate focus exercises. With these exercises, each partner

(continued)

Sexual pain disorders (continued)

takes turns paying increased attention to his own physical sensations.

Vaginismus

With vaginismus, involuntary spasmodic muscle contractions occur at the entrance to the vagina when the male tries to insert his penis. Pain occurs if intercourse is attempted despite these contractions.

This condition makes intercourse extremely painful or impossible. However, women with vaginismus are capable of becoming sexually aroused and achieving lubrication and orgasm through clitoral or other alternative stimulation.

Vaginismus can be primary or secondary. With primary vaginismus, the person has never been able to have intercourse with penetration (resulting, for example, in an unconsummated marriage). In secondary vaginismus, the service user previously experienced normal intercourse before developing the condition.

Causes

Most authorities believe vaginismus is a learned response commonly stemming from dyspareunia. Women who have had frightening, unsatisfying or painful sexual experiences may fear that penetration and intercourse will cause pain. A strict cultural or religious background can have the same effect. This fear and anticipation of pain may lead to a pattern of sexual anxiety, causing vaginal dryness and tightness before intercourse.

Other psychological factors that may cause or contribute to vaginismus include fears of pregnancy, of being controlled by a man or of losing control.

Physical causes of vaginismus include vaginal infection, physical after-effects of childbirth and fatigue.

Treatment

Treatment for vaginismus stemming from psychological causes may include a combination of:

- couples therapy
- Kegel exercises to strengthen the pubococcygeal muscle
- sensate focus exercises for the couple
- progressive use of a plastic dilator or finger, which is inserted into the vaginal opening to progressively stretch the contracted muscles.

When treated by a professional using these or similar techniques, vaginismus has a cure rate of about 80–100%.

In some people, a sexual dysfunction is present at the onset of sexual functioning and activity. In others, it follows a period of normal sexual functioning.

Sexual dysfunctions are commonly linked to psychological factors, medical conditions, substance use or a combination of these factors.

Categorising sexual dysfunctions

Sexual dysfunctions fall into several categories:
- sexual arousal disorders
- sexual desire disorders
- orgasmic disorders
- sexual dysfunction caused by a medical condition
- sexual pain disorders. (See *Types of sexual dysfunctions*, page 477.)

Generalised vs. situational dysfunction

A sexual dysfunction may be generalised or situational. In the generalised type, the dysfunction occurs with all types of stimulation, situation and partners. In

Types of sexual dysfunctions

The *Diagnostic and Statistical Manual of Mental Disorders*, Fourth Edition, Text Revision, classifies sexual dysfunctions (other than paraphilias and gender identity disorder) as described below.

Sexual desire disorders: Hypoactive sexual desire disorder, sexual aversion disorder

The key feature of hypoactive sexual desire disorder is a deficiency or absence of sexual fantasies or desire for sexual activity. The person rarely initiates sexual activity, but may engage in it reluctantly when the partner initiates it.

With sexual aversion disorder, the person dislikes and avoids genital sexual contact with a sexual partner.

Sexual arousal disorders: Female sexual arousal disorder, male erectile disorder

With female sexual arousal disorder, the woman has a persistent or recurrent inability to attain or maintain (until the completion of sexual activity) an adequate lubrication-swelling response of sexual excitement.

With male erectile disorder, the man has a persistent or recurrent inability to attain or maintain (until the completion of sexual activity) an adequate erection.

Orgasmic disorders: Female orgasmic disorder, male orgasmic disorder, premature ejaculation

With male and female orgasmic disorders, the person experiences a persistent or recurrent delay in, or absence of, orgasm following a normal sexual excitement phase.

Premature ejaculation refers to a persistent and recurrent onset of orgasm and ejaculation with minimal sexual stimulation.

Sexual dysfunction due to a general medical condition

With sexual dysfunction due to a general medical condition, the person's sexual dysfunction is fully explained by the direct physiological effects of a general medical condition. This category includes sexual dysfunction caused by substance use, such as alcohol, prescription drugs or street drugs.

Sexual pain disorders: Dyspareunia, vaginismus

The essential feature of dyspareunia is genital pain associated with sexual intercourse. Vaginismus refers to a recurrent or persistent involuntary contraction of the perineal muscles surrounding the outer third of the vagina when vaginal penetration is attempted. With some people, even the anticipation of vaginal insertion may result in muscle spasm.

---

the situational type, the dysfunction is limited to certain types of stimulation, situation or partners.

Prognosis
The prognosis is good for temporary or mild sexual dysfunctions stemming from misinformation or situational stress. It's guarded for dysfunctions that result from intense anxiety, chronically discordant relationships, psychological disturbances or drug or alcohol abuse in either partner.

Female sexual arousal disorder and female orgasmic disorder

Defined as the inability to achieve or maintain an adequate lubrication-swelling response of sexual excitement, female sexual arousal disorder is one of the most severe sexual dysfunctions in women.

Female orgasmic disorder, the most common sexual dysfunction in women, is the inability to achieve orgasm. Unlike a woman with sexual arousal disorder, one with orgasmic disorder may desire sexual activity and become aroused, but feels inhibited as she approaches orgasm.

Primary and secondary categories

These disorders can be primary or secondary. They're primary when they occur in someone who has never experienced sexual arousal or orgasm. They're secondary when a physical, mental or environmental condition inhibits or prevents previously normal sexual functioning.

Causes

Factors that may cause or contribute to female sexual arousal or orgasmic disorder include:
- depression
- drug use (such as CNS depressants, antidepressants, hormonal contraceptives, alcohol or street drugs)
- discordant relationships (poor communication, hostility or ambivalence towards the partner or fear of abandonment or of asserting independence)
- diseases (general systemic illness, endocrine or nervous system disorders or diseases that impair muscle tone or contractility)
- fatigue
- gynecological factors (chronic vaginal or pelvic infection or pain, congenital anomalies or genital cancer, trauma or surgery)
- inadequate or ineffective sexual stimulation
- lifestyle disruptions
- psychological factors (such as stress, anxiety, anger, hostility, boredom with sex, guilt, depression, unconscious conflicts about sexuality or fear of losing control of one's feelings or behaviour)
- pregnancy
- religious or cultural taboos that reinforce guilt feelings about sex.

Signs and symptoms

Assessment findings in service users with sexual dysfunctions vary with the specific dysfunction.

Female sexual arousal disorder

A woman with sexual arousal disorder usually reports limited or absent sexual desire and little or no pleasure from sexual stimulation. Her history may include:
- decreased sexual desire
- individual or family stress or fatigue, as occurs in many working mothers with children under age 5 who are too exhausted to care about sex
- misinformation about sex and sexuality
- a pattern of dysfunctional sexual response

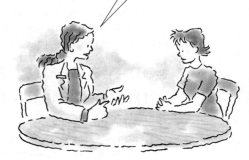

Sexual arousal disorder commonly occurs in working mothers with young children. Maybe you're just too exhausted to care about sex.

- conceptual problems during childhood and adolescence about sex in general and, specifically, about masturbation, incest, rape, sexual fantasies and homosexual or heterosexual practices
- concerns about contraception and reproductive ability
- problems in the current sexual relationship
- poor self-esteem and body image.

Physical indications of sexual arousal disorder include the lack of vaginal lubrication and the absence of signs of genital vasocongestion.

Female orgasmic disorder

A woman with orgasmic disorder may report an inability to achieve orgasm, either totally or under certain circumstances.

Diagnosis

A thorough physical examination, laboratory tests and medical history can rule out physical causes of female sexual arousal or orgasmic disorder.

A sexual dysfunction is diagnosed if the person fulfills the criteria in the *DSM-IV-TR*. (See *Diagnostic criteria: Female sexual arousal disorder*, and *Diagnostic criteria: Female orgasmic disorder*, page 480.)

Treatment

Treatment varies with the specific dysfunction.

Treating sexual arousal disorder

Female sexual arousal disorder can be challenging to treat – especially if the woman has never experienced sexual pleasure. The goal of therapy is to help her relax, become aware of her feelings about sex and eliminate guilt and fear of rejection. Some women and their partners need reassurance about their activities, while others need suggestions and more intensive therapy.

Diagnostic criteria: Female sexual arousal disorder

The diagnosis of female sexual arousal disorder is confirmed when the woman meets the following criteria from the *Diagnostic and Statistical Manual of Mental Disorders*, Fourth Edition, Text Revision.

- The woman experiences persistent or recurrent, partial or complete failure to attain or maintain (until the completion of sexual activity) the lubrication-swelling response of sexual excitement.
- The disturbance causes marked distress or interpersonal difficulty.
- The disorder doesn't occur exclusively during the course of another Axis I disorder such as major depression.

Subtypes

Female sexual arousal disorder may be:

- lifelong or acquired
- generalised or situational
- caused by psychological factors or combined factors.

Diagnostic criteria: Female orgasmic disorder

The diagnosis of female orgasmic disorder is confirmed when the woman meets the following criteria from the *Diagnostic and Statistical Manual of Mental Disorders*, Fourth Edition, Text Revision.

- The woman experiences a persistent or recurrent delay in or absence of orgasm after a normal sexual excitement phase, during sexual activity deemed to be adequate. (Some women experience orgasm during noncoital clitoral stimulation but not during coitus without manual clitoral stimulation. For most of them, this is a normal variation of the sexual response and doesn't justify the diagnosis. In others, this represents a psychological inhibition that *does* justify the diagnosis. A thorough sexual evaluation can aid this difficult judgement.)

- The woman suffers marked distress or interpersonal difficulty because of the disturbance.
- The disorder doesn't occur exclusively during the course of another Axis I disorder such as major depression.

Subtypes

Female orgasmic disorder may be:

- lifelong or acquired
- generalised or situational
- caused by psychological factors or combined factors.

For some women, psychotherapy or behavioural therapy is indicated. Psychotherapy may consist of free association, dream analysis and discussion of life patterns to achieve greater sexual awareness. One behavioural approach attempts to correct maladaptive patterns through systematic desensitisation to situations that provoke anxiety – for example, by encouraging the woman to fantasise about these situations.

Sensate focus exercises

Many people with sexual arousal disorder benefit from sensate focus exercises. These exercises minimise the importance of intercourse and orgasm while emphasising touching and awareness of sensual feelings over the entire body (not just genital sensations).

Sensate focus exercises are done with a partner. Each partner takes turns giving and then receiving touch and massage. At first, they're instructed to give pleasure without touching the breasts or genitals. The person receiving the pleasure places his or her hand over the giver's to show where the touch should be and what it should feel like. This improves communication and teaches the couple what they *can* achieve rather than what they *can't*.

Later, the ban against genital touching and orgasm is reduced as the couple realises that mutual pleasure can be derived from simple touching. A sensate focus programme may also include masturbation, either alone or together.

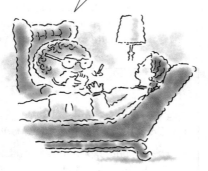

To treat sexual arousal disorder, I recommend that you fantasise about the situations that cause you anxiety.

Treating orgasmic disorder

In treating orgasmic disorder, the goal is to decrease or eliminate involuntary inhibition of the orgasmic reflex. Treatment may include experiential therapy, psychoanalysis or behaviour modification. Individual therapy, marital or couples therapy or sex therapy may be indicated.

Medications may be prescribed to decrease symptoms, if appropriate. Any underlying physical disorder should be treated.

Managing primary orgasmic disorder

For primary orgasmic disorder, treatment may include teaching the person self-stimulation and distraction techniques, such as focusing on fantasies, breathing patterns and muscle contractions to relieve anxiety. Thus, the person learns new behaviour through exercises she does at home between sessions. Eventually, the therapist involves the person's sexual partner in treatment sessions (although some therapists treat the couple as a unit from the beginning).

Strategies for secondary orgasmic disorder

For secondary orgasmic disorder, the goal of treatment is to decrease anxiety and promote the factors necessary for the person to experience orgasm. The therapist communicates an accepting and permissive attitude and helps the person understand that satisfactory sexual experiences don't always require coital orgasm.

Nursing interventions

Nursing interventions for female sexual arousal or orgasmic disorder are the same for other sexual disorders. (See *Nursing interventions for people with sexual disorders*, pages 474 and 475.)

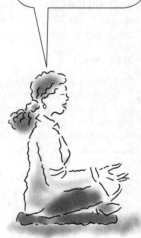

Focusing on breathing patterns or muscle contractions is therapeutic for some service users with primary orgasmic disorder.

Premature ejaculation

Premature ejaculation refers to a male's inability to control the ejaculatory reflex during sexual activity. The condition causes ejaculation to occur before or immediately after penetration or before the wishes of both partners.

This disorder affects men of all ages. Unlike male erectile disorder, premature ejaculation doesn't affect the ability to have or maintain an erection. (See *Understanding male erectile disorder*, page 482.)

Prematurity perils

Premature ejaculation can seriously disrupt intimate relationships. It may lead to generalised anxiety disorder or pervasive feelings of inadequacy, guilt and self-doubt.

Causes

Psychological factors, such as stress, performance anxiety or limited sexual experiences, typically play a key role in premature ejaculation. Other psychological factors that may cause or contribute to this disorder include:
• ambivalence towards or unconscious hatred of women
• negative sexual relationships in which the man unconsciously denies his partner sexual fulfillment
• guilt feelings about sex.

Understanding male erectile disorder

Male erectile disorder (commonly called *impotence*) refers to the inability to attain or maintain penile erection long enough to complete sexual intercourse. The man's history may reveal a long-standing inability to achieve erection, sudden loss of erectile function or a gradual decline in function. It may also include a medical condition, drug therapy or psychological trauma that could contribute to erectile disorder.

When the cause of the disorder is psychogenic rather than organic, the man may report that he can achieve erection through masturbation but not with a partner. He may show signs of anxiety when discussing his condition, such as sweating and palpitations – or he may appear disinterested. Depression, another common complaint, may be either a cause or an effect of erectile disorder.

Treatment

Sex therapy designed to reduce performance anxiety may effectively cure psychogenic impotence.

Treatment for organic impotence focuses on eliminating the underlying cause. If this isn't possible, counselling may help the couple deal with their situation realistically and explore alternatives for sexual expression. Some men may benefit from a surgically inserted inflatable or semi-rigid penile prosthesis. Others may benefit from such medications as sildenafil (Viagra).

However, the disorder can occur in emotionally healthy men with stable, positive relationships.

In some men, premature ejaculation is linked to an underlying degenerative neurological disorder such as multiple sclerosis or an inflammatory process, such as posterior urethritis or prostatitis. Other physical factors associated with premature ejaculation include drug or alcohol use and genital surgery or trauma.

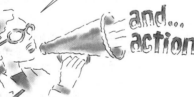

Next time, wait until I yell 'Action!'

Signs and symptoms

The man's history may reveal that he can't prolong foreplay or that he ejaculates as soon as he inserts his penis into the vagina. In some cases, the partner seeks mental health treatment, complaining that the man is indifferent to her sexual needs.

Other assessment findings may include:
• anxiety
• depression
• disturbance in body image
• frustration and feelings of being unattractive
• ineffective coping
• pain during sexual intercourse
• poor self-concept
• social isolation.

Diagnosis

Diagnostic tests can rule out medical causes of premature ejaculation. The disorder is diagnosed if the man meets the criteria in the *DSM-IV-TR*. (See *Diagnostic criteria: Premature ejaculation*, page 483.)

Diagnostic criteria: Premature ejaculation

The diagnosis of premature ejaculation is confirmed when the man meets the following criteria from the *Diagnostic and Statistical Manual of Mental Disorders*, Fourth Edition, Text Revision.

* The man persistently or recurrently ejaculates with minimal sexual stimulation before, on or shortly after penetration and before he wishes it. (The clinician considers factors that affect the duration of the sexual excitement phase, such as age, novelty of the sex partner and recent frequency of sexual activity.)
* The disturbance causes marked distress or interpersonal difficulty.
* The disorder doesn't result exclusively from the direct effects of a substance (as from opioid withdrawal).

Subtypes

Premature ejaculation may be:

* lifelong or acquired
* generalised or situational
* caused by psychological factors or combined factors.

Treatment

Masters and Johnson developed a highly successful intensive treatment programme for premature ejaculation that helps the man focus on sensations of impending orgasm. The programme combines insight therapy, behavioural techniques and experiential sessions involving both partners.

Explore, caress, squeeze

Therapy sessions, which last 2 weeks or longer, typically include:
* mutual physical exploration to enhance the couple's awareness of anatomy and physiology while reducing shameful feelings about sexual body parts
* sensate focus exercises, which allow each partner to caress the other's body without intercourse and to focus on pleasurable touch sensations
* the squeeze technique, which helps the man gain control of ejaculatory tension. (See *Squeeze play for premature ejaculation*, page 484.)

Start, stop, start, stop

The stop-and-start technique also helps to delay ejaculation. Performed with the woman in the superior position, this method involves pelvic thrusting until orgasmic sensations begin. Thrusting then stops and is restarted to promote control of ejaculation. Eventually, the couple is allowed to achieve orgasm.

Nursing interventions

Nursing interventions for men with premature ejaculation resemble those used for other sexual disorders. (See *Nursing interventions for people with sexual disorders*, pages 474 and 475.)

> In the stop-and-start technique, the couple starts and stops pelvic thrusting repeatedly to help the man learn to control his ejaculation.

Advice from the experts

Squeeze play for premature ejaculation

The squeeze technique, used to overcome premature ejaculation, may be practised either with a partner or alone during masturbation. Advise the man or his partner to position the fingers correctly around the penis and apply the right amount of pressure. When the man feels the urge to ejaculate, he or his partner should place a thumb on the frenulum of the penis and place the index and middle fingers above and below the coronal ridge, as shown here.

Then the man or partner should squeeze the penis from front to back – more firmly for an erect penis and less firmly for a partially flaccid one. They should apply and release pressure every few minutes during a touching exercise. The goal is to delay ejaculation by keeping the man at an earlier phase of the sexual response cycle.

The man should feel pressure but no pain. After several squeezes, he should have a more intense ejaculation than usual.

Anatomic structures

Urethral meatus
Glans
Frenulum
Coronal ridge
Shaft

Hand position

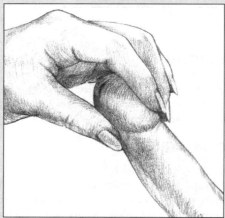

Gender identity disorder

Gender identity disorder is marked by discomfort with one's apparent or assigned gender and a strong, persistent identification with the opposite sex. Someone with this disorder (sometimes called a *transsexual*) wants to be like or to become the opposite sex and is extremely uncomfortable with his or her assigned gender role.

Gender identity – the intimate, personal feeling one has about being male or female – includes three components: self-concept, perception of an ideal partner and external presentation of masculinity or femininity through behaviour, dress and mannerisms. People with gender identity disorder may have a problem with one or all of these components. Typically, they behave and present themselves as a person of the opposite sex.

Gender identity disorder shouldn't be confused with the far more common phenomenon of feeling inadequate in meeting the expectations normally associated with a particular sex.

Childhood rejection

Children with gender identity disorder, particularly boys, are likely to be rejected by their peer group. Girls may not experience social difficulties until early adolescence.

Impaired and despairing

Gender identity disorder may seriously impair social and occupational functioning – not just because of the psychopathology but also because of the problems associated with trying to live as the opposite sex. Anxiety and depression are common among those with this disorder and may lead to suicide attempts.

With or without treatment, females with gender identity disorder have shown more stable adjustment patterns than males.

Prevalence and onset

The prevalence of gender identity disorder is unknown. Relatively recent data suggest that it occurs in approximately 1 of 11,900 adult males and 1 of every 30,400 adults.

Gender identity disorder usually arises during childhood. Onset after marriage may significantly disrupt the marital relationship.

Causes

Current theories about the cause of gender identity disorder suggest a combination of predisposing factors, including:
* chromosomal anomalies
* hormonal imbalances (particularly in utero during brain formation)
* pathological defects in early parent–child bonding and child-rearing practices. For example, parents who treat their child as a member of the opposite sex may contribute to gender identity disorder.

Contributing factors may include:
* concurrent paraphilias, especially transvestic fetishism
* feelings of sexual inadequacy
* generalised anxiety disorder
* personality disorders.

> Parents who treat their child like a member of the opposite sex may contribute to gender identity disorder.

Signs and symptoms

Signs and symptoms of gender identity disorder differ among adults, adolescents and children.

Assessment findings in adults and adolescents

Adults and adolescents with this disorder typically believe they were born the wrong sex. They're preoccupied with eliminating primary and secondary sex characteristics. Some people request hormones, surgery or other procedures to physically alter their sexual characteristics.

Males may describe a lifelong history of feeling feminine and pursuing feminine activities. Females exhibit similar propensities for opposite-sex activities and discomfort with the female role.

Other assessment findings may include:
- anxiety
- attempts to mask or remove the sex organs
- cross-dressing
- depression
- disturbances in body image
- dreams of cross-gender identification
- fear of abandonment by family and friends
- finding one's genitals 'disgusting'
- ineffective coping strategies
- peer ostracism
- preoccupation with appearance
- self-hatred
- self-medication such as with hormonal therapy
- strong attraction to stereotypical activities of the opposite sex
- suicide attempts or ideation.

The puberty predicament

In both sexes, the crisis seems especially acute during puberty. Development of secondary sex characteristics (breasts and pubic hair in the female, and enlarged penis and testes in the male) may trigger intense distress or intensify the feeling that one is a misfit.

Assessment findings in children

Children with gender identity disorder may express the desire to be – or insist that they are – the opposite sex. They may express disgust with their genitalia, along with an ardent hope to become the opposite sex when they grow up.

Diagnosis

Diagnostic test results suggesting gender identity disorder include:
- karyotyping for sex chromosomes, which may show abnormalities
- psychological tests, which reveal cross-gender identification or behaviour patterns
- sex hormone assay, which may reveal an abnormality.

The diagnosis of gender identity disorder is confirmed if the person meets the criteria in the *DSM-IV-TR*. (See *Diagnostic criteria: Gender identity disorder*, page 487.)

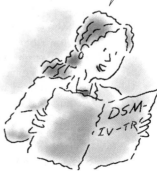

The criteria in this book determines whether the person qualifies for an official diagnosis of gender identity disorder.

Diagnostic criteria: Gender identity disorder

The diagnosis of gender identity disorder is confirmed when the person meets the following criteria from the *Diagnostic and Statistical Manual of Mental Disorders*, Fourth Edition, Text Revision.

Cross-gender identification

The person has a strong, persistent identification with the opposite sex, not just a desire for any perceived cultural advantages of being the other sex.
In an adolescent or adult, the disturbance manifests as:

- a stated desire to be the opposite sex or to live or be treated as the opposite sex
- frequent passing as the opposite sex
- belief that he or she has typical feelings and reactions of the opposite sex.

In a child, the disturbance manifests as four or more of the following behaviours:

- a repeatedly stated desire to be, or an insistence that he or she is, the opposite sex
- in a male, a preference for cross-dressing or simulating female attire; in a female, insistence on wearing only stereotypical masculine clothing
- strong, persistent preference for cross-sex roles in make-believe play or persistent fantasies of being the opposite sex
- intense desire to engage in the stereotypical games and pastimes of the opposite sex
- strong preference for playmates of the opposite sex.

Discomfort with one's own sex

The person has a persistent discomfort with his or her own sex or a sense that the assigned gender role is inappropriate for himself or herself.
In adolescents and adults, this manifests as:

- preoccupation with eliminating primary and secondary sex characteristics – for example, requesting hormones, surgery or other procedures to physically alter one's sexual traits and thus simulate the opposite sex
- belief that he or she was born the wrong sex.

In children, the disturbance manifests as any of the following behaviours:

- in a male, asserting that the penis or testes are disgusting or will disappear, or that he would be better off not having a penis; or an aversion for rough-and-tumble play and rejection of stereotypical male toys, games and activities
- in a female, rejection of urinating in a sitting position, assertions that she has or will grow a penis and doesn't want to grow breasts or menstruate or a marked aversion for stereotypical feminine clothing.

Other criteria

- The disturbance isn't concurrent with a physical intersex condition (being born with anatomic or physiological traits that differ from contemporary ideals of what constitutes a 'normal' male or female).
- It causes clinically significant distress or impairment in social, occupational or other important areas of functioning.

Subtypes

In sexually mature people, subtypes of gender identity disorder include:

- sexual attraction to males
- sexual attraction to females
- sexual attraction to both males and females
- sexual attraction to neither males nor females.

Treatment

Individual and couples therapy may help an adult cope with the decision to live as the opposite sex or, depending on the circumstances, to cope with the knowledge that he or she won't be able to live as the opposite sex.

Mental health management, including hospitalisation, may be indicated if the person has the potential for violence, such as suicidal ideation or self-mutilation fantasies. Group or individual psychotherapy may also be appropriate.

For a child, individual and family therapy are indicated. Having a therapist of the same sex may be useful for role-modelling purposes. The earlier the problem is diagnosed and treatment begins, the better the prognosis.

Sex reassignment surgery

For some people, sex reassignment through hormonal therapy and sex-change surgery may be an option. However, sex reassignment hasn't been as beneficial as first hoped. Severe psychological problems may persist afterwards – sometimes even leading to suicide.

Also, people who seek sex reassignment may have a larger pattern of depression and concomitant personality disorders such as borderline personality disorder.

Nursing interventions

Nursing interventions for people with gender identity disorder resemble those for other sexual disorders. (See *Nursing interventions for people with sexual disorders*, pages 474 and 475.)

Quick quiz

1. The phase of the sexual response cycle involving fantasy and expectation is the:
    A. desire phase.
    B. excitement phase.
    C. orgasm phase.
    D. resolution phase.

Answer: A. The desire phase of the sexual response cycle involves fantasy and expectation.

2. What may cause or contribute to sexual dysfunction?
    A. Drug use
    B. Dissociative disorders
    C. Supplemental vitamin use
    D. Exercise

Answer: A. Sexual dysfunctions sometimes stem from transient conditions, such as drug or alcohol use.

3. A persistent urge to show one's private parts to a stranger occurs in:
    A. fetishism.
    B. paedophilia.
    C. exhibitionism.
    D. transsexualism.

Answer: C. An exhibitionist has sexual fantasies, urges or behaviours involving exposing the genitals to strangers.

4. Treatments commonly recommended for a female with orgasmic disorder include:
   A.   taking soothing bubble baths.
   B.   touching her partner.
   C.   having sexual intercourse more often.
   D.   increasing the degree of sexual arousal.

Answer: B. Sensate focus exercises are recommended for female orgasmic disorder. These exercises emphasise touching and awareness of sensual feelings throughout the entire body while minimising the importance of intercourse and orgasm. The couple takes turns giving and receiving touch.

5. A nonliving object may replace a human partner in a service user with:
   A.   fetishism.
   B.   gender identity disorder.
   C.   transsexualism.
   D.   sexual desire disorder.

Answer: A. In one form of fetishism, a nonliving object completely replaces a human partner. The object may be undergarments, shoes or a fabric, such as velvet or silk.

6. Gender identity disorder should be suspected if the person:
A. has a strong desire to be of the same sex.
B. insists that he or she is of the opposite sex.
C. prefers the opposite sex.
D. engages in games with the same sex.

Answer: B. Gender identity disorder is marked by a repeatedly stated desire to be the opposite sex or an insistence that one is the opposite sex.

7. Sexual attraction to children is termed:
A. sadism.
B. necrophilia.
C. exhibitionism.
D. paedophilia.

Answer: D. In paedophilia, the person has sexual fantasies, urges or activity involving a child.

Scoring

☆☆☆ If you answered all seven items correctly, intense! Your dedication to understanding sexual disorders has climaxed in a perfect score!

☆☆ If you answered five or six items correctly, you deserve a pat on the back, if not a full-body massage! You've nearly mastered Masters' and Johnson's favourite topic.

☆ If you answered fewer than five items correctly, that's OK. We're sure you have the desire to understand sexual disorders and may even find the subject arousing. To reach peak comprehension, just read the chapter again.

Appendices and index

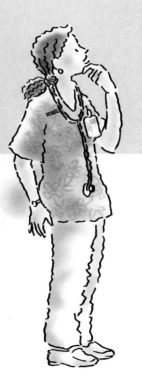

Glossary

acetylcholine: a neurotransmitter

acting out: repeatedly performing actions without weighing the possible results of those actions

ambivalence: coexisting, strong positive and negative feelings, leading to emotional conflict

amphetamine: stimulant drugs used to increase alertness, relieve fatigue and feel stronger and more decisive; used for euphoric effects or to counteract the 'down' feeling of tranquillisers or alcohol

anhedonia: a diminished capacity to experience pleasure; may be reflected by a lack of interest in activities with substantial time spent in purposeless activity

antisocial personality disorder: a pervasive lack of remorse or lack of exhibiting feelings that leads to a total disregard for the rights of others

asociality: a lack of interest in relationships

attention level: ability to concentrate on a task for an appropriate length of time

aversion therapy: application of a painful stimulus that creates an aversion to the obsessed thought, leading to the undesirable behaviour

avoidant personality disorder: negativity, poor self-esteem and issues surrounding social interaction; difficulty looking at situations and interactions in an objective manner

Beck Depression Inventory: helps diagnose depression and determine its severity

blunted affect: a flattening of emotions in which the person's face may appear immobile with poor eye contact and lack of expressiveness

body dysmorphic disorder: preoccupation with an imagined or an actual slight defect in physical appearance; perceived thoughts are often distorted, making the problem, or perceived problem, bigger than it actually is; in many cases, the flaw doesn't exist

borderline personality disorder: a pattern of instability or impulsiveness in a person's mood, interpersonal relationships, self-esteem, self-identity, behaviour and cognition; originates in early childhood

clang association: words that rhyme or sound alike used in an illogical, nonsensical manner – for example, 'It's the rain, train, pain.'

clanging: the choice of a word based on the sound rather than the meaning

cocaine: a narcotic and stimulant which may be ingested, injected, sniffed or smoked to obtain its effects; street names include coke, flake, snow, nose candy, hits, crack (hardened form), rock and crank

Cognitive Assessment Scale: measures orientation, general knowledge, mental ability and psychomotor function

comorbidity: the coexistence of two disorders, such as mental and somatic disorders occurring together in a person

compensation: hiding a weakness by stressing too strongly the desirable strength

comprehension: the ability to understand, retain and repeat material

compulsion: a preoccupation that's acted out, such as constantly washing one's hands

concept formation: testing the person's ability to think abstractly

concrete thinking: inability to form or understand abstract thoughts

confabulation: unconscious filling of gaps in memory with fabricated facts and experiences

conversion disorder: (previously called hysterical neurosis, conversion type) disorder in which people resolve psychological conflicts through the loss of a specific physical function; examples include paralysis, blindness or the inability to swallow; people exhibit symptoms that suggest a physical disorder, but evaluation and observation can't determine a physiological cause

delusions: false ideas or beliefs accepted as real by the person; somatic illness, depersonalisation and delusions of grandeur, persecution and reference are common in schizophrenia

denial: protecting oneself from unpleasant aspects of life by refusing to perceive, acknowledge or deal with them

dependent personality disorder: an extreme need to be taken care of that leads to submissive, clinging behaviour and fear of separation; pattern begins by early adulthood, when behaviours designed to elicit caring from others become predominant

depersonalisation: the feeling that one has become detached from one's mind or body or has lost one's identity

derailment: speech that vacillates from one subject to another; the subjects are unrelated; ideas slip off the track between clauses

displacement: misdirecting pent-up feelings towards something or someone that's less threatening than that which triggered the response

dissociation: separating objects from their emotional significance

echolalia: meaningless repetition of words or phrases

echopraxia: involuntary repetition of movements observed in others

extinction: a technique that simply ignores undesirable behaviour, provided that the behaviour isn't dangerous or illegal

fantasy: creation of unrealistic or improbable images to escape from daily pressures and responsibilities

flat affect: unresponsive range of emotion, possibly an indication of schizophrenia or Parkinson's disease

flight of ideas: rapid succession of incomplete and poorly connected ideas

flooding: a frequent full-intensity exposure, possibly through the use of imagination, to an object that triggers a symptom; produces extreme discomfort

fluid intelligence: a form of intelligence defined as the ability to solve novel problems

focusing: a technique in which the nurse assists the person in redirecting attention towards something specific, especially if the person is vague or rambling

Functional Dementia Scale: measures orientation, affect and the ability to perform activities of daily living

Global Deterioration Scale: assesses and stages primary degenerative dementia based on orientation, memory and neurological function

hallucinations: false sensory perceptions with no basis in reality; usually visual or auditory, hallucinations also may be olfactory (smell), gustatory (taste) or tactile (touch)

hallucinogens: drugs that produce behavioural changes that are often multiple and dramatic; no known medical use; however, some block sensation to pain and use may result in self-inflicted injuries; an example is lysergic acid diethylamide that has street names such as acid, green or red dragon, microdot, sugar and big D; mescaline, peyote, psilocybin and phencyclidine; designer drugs (Ecstasy-PCE) are made to imitate certain illegal drugs and are often many times stronger than the drugs they imitate

histrionic personality disorder: a pervasive pattern of excessive emotionality and attention seeking; often begins in early adulthood and may be present in a variety of contexts

hypochondriasis: misinterpretation of the severity and significance of physical signs or sensations or the fear of contracting a disease; leads to the preoccupation with having a serious disease, which persists despite medical reassurance to the contrary; significant distress or impairment in functioning occurs

ideas of reference: misinterpreting acts of others in a highly personal way

identification: unconscious adoption of the personality characteristics, attitudes, values and behaviour of another person

implicit memory: information that can't be brought to mind but can be seen to affect behaviour

illusions: false sensory perceptions with some basis in reality; for example, a car backfiring mistaken for a gunshot

implosion therapy: a form of desensitisation; requires repeated exposure (that increases in graduated levels) to a highly feared object, and strong interpersonal support or anxiolytic medication

inappropriate affect: inconsistency between expression (affect) and mood (for example, a person who smiles when discussing an anger-provoking situation)

incoherence: incomprehensible speech

intellectualisation: hiding feelings about something painful behind thoughts; keeping opposing attitudes apart by using logic-tight comparisons

introjection: adopting someone else's values and standards without exploring whether or not they actually fit; often responds to 'should' or 'ought to'

lability of affect: rapid, dramatic fluctuation in the range of emotion

loose associations: not connected or related by logic or rationality

magical thinking: belief that thoughts or wishes can control other people or events

magnetoencephalography: measures the brain's magnetic field

mini–mental status examination: measures orientation, registration, recall, calculation, language and graphomotor function

modelling: provides a reward when the person imitates the desired behaviour

narcissistic personality disorder: projecting an image of perfection and personal invincibility because of a fear of personal weakness and imperfection; often projecting an inflated sense of self to hide low self-esteem

negative reinforcement: involves the removal of a negative stimulus only after the person provides a desirable response

neologisms: distorted or invented words that have meaning only for the person

NICE: National Institute for Clinical Excellence; produces guidelines for treatment and management of mental illness in primary and secondary care

nonverbal communication: eye contact, posture, facial expression, gestures, clothing, affect, silence and other body movements that can convey a powerful message

obsessive–compulsive personality disorder: a lack of openness and flexibility in daily routines, as well as in interpersonal relationships and expectations; a preoccupation with orderliness and perfectionism; treatment options that don't fit in with the person's cognitive schema will be rejected quickly

obsessions: intense preoccupations that interfere with daily living

opiates: narcotics and depressants used medicinally to relieve pain, but have a high potential for abuse; cause relaxation with an immediate 'rush', but also have initial unpleasant effects, such as restlessness and nausea; include codeine, heroin, meperidine and opium; street names include junk, horse, H and smack

paranoid personality disorder: extreme distrust of others and an avoidance of relationships in which the person isn't in control or has the potential of losing control

pharmacodynamics: the drug's effect on its target organ

phencyclidine or PCP: a hallucinogen that produces behavioural changes that are often multiple and dramatic; flashbacks may occur long after use; street names include hog, angel dust, peace pill, crystal superjoint, elephant tranquilliser and rocket fuel

phobia: an irrational and disproportionate fear of objects or situations

positive reinforcement: increase of the likelihood of a desirable behaviour being repeated by promptly praising or rewarding the person when performing it

poverty of speech: diminution of thought reflected in decreased speech and terse replies to questions, creating the impression of inner emptiness

processing capacity: understanding text, making inferences and paying attention, which all depend on working memory capability

prospective memory: remembering things that one needs

projection: displacement of negative feelings onto another person

punishment: discouraging of problem behaviour by inflicting a penalty, such as temporary removal of a privilege

rationalisation: substitution of acceptable reasons for the real or actual reasons motivating behaviour

reaction formation: conduct in a manner opposite from the way the person feels

recent memory: an event experienced in the past few hours or days

regression: return to an earlier developmental stage

remote memory: ability to remember events in the more distant past, such as birthplace or school days

repression: unconsciously blocking out painful thoughts

response prevention: a form of behaviour therapy that may require hospitalisation as well as family involvement to be effective

schizoid personality: a pervasive pattern of detachment from social relationships and restricted range of expression of emotions in interpersonal settings

schizotypal personality disorder: a pervasive pattern of social and interpersonal deficits marked by acute discomfort with, and reduced capacity for, close relationships, as well as by cognitive or perceptual distortions and eccentricities of behaviour; begins in early adulthood and is present in a variety of contexts

self-efficacy: a personality measure defined by the ability to organise and

execute actions required to deal with situations likely to happen in the future

shaping: initially rewards any behaviour that resembles the desirable one; then, step by step, the behaviour required to gain a reward becomes progressively closer to the desired behaviour

sharing impressions: the nurse attempts to describe the person's feelings and then seeks corrective feedback from the person

somatisation disorder: experiencing multiple signs and symptoms that suggest a physical disorder, but no verifiable disease or pathophysiological condition exists to account for them; unexplained symptoms appear to represent an unconscious somatised plea for attention and care; often familial with unknown aetiology

sublimation: transforming unacceptable needs into acceptable ambitions and actions; for instance, a person can funnel anger and resentment into an obsession to excel in a lucrative career

substance abuse: a maladaptive pattern of substance use coupled with recurrent and significant adverse consequences

substance dependence: physical, behavioural and cognitive changes resulting from persistent substance use; persistent drug use results in tolerance and withdrawal

substance intoxication: the development of a reversible substance-specific syndrome due to the ingestion of or exposure to a substance; the clinically significant maladaptive behaviour or psychological changes vary from substance to substance

thematic apperception test: test in which, after seeing a series of pictures that depict ambiguous situations, the person tells a story describing each picture

thought blocking: sudden interruption in the person's train of thought

thought replacement or switching: replacement of fear-inducing self-instructions with competent self-instructions, which teaches the person to replace negative thoughts with positive ones until the positive thoughts become strong enough to overcome the anxiety-provoking ones

thought stopping: method that breaks the habit of fear-inducing anticipatory thoughts; to stop unwanted thoughts by saying the word 'stop' and then focus attention on achieving calmness and muscle relaxation

tolerance: an increased need for a substance or need for an increased amount of the substance to achieve an effect

undoing: trying to superficially repair or make up for an action without dealing with the complex effects of that deed; also called *magical thinking*

withdrawal: becoming emotionally uninvolved by pulling back and being passive

word salad: illogical word groupings; the extreme form of loose associations; for example, 'She had a star, barn, plant.'

working memory: the part of the brain that enables not paying attention to irrelevancies

Selected references

American Psychiatric Association. *Diagnostic and Statistical Manual of Mental Disorders*, 4th ed., Text Revision. Washington, D.C.: American Psychiatric Association, 2000.

BMJ Group and RPS. *British National Formulary 55*. London: BMJ Group and RPS Publishing, March 2008.

Boyd, M.A. *Psychiatric Nursing Contemporary Practice*, 2nd ed. Philadelphia: Lippincott Williams & Wilkins, 2002.

Brown, E.L., et al. 'Assessing Behavioral Health Using OASIS Part 1 Depression and Suicidality,' *Home Healthcare Nurse* 20(3):154–61, March 2002.

Copel, L.C. *Nurse's Clinical Guide: Psychiatric and Mental Health Care*, 2nd ed. Springhouse: Lippincott Williams & Wilkins, 2000.

Gallop R., and O'Brien, L. 'Re-establishing Psychodynamic Theory as Foundational Knowledge for Psychiatric/Mental Health Nursing,' *Issues in Mental Health Nursing* 24(2):213–27, January–February 2003.

Keltner, N.L., et al. *Psychiatric Nursing*, 4th ed. St. Louis: Mosby–Year Book, Inc., 2003.

Kemppainen, J.K., et al. 'Psychiatric Nursing and Medication Adherence,' *Journal of Psychosocial Nursing and Mental Health Services* 41(2):38–49, February 2003.

Killeen, M. 'Private Matters,' *Journal of Child and Adolescent Psychiatric Nursing* 15(4):141–42, October–December 2002.

Kools, S., and Spiers, J. 'Caregiver Understanding of Adolescent Development in Residential Treatment,' *Journal of Child and Adolescent Psychiatric Nursing* 15(4):151–62, October–December 2002.

McAllister, M., et al. 'Dissociative Identity Disorder and the Nurse-Patient Relationship in the Acute Care Setting: An Action Research Study,' *Australian and New Zealand Journal of Mental Health Nursing* 10(1):20–32, March 2001.

McAllister, M., and Walsh, K. 'CARE: A Framework for Mental Health Practice,' *Journal of Psychiatric and Mental Health Nursing* 10(1):39–48, February 2003.

Mohr, W., ed. *Johnson's Psychiatric-Mental Health Nursing Adaptation and Growth*, 5th ed. Philadelphia: Lippincott Williams & Wilkins, 2002.

Murphy, C.F., et al. 'Assessing Behavioral Health Using OASIS: Part 2: Cognitive Impairment, Problematic Behaviors, and Anxiety,' *Home Healthcare Nurse* 20(4):230–235, April 2002.

National Institute for Clinical Excellence. *Schizophrenia: The Treatment and Management of Schizophrenia in Primary and Secondary Care* (Clinical Practice Algorithms and Pathways to Care). London: National Institute for Clinical Excellence, 2002.

National Institute for Clinical Excellence. *Guidance on the Use of Electroconvulsive Therapy* (Technology Appraisal 34). London: National Institute for Clinical Excellence, 2003.

National Institute for Clinical Excellence. *Depression: Management of Depression in Primary and Secondary Care* (Clinical Guideline 23). London: National Institute for Clinical Excellence, 2004.

National Institute for Clinical Excellence. *Eating Disorders: Core Interventions in the Treatment and Management of Anorexia Nervosa, Bulimia Nervosa and Related Eating Disorders* (Clinical Guideline 4). London: National Institute for Clinical Excellence, 2004.

National Institute for Clinical Excellence. *Obsessive-Compulsive Disorder: Core Interventions in the Treatment of Obsessive-Compulsive Disorder and Body Dysmorphic Disorder* (Clinical Guideline 31). London: National Institute for Clinical Excellence, 2005.

National Institute for Clinical Excellence. *Bipolar Disorder: The Management of Bipolar Disorder in Adults, Children and Adolescents, in Primary and Secondary Care* (Clinical Guideline 38). London: National Institute for Clinical Excellence, 2006.

Piaget, J. 'Stages of Intellectual Development of the Child,' *Bulletin of the Menninger Clinic* 26(4103):120–32, 1962.

Rinomhota, A.S., and Marshall, P. *Biological Aspects of Mental Health Nursing*. St. Louis: Mosby–Year Book, Inc., 2001.

Silberg, J.L. 'Fifteen Years of Dissociation in Maltreated Children: Where Do We Go from Here?' *Child Maltreatment* 5(2):119–36, May 2000.

Steinberg, M. 'Advances in the Clinical Assessment of Dissociation: The SCID-D-R,' *Bulletin of Menninger Clinic* 64:146–64, 2000.

Stuart, G., and Laraia, M. *Principles and Practice of Psychiatric Nursing*, 7th ed. St. Louis: Mosby–Year Book, Inc., 2001.

Szczesny, S., and Miller, M. 'PRN Medication Use in Inpatient Psychiatry,' *Journal of Psychosocial Nursing and Mental Health Services* 41(1):16–21, January 2003.

Townsend, M.C. *Psychiatric/Mental Health Nursing: Concepts of Care*, 4th ed. Philadelphia: F.A. Davis Company, 2003.

Wright, M. 'Violence Against Psychiatric Nurses: Team Approach Is Needed,' *Journal of Psychosocial Nursing and Mental Health Services* 41(1):8, January 2003.

Index

i refers to an illustration; t refers to a table

i refers to an illustration; t refers to a table

i refers to an illustration; t refers to a table

i refers to an illustration; t refers to a table